The Mammoth Book of the

Kama Sutra

↳ They said it,
and you read it right.
And now th[...]
written i[...]
return[...] [...] it!

Hope you're
hungry.

Love,
Your lover

Also available

MAXIM JAKUBOWSKI is a London-based novelist and editor. He was born in the UK and educated in France. Following a career in book publishing, he opened London's world-famous Murder One bookshop in 1988 and has since combined running it with his writing and editing career. He has edited a series of 12 bestselling erotic anthologies and two books of erotic photography, as well as many acclaimed crime collections. His novels include *It's You That I Want To Kiss, Because She Thought She Loved Me* and *On Tenderness Express*, all three recently collected and reprinted in the USA as *Skin In Darkness*. Other books include *Life In The World of Women, The State of Montana, Kiss Me Sadly* and *Confessions Of A Romantic Pornographer*. In 2006 he published a major erotic novel which he directed and on which 15 of the top erotic writers in the world have collaborated, *America Casanova*, and his collected erotic short stories as *Fools For Lust*. He is a winner of the Anthony and the Karel Awards, a frequent TV and radio broadcaster, crime columnist for the *Guardian* newspaper and Literary Director of London's Crime Scene Festival.

Constable & Robinson Ltd
3 The Lanchesters
162 Fulham Palace Road
London W6 9ER
www.constablerobinson.com

First published in the UK by Robinson,
an imprint of Constable & Robinson, 2008

A copy of the British Library Cataloguing in Publication
Data is available from the British Library

UK ISBN 978-1-84529-822-7

1 3 5 7 9 10 8 6 4 2

First published in the United States in 2008 by Running Press Book Publishers. All rights
reserved under the Pan-American and International Copyright Conventions

9 8 7 6 5 4 3 2 1
Digit on the right indicates the number of this printing

US Library of Congress number: 2008929938
US ISBN 978-0-7624-3393-3

Running Press Book Publishers
2300 Chestnut Street
Philadelphia, PA 19103-4371

Visit us on the web!

www.runningpress.com

Printed and bound in the EU

The Mammoth Book of the
Kama Sutra

Edited by Maxim Jakubowski

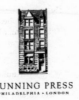

ROBINSON

RUNNING PRESS
PHILADELPHIA · LONDON

Contents

Contents

Picture Acknowledgements

By Carolyn Weltman

The Swing; The Lotus (1); Supported Congress; The Rising Position; The Half-pressed Position; Congress of the Cow; The Yawning; The Spit-roast; The Packed Position; The Clasping Position; The Turning Position; Face-to-Face; One Knot; The Swan; The Dog; The Fish; The Ass; The Foot Yoke; Sky Foot; Driving the Peg; The Ascending Position; The Lute; The Lotus (2).

By Louisa Minkin

The Tiger; The Spinning Top, The Full-pressed Position; The Flower in Bloom; Mouth Congress; The Bee; The Creeper; The Pair of Tongs; The Open Pincer; The Mixture of Sesame Seeds and Rice; The Crab; Suspended Congress; Churning; The Crow; Splitting Bamboo; The Herd; The Thunderbolt; The Tree; The Posture of Indrani; The Knee Elbow; The Encircling Position; The Wheelbarrow; The Cat; The Svastika; The Elephant; The Cobra; The Curved Knot; The Snake Trap.

Introduction

Everyone has heard of the *Kama Sutra*. But how many people have actually read it, in whatever translation or version, and realize that this legendary Indian book of love is not just a sex manual, an antique and exotic version of *The Joy of Sex* or any of the other how-to manuals that now populate the shelves of modern bookstores? And it is even less a pornographic work, as sadly, too many uninformed people still believe.

As Indra Sinha – whose contemporary translation is both poetic and faithful and outlined in five-line prose stanzas – points out in his introduction to *The Love Teachings of the Kama Sutra*, no two Sanskrit words, apart from svastika, are more widely known and misunderstood than *Kama Sutra*. "In the West the work is commonly believed to be a salacious, anecdotic account of exotic lovemaking, yet in India it is often given to young brides to read before their weddings."

In her own section examining both the book's genesis and its complex heritage and purpose, Trisha Telep explains where the book originated and why it actually contains no anecdotes and is much more than just a sex manual. In fact, only one of its seven books actually deals with the techniques of physical lovemaking. There is much more to it and I urge all of you curious readers to get hold of a copy in a modern translation and delve further.

The present volume is not yet another variation of the basic texts of the *Kama Sutra*, but a digest of some of its positions, with attractive illustrations by the talented artists Louisa Minkin and Carolyn Weltman. To this, we have taken the bold step of adding 24 brand new stories based on some of the selected positions, which I believe bring the *Kama Sutra* to life as never before. These stories are tales from the pens of provocative and exciting modern writers who have made it their mission to interpret the spirit of *Kama Sutra* for the modern reader. Some are deadly serious, some are humorous, while others are either sexy or even melancholy, but I feel they all add another dimension and make this *Mammoth Book of the Kama Sutra* more than just another familiar trawl down traditional roads.

So how did an ancient Hindu treatise come to be the world's best-known sex manual? Written in Northern India in the third century AD, when erotic culture lay at the heart of an exquisite civilization, the *Kama Sutra* is a unique document, the discovery of by which the West was brought about by Victorian scholars. It also almost created a revolution when first translated by that hardy explorer and visionary Sir Richard Burton in 1883. For decades it was almost an underground book, forced into the hands of publishing pornographers before being thrust once and for all into respectable daylight in the wake of the publication of *Lady Chatterley's Lover*.

   Now, of course, it has become part of the fabric of our sexual and cultural life and a plethora of editions, variations, adaptations can be easily found. But I believe it still remains a misunderstood book, and those two Sanskrit words have become a strange form of shorthand for sex or matters sexual amongst the majority of us. We think of ourselves as modern and educated, but then we realize that ancient Indian civilization knew more than we did about sexual matters and did so with more refinement and elegance. Which is why the *Kama Sutra* remains modern and apposite.

   Of course, the *Kama Sutra* in its unadorned version is an awkward book to summarize and understand, balancing the erotic arts with an almost mystical view of the bonds and relationships and contacts between men and women (as well as, surprisingly, in some instances, contacts between same-sex partners) and many a young person, at first intrigued if not titillated by the reputation of the book, has no doubt given up on it rather prematurely upon realizing it is not a fount of dirty words and is actually deadly serious in its intentions. I know that, as a teenager, I was one such defeated by the old-fashioned values and promises of the *Kama Sutra*. Ah, the folly of youth!

My wish is for this modest attempt to encapsulate its charm, heritage and knowledge and send many more readers out to sample the whole thing with a broad, open mind. I have no doubt it will make a better man or woman out of you, and not just in bed, or wherever you enjoy practising your sensuality.

Maxim Jakubowski

What is the Kama Sutra?

The *Kama Sutra* was initially written for the privileged castes of ancient India by a nobleman, Mallanaga Vatsyayana. Most historians and experts generally place Vatsyayana in the middle of the fourth century, during the reign of Gupta Emperor Samudragupta. Little is known of the now legendary author, aside from the fact that he was a celibate yogi who had attained *samadhi*, which would now be construed as enlightenment. In his day, he was likely to have been famous as a teacher, and he has indeed been called Maharishi (spiritual leader) in India over the past centuries since his death. He wrote the book for no other reason than to enable people to understand *Kama* and to use and enjoy it properly.

It is, in fact, not an original work, but a massive collection and distillation of treatises on love that originated in the early passages of Indian history. The first such writings were claimed to have been made by the bull-god Nandi, who recorded what he eavesdropped on as he stood guard outside the bedchamber of the God Shiva and the Goddess Parvati. For 1,000 years, according to the legend, the two remained locked in passionate embrace, with bystanding Nandi carefully absorbing every pearl of the lovers' wisdom and then passing the message on to the waiting eyes and ears of mere humanity.

"If men and women act according to each other's liking, their love for each other will not be lessened even in one hundred years."

Nandi's *Kama Shastra* was allegedly a huge work of more than 1,000 chapters. Over the course of time, it was reduced to 500 chapters, then further abridged to 150 chapters in the fifth century by separating and reworking the text into seven distinct books, which covered general social topics; amorous embraces;

union of males and females; on one's own wife; on the wives of other people; about courtesans; on the arts of seduction and aphrodisiacs; occult practices are even mentioned. By the fourth century, the 150 chapters, possibly because they were each written by a different scholar, or were in a different place, or were in differing states of repair, were unable to be found as a complete work. The work was in danger of being forgotten when Vatsyayana decided to compile and rework the still cumbersome books of the *Kama Sutra* into a new, definitive edition that would be understandable by everyone.

This is the version that has survived to this day.

Kama Sutra has now become the main text on love in Sanskrit. It affirms that sex is as necessary as water and as nourishing as food. We should be clear in understanding the *Kama Sutra* as a book of conduct, not merely a sex manual. It is a guide to the complexities of ancient Indian social relations. It contains a lengthy philosophical section on the role of pleasure in life, as well as wonderful, time-capsule descriptions of the ideal ancient Indian lover. There are rich sections on how a man-about-town enjoys and seduces all different types of women: from virgins, to his wife, to other men's wives, to courtesans, and – after a short stop at the local masseuse – to men disguised as women for oral delights. The book on aphrodisiacs and drugs is tantamount to spell-casting and sex magic. It is of course these specific sections that have made the strongest impact and which are responsible for the *Kama Sutra*'s reputation and inevitable association with the sexual arts.

Kama Sutra is the earliest attempt to define the entire relationship between a man and a woman, at the heart of which, of course, is the sexual act. It attempts to give answers to questions of who one should have sex with, under which circumstances and how. It meant cultivating the raw material of sex (this is *alamkara*, the aesthetic ideal) and turning it into a science. When the senses are conquered and under the individual's personal, considered control, then sex is in essence a microcosm of civilization. Sex becomes mannered, moral and social.

The essence of *Kama Sutra* is that sensual pleasures should be approached as a science. There are all sorts of sensual requirements to be done in order to fulfil the art of love to a suitable level of satisfaction. All the senses have to be taken into account. There should be soft music, beautiful clothes and food, sparkling conversation. A man and a woman depend on each other in sex, so there must be a method to ensure harmony in the union. Sexual relations cannot be left to instinct, although animals and unschooled people manage a basic form easily. All these are rules that might today be considered self-evident, but were not always so. Thus, the *Kama Sutra* provides a guide-book to teach both parties the appropriate ways to conduct themselves sexually.

Guidelines For Living

There are four main aims (*purusharthas*) in Hindu life. These aims were expounded by Brahma, the creator, and member of the Hindu Trinity, and relate to man's spiritual, physical and emotional needs, so regulating his existence.

Dharma is a doctrine that encompasses religious, moral and social duty, and is set out in the *Dharma Shastra*. Every person has their own specific *dharma* that they must fulfil. This personal *dharma* takes into account social contexts such as caste and gender. Because everyone has different circumstances, everyone's *dharma* is different. It is a teacher's *dharma* to teach his students, a member of parliament's *dharma* to represent his constituency and an actor's *dharma* to entertain his audience. *Dharma* is considered to be the most important of the four *purusharthas*, and fulfilment of your *dharma* means freedom from the cycle of rebirth.

Artha, the second aim, has to do with a citizen's duties as a member of society (its text is the *Arthashastra*). There is a responsibility to secure fame and fortune, to better yourself socially and to promote the worldly success of your family through acquired wealth and power. *Artha* is tempered by *dharma* (or it would merely become opportunism). The pursuit of money allows for the pursuit of spirituality, by fulfilling one's earthly requirements, thus also liberating a person to seek pleasure.

Kama is the third aim. Think of Kama as the Hindu Cupid. In ancient Indian texts, Kama is depicted as a handsome young man with wings, never without his sugarcane bow and quiver full of flower-festooned arrows. According to some sources he may be one of the sons of Brahma, the Creator of the Universe. He is associated with springtime, gentle spring breezes and birds such as parrots and cuckoos. He is identified as the beginning of life, the desire to create and procreate. *"Kama"* means desire or, more explicitly, sexual desire, though some say its meaning is broader, meaning all pleasures experienced by the senses. Because it is the *dharma* of a married man to make love to his wife, *kama*, though relegated by some to the inferior position of the three mortal *purusharthas*, has an amazing amount of weight. The *Kama Sutra* is therefore a book that teaches how to make love well, how to do your duty to the utmost of your ability. In essence, the *Kama Sutra* was written to create masters of sensuality.

Within the four main aims of life, *kama* is certainly the most dangerous, the one that can easily overturn the apple cart and leave its practitioner firmly in reincarnation's grip, and with no hope of moving into a higher caste for the next life. The *shastras* (teachings) of *dharma* and *artha* are quite hostile to *kama* (despite the idea that they should all be pursued in harmony). Kama contradicts *dharma* and *artha* by giving advice on immoral (but likely pleasurable) activities such as adultery. *Kama*'s very existence contradicts the other two and causes many ambiguities and moral problems. But *kama* is a reward for the religion and power found in *dharma* and *artha*, though *kama* is also riddled with possible temptations that can lead to weakness. With such a complex web of concepts and tenets the *Kama Sutra* is teaching its reader that you can't live a life based purely on pleasure.

The above aims are, of course, closely associated with the four stages of Hindu life. A young man should gain knowledge and study classical texts – and the *Kama Sutra* (he should, however, only learn the text in theory, remaining celibate). In middle age, he should acquire wealth through the practice of *artha* and sensual experience through *kama*. In old age he should perform *dharma*, and thereby, gain *moksha* (the fourth and final aim), enlightenment and release from rebirth.

The *Kama Sutra*'s Audience

Vatsyayana's *Kama Sutra* came into the Indian world as it was experiencing a Renaissance-like Golden Age, with patronage for the arts and sciences at an all-time high. The cities were characterized by sophistication and fast living, and were full of wealthy individuals pursuing sensuous lives, especially those men in their second stage of life, called *nagarakas*, whose lives were principally devoted to pleasure. Success with women was a defining characteristic of these types of gentlemen. It was mainly for these erstwhile playboys that Vatsyayana compiled his *Kama Sutra*.

At different times in their lives, *nagarakas* would be seducers of virgins, ideal husbands, the pursuers of other men's wives, clients of courtesans and, finally, men requiring aphrodisiacs and sexual stimulants to perform. The *Kama Sutra* sets out the rules for living the life of a gentleman. Vatsyayana instructs them how to perfume and pamper themselves, how to spend idle days with friends and how to outfit the ideal bachelor pad for seductions. The study of the *Kama Sutra* was, in its own right, an exercise in self-improvement for the aspiring *nagaraka*. It was also simply not possible to afford all of the *Kama Sutra*'s prescribed luxuries and pleasures without a lot of money.

For these gentlemen, sex should be elevated to a level of civilized humanity, over and above the basic, instinctual mating of animals, and sexual expertise was a social and moral obligation. Becoming masters of sensuality meant success in all areas of life. The mastery of the 64 arts of love (of which more later) guaranteed a man the respect of the learned, made him a leader in society and earned him the love of his wife, other men's wives and courtesans.

Although the *Kama Sutra* wasn't specifically written for women, the book teaches women the roles they are expected to play in a sexual relationship. It lets them know what they can expect when being seduced, married or losing their virginity. They are not expected to be passive. The *Kama Sutra* seeks reciprocity in sex, and not the ravishing of a virgin by an experienced male. Women have an active role to play and their pursuit of their own pleasure is a necessity (it was believed that successful conception would not take place unless the woman achieved orgasm). Women were expected to know the *Kama Sutra*, while for men it was mandatory. According to the book, throughout their lives women play the roles of virgins, wives, other men's wives and courtesans. The *Kama Sutra* also mentions unmarried and lower-caste women as females to whom a man may or may not resort purely for sexual congress.

The Erotics of the *Kama Sutra*

The *Kama Shastra* tradition is a venerable tradition of erotic science, of which the *Kama Sutra* is an addition. A *shastra* is a learned teaching on a particular topic. Vatsyayana was contributing in form to the idea that drove these ancient texts from the very beginning: the art of love is also a science, a thing to be studied, practised and perfected.

These works were written in *sutras*: distinctly Hindu compositions much like aphorisms, designed to make complex scientific ideas easy to remember and pass on by word of mouth. The *sutras* were essentially written to instruct teachers in the teaching of others. These short aphoristic texts were always meant to be accompanied by commentaries in order to make their slightly cryptic, often poetical verses clear and understandable. A written commentary was added to the *Kama Sutra* by Yashodhara in the thirteenth century, and another, much later one, by Devadutta Shastri in 1964. Most translations are an abridgement or mix of Vatsyayana's *sutras* and the accompanying commentary. The translation by Alain Danielou, however, presents the *sutras* alone, and includes both the above commentaries separately.

After the *Kama Sutra* came a host of other texts in the same erotic tradition. Some were better than others. These texts mainly concentrated on the sexual positions and ambitiously competed against one another to come up with the most gymnastic ways to make love. Some of the more famous of the inspired texts are the *Ananga Ranga*, which was written by a sixteenth-century poet for his wealthy patrons, and the eleventh-century *Ratirahasya*, often called the *Koka Shastra* or *Koka's Book*. The rest of the later love texts are quite forgettable, but some, like the undated *Ratikallolini* (River of Love), the small, fifteenth-century *Ratimanjari*, the fourteenth-century *Smaradipika* by Sri Minanath and Harihara's *Srngararasaprabandhadipika* (The Light of Love) feature fun variations on traditional sexual postures that are a worthwhile study by lovers.

The Chequered History of the *Kama Sutra*

By the sixteenth century, the *Kama Sutra* was largely forgotten in India. Amid disapproval by religious scholars and, in a larger sense, because of the now sizeable Muslim presence in the country, texts having to do with erotic science were deliberately allowed to languish and be lost completely. In addition, erotic literature had always been the creation of princes, poets and royal patronage, and all those things were slowly disappearing from Indian tradition.

Contrary to popular belief, India has always had a love/hate relationship with pleasure (one only has to devote a closer examination to the four main aims of Hindu life and their myriad contradictions). There has always been a virtual tug of war between the sensualist and the ascetic. Even from as early as the tenth century, all the *Kama Shastra* texts, their origins now cloudy and forgotten, were hijacked by the ascetic. Tantric sex acted like a precarious bridge between the world of human pleasures and spiritual contemplation. Then, suddenly, the *Kama Sutra* was reinvented as sensual and sexual pleasure in pursuit of union with the Divine. Much later, an English-educated Mahatma Gandhi was certainly no friend to an indulgence in earthly, sensual pleasures. Neither was the British Raj, responsible in 1860 for an Indian Penal Code that punished all "non-procreative sex" as criminal (this penal code, interestingly enough, was based on the ancient laws of *dharma*).

Richard Burton was in the British army in India at the height of Britain's imperialist phase. The *Kama Sutra* was almost impossible to find in India at that time. Under the Raj, because court patronage for the erotic sciences (and their libraries) had ended, manuscripts tended to disappear. Burton was also a consummate libertine, knew many Indian languages and dialects (though not Sanskrit to a level of translation), and was already a pioneering erotic anthropologist who hated all the sexual hypocrisy of Victorian Britain, and delighted in transgression (he was also the proud founder of a debating and pro-flagellation group called The Cannibal Club). Here was the perfect Westerner to champion and resurrect the *Kama Sutra*.

Although many Indologists in Britain were translating Indian texts for Western readers, they had all carefully been ignoring the erotic texts. This might be an indication of the prudery of Victorian Britain or it might simply be that the erotic sciences were not given the same respect in Western society as they were in ancient India. Many of these serious translators felt that the *Kama Shastra* texts were mere frippery compared to the more academic Indian texts waiting to be given a Western audience.

But Burton thought differently. He knew that the combination of Indian exoticism and forbidden erotica was a goldmine in the West. He set up a *Kama Shastra* society that was simply a clandestine publishing operation to get round the strict censorship of Victorian Britain's Obscene Publications Act. Under this act, the *Kama Sutra*, with its ancient pedigree, high ideals and honourable aims would be treated in exactly the same way as any other work, fictional or not, dealing with sex and sexuality. The fact that the Victorian erotica being produced, and prosecuted, at that time came under titles such as *The Voluptuous Experiences of an Old Maid*, *The Lustful Turk* and *The Amatory Experiences of a Surgeon* (to our modern eyes all prime examples of dated pornography full of naughty school-girls, fierce headmistresses with lesbian tendencies and large doses of upstairs-downstairs forms of corporeal punishment) is an indication of the unhealthy Victorian sexual attitudes with which the new, English-translated *Kama Sutra* was rubbing shoulders. The book, however, was tremendously well received by the proprietors of London's Holywell Street (aka 'Erotica Row') in 1883, the year Burton's translation appeared.

Once published, Burton exploited the markets of scholarship as well as the markets of pornographic material. The *Kama Sutra* became a great success. It even helped that no copyright had been established. Because of this, it was pirated until 1963 and multiplied in all sorts of editions around the world (the bestselling version came from Olympia Press). After the success of the *Kama Sutra*, Burton also later published the *Arabian Nights*, *Ananga Ranga*, *The Perfumed Garden* and many other texts in the *Kama Shastra* tradition.

The Heart of the *Kama Sutra*

Let us now take a detailed trip through the *Kama Sutra* and study and explain its precepts and many divisions.

The notion that the *Kama Sutra* instructs on 64 distinct sex positions is mistaken. There are only 21 actual sexual positions in the text, the rest are types of strokes to be used by the man during intercourse, kisses, love bites and embraces. In Burton's translation, Vatsyayana explains that it's famously called 64 because it contains eight subjects: embraces, kissing, scratching, biting, lying down, making various sounds, playing the part of a man and mouth congress, and these eight subjects each contain eight parts, giving a total of 64 instructions. These 64 arts are not to be confused with the 64 sensual skills to be mastered by men and women, including singing, dancing, playing a musical instrument and cooking, as well as other fascinating skills that reveal the *Kama Sutra*'s ancient Indian setting, such as performing magic and sorcery, and teaching parrots and starlings to speak.

Many of these teachings are simply universal ways to embrace a life of pleasure, to master things that have no other aim than creating beauty. Man is seen as having a duty to engage the five senses with beauty at every opportunity and to create a life of sensual pleasure for himself and those around him. *Kama Sutra* encourages taking responsibility and choosing a sensual, life-affirming environment to live in.

According to the *Kama Sutra*, a man employing the 64 arts attains the object of his desire, and enjoys women of the first quality. If he does not know the 64 arts, even if he speaks well on other subjects, no great respect is paid to him in the assembly of the learned. A man, devoid of other knowledge, but well acquainted with the 64 divisions, becomes a leader in any society of men and women. The 64 arts are dear to women because they respect and are charmed by the men who know them.

The mere fact that across the modern world the entire *Kama Sutra* has been neglected in favour of the section on sexual union and the 64 arts, simply confirms that the love relationship is at the heart of this book. The 64 moods and modes of lovemaking are contained in part two of the *Kama Sutra* called "On Sexual Union", and are presented below according to the Burton translation (minus the section called "Lying down", with its 21 sexual positions, which are detailed later in this book).

Man is divided into three classes: the hare man, the bull man and the horse man, according to the size of his *lingam*. Women also, according to the depth of their *yoni*, are either a female deer, a mare or a female elephant. There are thus three equal unions between persons of corresponding dimensions, and there are six unequal unions when the dimensions do not correspond. The sizs are given thoughtful consideration in the *Kama Sutra* so that every size will be able to reach orgasm with every other size (and therefore every size can be satisfied sexually with every other size).

Throughout the breakdown of these 64 arts, Vatsyayana qualifies these rules (as he does, charmingly, through the whole book) by saying that love and passion dictate what happens when. The more rigid rules seem to be for the conscious application of a less-impassioned sex: married sex which has a feel of duty, perhaps. The truth is that the conscious application of these elegant rules can awaken passion in a familiar routine. It is simply a fact that putting two bodies together will cause a physical reaction. So, the 64 arts can be used to facilitate familiar sex and love just as they can be used in erotic play for impassioned lovers.

Congress

There are seven kinds of congress. "Loving congress" is when a man and a woman who have been in love with each other for some time come together at last with great difficulty, or when one of the pair returns from a journey, or are reconciled after having been separated because of a quarrel. This kind of congress is carried on according to the liking of the lovers, and for as long as they choose. The next type of congress is when two persons come together while their love is still in infancy. This is the "congress of subsequent love". The "congress of artificial love" is when a man carries on the congress by exciting himself by means of the 64 ways, or when a man and a woman come together who are attached to others. When the man, while having sex with the woman, is thinking of someone else, that's "congress of transferred love", and congress with a lower caste for the simple aim of sexual release is "congress like that of eunuchs". "Deceitful congress" is that congress between unequal partners. The congress that takes place between two persons who are attached to one another, and which is done according to their own liking is called "congress of spontaneous love".

Generally, before sexual union takes place, and in no fixed order, the embrace, the kiss and the pressing or scratching with the nails or fingers should be done.

Embracing

The first of the eight parts of the 64 acts concerns embraces, and this is a very important part of the *Kama Sutra*. Embracing can increase sensual enjoyment and can also be used while actually having sex. They are useful if the man's passion is not strong. There are four kinds of embraces that indicate the mutual love of a man and woman. There are also four embraces that are more like physical positions, used at the time that a man and a woman meet for love. As well, there are four ways of embracing single parts of the body during these embraces. The last two sets of embraces could be considered sexual positions and might be incorporated into lovemaking before, during or after sexual congress.

The first four embraces are the "touching embrace", the "piercing embrace", the "rubbing embrace" and the "pressing embrace". The first embrace is when the man, under some pretext or other, goes in front or alongside a woman and touches her body with his own. The "piercing embrace" is when a woman contrives to tantalize a man by bending down and displaying her cleavage or some other sexually suggestive area of her body. The "rubbing embrace" takes place when two lovers are walking slowly together, either in a dark, lonely place or a public place, and they rub their bodies against each other. The "pressing embrace" is when, on the same occasion, one of the lovers presses the other's body forcibly against a wall or a pillar.

Then come the four embraces that are more similar to physical positions. They are *jataveshtitaka*, or the twining of a creeper; *vriskshadhirudhaka*, or climbing a tree; *tila-tandulaka*, or the mixture of sesame seed with rice; and *kshiraniraka*, or the milk-and-water embrace. These are explained later.

The last four embraces are basically variations of the position embraces above. The "embrace of the thighs" occurs when one of the two lovers forcibly presses one or both of the thighs of the other between his or her own. The "embrace of the *jaghana*", that is, the part of the body from the navel downwards to the thighs, is when the man presses this part of the woman against his own midsection, and mounts upon her, as if practising penetrating her, all the while scratching with his nails or fingers, or biting, striking or kissing. On this occasion, the hair of the woman should be loose and flowing. The next embrace is the "embrace of the breasts", where a man places his breast between the breasts of the woman and presses her with it. Finally, when either of the lovers touches the mouth, eyes and the forehead of the other with his or her own, it's called the "embrace of the forehead".

The Art of Kissing

The second part of the book discusses the art of kissing. The essential places to kiss are the forehead, the eyes, the cheeks, the throat, the breasts, the lips and the interior of the mouth. Vatsyayana gives us some regional variations which have arisen because of the intensity of the love of people living in different areas of the country. What is good for some, however, is not good for all. Regional variations include kissing the joints of the thighs (hips) the arms and the navel. Throughout the book, Vatsyayana provides us with ideas of practices that are acceptable and pleasant only to people in certain areas.

There are three sorts of kisses with a young woman. The "nominal kiss" is when a girl touches only the mouth of her lover with her own, but doesn't do anything else. The "throbbing kiss" is a continuation of the nominal kiss. When she sets aside her bashfulness a little, the girl desires to touch the lip that is pressed into her mouth, so she moves her lower lip, but not her upper one. The "touching kiss" is another continuation of the two previous kisses, in the sense that the girl is getting a little bolder, and touches her lover's lip with her tongue and, having shut her eyes, places her hands on those of her lover.

Vatsyayana admits that the objects of affection are often young. They are not yet skilled in the arts of love. They must be coaxed and petted and introduced skilfully and carefully. The *Kama Sutra* assures us that pouncing on an inexperienced girl and doing what you please is not a good thing to do. An unskilled, unpractised, inexperienced lover needs to be handled with care. The pleasure of sex can be snuffed out for an individual by one careless first lover. Sex and eroticism are powerful. Letting go and giving yourself to your partner, being open and vulnerable, can be scary. Vatsyayana reminds us that new partners should go very slowly and gain each other's confidence and trust. And that's when real lovemaking can begin.

Other authors who worked on the predecessor texts of the *Kama Sutra*, Vatsyayana says, describe five other types of kisses. The "straight kiss" is when the lips of two lovers are brought into direct contact with each other. When the heads of two lovers are bent towards each other and kissing takes place, it is called the "bent kiss". The "turned kiss" is when one of the lovers turns up the face of the other by holding the head and chin, and then kissing. When the lower lip is pressed with a good deal of force, it is the "pressed kiss". The fifth kiss, the "greatly pressed kiss", is effected by taking hold of the lover's lower lip between the fingers and then, after touching it with the tongue, pressing it with great force with the lip.

But then at the end of these further kisses, we are treated to three more. (This 64 is not looking much like 64 any more.) The "kiss of the upper lip" is when a man kisses the upper lip of the woman, while she in return kisses his lower lip. When one of the lovers takes both the lips of the other between his or her own, that's a "clasping kiss". This type of kiss will only be welcomed by the woman if the man has no moustache. This kiss is also sometimes accompanied by "the fighting of the tongue", which is when, during this kiss, one of the couple touches the teeth, tongue and palate of the other with his or her tongue. The "pressing of the teeth" against the mouth of the lover is also encouraged.

Different kinds of kisses are appropriate for different parts of the body and go from moderate to contracted, and from pressed to soft. There are also specific types of kisses for specific instances. The "kiss that kindles love" is when a woman looks at the face of her lover while he is asleep, and kisses it to show her intention or desire. When a woman kisses her lover while he is engaged in business, or while he is quarrelling with her, or while he is looking at something else, so that his mind may be turned away, that's a "kiss that turns away". The "kiss that awakens" is a rather theatrical kiss where the woman may be pretending to be asleep when her lover arrives home, even if she wants to get up and run into his arms. She keeps pretending to be asleep so he can employ this kiss and show his intention. The erotic qualities of waiting are often explored in the *Kama Sutra*; a central theme is the deliciousness of patience.

Add to these kisses three more, and we finally have them all. The "kiss showing intention" is when a person kisses the reflection of the person he loves in a mirror, or water, or on a wall. The "transferred kiss" is when a person kisses a child, or an image or figure, in the presence of the beloved. When at night at a public place, a man comes up to a woman and kisses a finger of her hand if she's standing, or a toe of her foot if she's sitting, or when a woman in shampooing her lover's body places her face on his thigh so as to inflame his passion, that's the "demonstrative kiss".

All this specificity is just a reminder, an inspiration, of how many different ways there are to awaken desire in your lover. Two different people in different moods will not be in the same passion, perhaps at the same time. These exhausting, exhaustive menus are so intricate and conscious and erotic that, in spite of yourself, a person would become aroused by the sheer force of the attention, the attrition, the breaking down of will and subsiding into pleasure.

Vatsyayana talks about the quality and the tone of lovemaking. Sex is to be entered into as something of a play fight, with wagers and mock quarrels, mini-pseudo rages, and cajoling, coaxing and tenderness. The whole tone of lovemaking should be mocking and playful and teasing, he says, and gripped with the energy of a real argument: the victory of winning, the agony of defeat. It should be a passionate event. It is a piece of theatre. The *Kama Sutra* prescribes how the woman is expected to act during love quarrels, and how the man should then approach her. The woman has to know her part because while the man is trying his best to pacify her, she has to wait until his conciliatory words have reached their utmost, and not until then does she embrace him. It's all a game, and Vatsyayana teaches the participants how to play their roles.

Vatsyayana advises that these mock-arguments and games can also be applied to scratching, biting and striking, however, only with men and women of intense passion. This is perhaps because scratching, biting and striking are somewhat sadomasochistic and the use of these techniques can cause a bit of pain. Perhaps they should only be used when the couple is completely carried away by sexual excitement. These are intense physical sensations and may be best absorbed by lovers in the throes of passion. Perhaps passion is something of an anaesthetic. Kissing is gentle and playful. Scratching, biting and striking need passion as a guide so they can be used appropriately.

At the end of the chapter on kisses, Vatasyayana reminds the reader that there should always be reciprocity. There should not be things that one lover does to the other, that are not returned. There are two people involved in this act. The aim is to get both lovers inflamed with passion, and not just one passionate partner who envelops the other. As his talk of kissing speaks of "first times", it seems that he is moderating between experienced men and virgins, perhaps. Going slowly with young, inexperienced girls is necessary in order to get the object of your desire (the girl) into a fit state for reciprocal pleasure.

On Marking and Pressing With the Nails

Vatsyayana says that scratching happens when love becomes intense, and then only on certain occasions, of which there are five. On the first visit, at the time of setting out on a journey, on a return from a journey, at the time when an angry lover is reconciled or when the woman is intoxicated, these are the appropriate times for marking or pressing with the nails. Vatsyayana, as usual, follows this by mentioning again that love knows no rules and the *Kama Sutra* should be thrown out the window when passion is present.

There are eight kinds of pressing with the nails according to the marks produced. The first kind, "sounding" is the mark made when a person presses the chin, the breasts, the lower lip, or the *jaghana* of the other so softly that no scratch or mark is left. The hair on the body, however, becomes erect from the touch of the nails. The nails themselves also make a sound, hence the name "sounding". Vatsyayana says that this type of pressing is used in the case of a young girl when her lover shampoos her, scratches her head and wants to trouble or unnerve her.

The second mark is called the "half-moon". It is a curved mark made with the nails and is impressed on the neck and breasts. The "circle" results when two half-moons are impressed directly opposite each other. This mark is generally made on the navel, the small cavities around the buttocks and on the joints of the thighs. The next mark is the "line" and is basically just that: a mark made in the form of a short line, and can be made on any part of the body. The "line" may evolve into the fifth mark when it curves and becomes the "tiger's nail" or the "tiger's claw". A "peacock's foot" is a curved mark made on the breast by means of all five nails. This mark is difficult to make, requires a great deal of skill and is used in order to be praised. When five marks are made close to one another near the nipple with all five nails, it is called "the jump of a hare" and it is the seventh mark. Lastly, a mark like the many spiky leaves of the blue lotus blossom, when imprinted on the breast or hips, is called "the leaf of a blue lotus".

There are five places that can be pressed with the nails. These are the armpit, the breasts, the lips, the *jaghana*, and the thighs. And going even further, Vatsyayana describes the ideal male nails to make these marks. The nails should be bright, well set, clean, whole, convex, soft and glossy. He talks about regional differences in the look of men's nails and how nails can vary from place to place in size: from small to middling to large. It seems that Vatsyayana prefers large nails because they give grace to the hands and are attractive to women.

Again Vatsyayana advises that when passion and intensity are present, all rules should be ignored. At that time, marks should be made wherever passion dictates. Passion also dictates what marks are made, and he says that men should also just follow their inspiration, throw caution to the wind and come up with their own marks. No one can say exactly how many distinct marks exist because we can't visit everyone's bedrooms to see their favourites, their variations, and creative, original marks, says Vatsyayana. He encourages readers to use their imaginations. The rules are just a guide into your own creativity. Variety is the spice of life (and sex).

When a person is going on a journey, they make a mark on the lover they are leaving, or the lover makes a mark on them, on their thighs or breast. This mark is called "a token of remembrance", and it appears as three or four lines impressed close to one another on the skin. Marks leave memories of the lovemaking and the lover. Even if you haven't seen each other for a while, the marks remind the lover of the previous lovemaking and rekindle the love and desire all over again. A man seeing his marks on his woman, and a woman seeing her marks on her man, increases the lover's love for the other.

Marking, and biting (covered in the next section), are the two things that increase love the most. They leave memories on the skin that linger in the physical sense, not only in the mind. Marks, however, should not be made on married women in an adulterous situation (or if they are then only on their private parts for remembrance and the increase of love).

On Biting

In the chapter on biting, we are treated to ideas on the ideal teeth for biting. The qualities of good teeth are that they are equal, pleasingly bright, capable of being coloured, of proper proportions, unbroken and sharp ended. Defects are blunt, protruding, rough, soft, large and loosely set teeth. So, with these ideal teeth, all the places that can be kissed are also places that can be bitten, except the upper lip, the interior of the mouth and the eyes. There are eight different kinds of bite

Vatsyayana lets us in on the preferences of the women of different countries. He seems to be wanting to let his ideal readers (the *nagarakas* mentioned earlier) know what kind of sexual liaisons they can expect in different areas. Women of a certain area think that pressing with the nails and biting are disgraceful. Some women in certain countries are won over by striking, while still others are fond of foul pleasures and have no manners. Some like to talk dirty, and some show their likings only in secret. Some women are difficult to make passionate, and some take aphrodisiacs. In addition to regional variations, individual women, Vatsyayana says, often have different, individual preferences. It is a rule, however, that the things that increase passion (the things that really turn the woman on) should be done first. The things done just for variety and pleasure should be left for later.

pattern that can be made, and the places where they should be made are set out in the text so the reader can make no mistake. The bites escalate in intensity from one to eight. And as well as biting the beloved herself, you can mark with the nails or bite certain things worn by or belonging to the beloved. Doing this shows a desire for congress. Such acceptable things to bite are ornaments of the forehead, earrings, bunches of flowers, betel leaves and tamala leaves.

The "hidden bite" is shown only by the excessive redness of the skin which has been bitten. This type of bite is to be made on the lower lip. The "swollen bite" is also to be placed on the lower lip but can also be made on the left cheek. This type of bite occurs when the skin is pressed down between the teeth on both sides. Again, the lower lip is the prescribed spot to leave the third type of bite: the "point". When a small portion of the skin is bitten with two teeth only, you make this mark. The "line of points" takes the "point" one step further, and occurs when small portions of the skin are bitten with all the teeth. This type of bite is meant for the throat, armpit, joints of the thighs, forehead and the thighs themselves. The biting which is done by bringing together the teeth ("the jewel") and the lips ("the coral") is called "the coral and the jewel". The left cheek is the favoured place to leave this fifth type of bite. When biting is done with all the teeth, it is called the "line of jewels", and may be made on the throat, armpit, or the joints of the thighs. A "broken cloud" occurs when a bite is made by teeth that have a space between them, so the circle created by the bite is broken. This mark is only to be made on the breasts. The final bite is called "the biting of the boar" and consists of many broad rows of marks near to one another with inflamed, red intervals of skin between. This bite should also be made on the breasts. The last two bites are peculiar to people of intense passion.

Reciprocity is a sticking point. When a man bites a woman she should return the bite, but one level of intensity higher ("a point" should be returned as a "line of points"). Mock quarrels are often appropriate here. She should smile at the sight of

The *Kama Sutra* is written for the playboy but is also meant to be read by women. Women, as the objects of desire, are instructed on how to match the man. This is what you have to do, the text tells her, this is how you play the game. This will bring the two of you into a close union that will last forever. This is not a one-sided affair. The man needs a love partner. He wants an equal player in this game. That is when the *Kama* game is best.

marks she has made on her lover's body. This erotic, emotional, sexual reciprocity is the recipe for a lasting relationship.

Moaning and Striking

This chapter examines moaning and striking. As mentioned previously, sexual intercourse can be compared to a quarrel, as contradictory emotions are brought up and love naturally leads to disputes. It seems that it is not supposed to be easy and harmonious. There is supposed to be passion and heartbreak, followed by quarrels and making-up sex.

The special places to strike are the shoulders, the head, the space between the breasts, the back, the *jaghana* (below the navel) and the sides. These places should be struck using the four prescribed methods. Striking can occur with the back of the hand, with the fingers a little contracted, with the fist and, finally, with the open palm of the hand. Vatsyayana says when a couple becomes blind with passion, they might hurt each other and not feel it until later. That's why readers should study the *Kama Sutra*. It helps lovers to overcome animal passion and retain consciousness in sex. So, even when blinded with passion, they will not succumb to the realm of animals, and hurt each other unnecessarily.

Some translations of the *Kama Sutra* into English tell of four kinds of striking that can be done using objects or instruments. A wedge is mentioned as suitable for use on the bosom; scissors are acknowledged as something with which to strike your lover on the head; there is a piercing instrument to strike the cheeks with; and the breasts and sides can be attacked with pincer-like objects. These may be an endorsement of sadomasochistic practices in the *Kama Sutra*. Translators after Sir Richard Burton, however, claim that his sexual attitudes and sadomasochistic tendencies may have got in the way of a clear translation. His desire to confront and shock Victorian society might have muddied the true meaning of the text in this instance. Many translators have claimed that these are not instruments at all, but simply hand shapes to be applied with specific movements (e.g. striking the head in a scissor motion with the hands in a scissor shape). Vatsyayana, always the voice of reason, interjects that he doesn't endorse these particular striking tactics anyhow.

Because striking causes a little pain, it gives rise to sounds of two kinds: kissing and crying. Kissing sounds are the sounds a woman makes in reply to being kissed and pleasured by her lover as lovemaking proceeds. There are eight appropriate sounds of crying. The first is the sound "hin". The second sound is the "thundering sound", which may perhaps sound like low, rumbling thunder. The "cooing sound" is inspired by doves and other cooing birds. An imitation of tearfulness and crying is made using the "weeping sound". Then comes the "sound made by something falling into water" and the next, the "sound of bamboo being split". The seventh and eighth sounds, "sut" and "plat", are never really explained in the text (it is only said that they aren't "onomatopoeic"). It is very possible that these sounds were actually made and used during lovemaking. (In the 64 charms, at least five charming things to be learned by both men and women concern mimicry of sounds, of animals and things. Mimicry of the sounds of life was considered a sensually charming pleasure.)

The woman is also encouraged to cry out things like "mother", "father", "set me free", "stop", "enough", "release me", or praise for her skilful lover, intermingled with the eight crying sounds. To this, add the mimicry sounds of the dove, cuckoo, green pigeon, parrot, bee, sparrow, flamingo, duck or quail and you have the repertoire of sounds expected of the female of the couple.

The man is encouraged to make sounds too, in appropriate places. Again, reciprocity is encouraged. Blows with the fist should be given on the woman's back while she is sitting in her lover's lap, and she should return the blows, verbally abuse him as if she were angry, and make cooing or weeping sounds. While having sex, the space between a woman's breasts should be struck with the back of the hand, slowly at first, then getting faster as the level of excitement rises towards orgasm. Near orgasm, the breasts, midsection and sides of the woman should be pressed with the open palms with some force, until orgasm, and then followed by sounds of a quail or goose.

The Roles of Men and Women

The characteristics of man are given as roughness and impetuosity, while the woman's are weakness, tenderness, sensibility and the inclination to turn away from unpleasant things. The excitement of passion can upset this natural state, however (but in the end, the natural state is resumed). What happens in the bedroom, stays in the bedroom, it seems.

Role reversal occurs when the woman plays the man's part. A woman should only play the part of a man if her lover is fatigued by constant congress but not satisfied; if her lover is curious and asks her to; or when she herself simply desires some novelty. Though a woman is naturally reserved, she should show all her love and desire when she gets on top. When the woman is playing the man's role, she performs the sexual strokes that are usually attributed to him. She also has three positions of her own to perform. A man will find out a lot about a woman's desires when she is on top of him playing his role.

Whatever is done by a man for giving pleasure to a woman is called "the work of a man" and consists of nine seduction techniques and nine physical strokes used during intercourse. The man, while the woman is lying on the bed and absorbed with his conversation, should loosen the knot of her undergarments and, when she disputes with him, he should overwhelm her with kisses. When his *lingam* is erect he should touch her in various places. If the woman is bashful, and it is the first time that they have come together, he should place his hands between her thighs. He should take hold of her hair and hold her chin in his fingers for the purpose of kissing her. He should gather from the action of the woman what things would be pleasing to her during congress. While he is doing to the woman what he likes best during congress, he should always make a point of pressing those parts of her body on which she turns her eyes. These seem to be the prescribed roles to be learned by both the man and the woman. The seducer learns to seduce, but the seduced is also told what to expect and how to act so that she is a suitable object of seduction, and her seduction can be complete.

The man is commonly responsible for such things as bringing the sexual organs together, which is called "moving forward", and also holding his *lingam* with his hand and turning it all around in her *yoni* ("churning"). He may also strike only the upper part of the *yoni* with his *lingam*. This is called "piercing". Or he may concentrate his thrusts on only the lower part of his lover's *yoni* ("rubbing"). A variation on the previous two strokes is achieved when he presses his *lingam* against her *yoni* for a considered amount of time before proceeding ("pressing"). "Giving a blow" is when he withdraws his *lingam* to some distance from the woman's *yoni*, and then forcibly strikes it, burying himself inside her in one swift motion. When one part of the *yoni* is rubbed with the *lingam*, it's "the blow of a boar", and when both sides are rubbed, it's "the blow of a bull". The last stroke done by a man is "the sporting of a sparrow", which is when the *lingam* is moved up and down in the *yoni* without being taken out.

The signs of the woman's enjoyment and satisfaction with these strokes and with the actions of her lover are that she closes her eyes, puts aside her bashfulness, and shows increased willingness and passion during sex. The signs of her failing to be satisfied are that she shakes her hands, does not let the man get up from the bed to leave after he has finished, feels dejected, bites the man, or kicks him. If she continues to go on moving after the man has had his orgasm, she is obviously upset at not having climaxed. In such cases, the man should rub the woman's *yoni* with his hand and fingers until she is satisfied.

On Fellatio and Cunnilingus

One of the last chapters of the *Kama Sutra* looks at oral sex. This was a practice done in ancient India, it seems, only by two kinds of eunuch (those disguised as males and those disguised as females), wanton women, female attendants and serving maids (all three being kinds of unmarried women). Ancient authors say that oral sex is low practice and opposed to the orders of the Holy Writ, and that the man suffers spiritually by coming into contact with the mouths of these kinds of women and eunuchs. Vatsyayana, however, says that this practice is akin to using courtesans and so is agreeable by Holy Writ. He also says that it is a practice that happens in certain regions and that it is a matter of personal preference. According to his creed in all things connected with love, people should do what they are comfortable with. Some male servants have oral sex with their masters, some men have oral sex with each other, and some women give each other oral pleasure. Some men even do the same thing with women. Vatsyayana alludes to cunnilingus and says that it is performed in the same way as kissing the mouth, and that sometimes men and women lie inverted in a position known as "the congress of a crow".

The techniques of fellatio, well known to both types of eunuch, start with "the nominal congress", which is when, holding the man's *lingam* with his hand, and placing it between his lips, the eunuch moves his mouth all around. The second technique is called "biting the sides". Here the eunuch covers the end of the man's *lingam* with his fingers that he's formed together in the shape of a flower bud. After this, the eunuch presses the sides of the man's *lingam* with his lips and teeth. This is "Pressing outside", the third technique. Next the eunuch presses the end of the *lingam* with pursed lips and kisses it as if drawing it out. When the eunuch puts the *lingam* further into his mouth and presses it with his lips, then takes it out, it's called "pressing inside". "Kissing" is when the *lingam* is held in the hand and kissed with the kiss generally given to the lower lip. The next technique is called "rubbing", and involves the eunuch touching the *lingam* with his tongue everywhere, and passing his tongue over the end of it. Technique seven is when the eunuch puts half the *lingam* in his mouth, forcibly kisses and sucks it. This is "sucking the mango". When orgasm is near, the eunuch performs the final technique, called "swallowing up", where he puts the entire *lingam* into his mouth, and takes it to the very back of his throat as if he were going to "swallow it up".

Sex Aids

Magic played a large part in ancient India, as did drugs for increasing sexual prowess of success. When a person was unable to secure the object of his desires by normal means like good looks or charm, he could resort to other, artificial means to get what he wanted. The following are examples of magic that could be employed to win unattainble women:

- If a man, after anointing his *lingam* with a mixture of the powders of the white thorn apple, the long pepper and the black pepper, and honey, engages in sexual union with a woan, he makes her subject to his will.
- If a man cuts into small pieces the spourts of the *vajnasunhi* plant, and dips them into a mixture of red arsenic and sulphur, and then dries them seven times, and applies this powder mixed with honey to his *lingam*, he can subjugate a woman to his will directly after he has had sexual union with her; or if by burning these very sprouts at night and looking at the smoke, he sees a golden moon behind, he will then be successful with any woman; or if he throws some of the powder of these same spourts mixed with the excrement of a monkey upon a maiden, she will not be given in marriage to anybody else.

The *Kama Sutra* in the Twenty-first Century

Simply put, there is no definitive translation of *Kama Sutra*. The interpretation of Vatsyayana's original Sanskrit and its conveyance into English appears to cover a broad spectrum. Each translator brings their own interpretations and agendas to their version of the *Kama Sutra*. From Sir Richard Burton and his desire to destroy prudish Victorian society, to Indra Sinha, who hoped to more closely portray Vatsyayana's *sutra* style by using five-line prose stanzas, to Alain Danielou, who fashioned himself as a modern-day *nagaraka*, there are as many interpretations of the text as there are translators.

The *Kama Sutra* today seems to have a life of its own. From its royal beginnings, it has become a public domain nightmare of strange positions and varying degrees of faithfulness to the text. There are some *Kama Sutra* picture books interested in developing sexual relationships between loving couples that soften some of the more acrobatic positions and focus instead on the healthy eroticism of the lovemaking. Then there are the soft-porn websites of certain men's magazines featuring positions that rarely resemble the traditional postures (with updated names to go with them) and which distort anything traditional to pornographic extremes. These seem to just use the *Kama Sutra* as a dirty book to provide inspiration for sex. That would probably be perfectly acceptable to Vatsyayana, as long as he could believe that men and women were being encouraged to engage in loving relationships at the behest of his book.

Even when separated from sex, however, the *Kama Sutra* offers an incredibly inspiring call to pay attention to creating the foundations of a sensuous life. It is also fascinating as a time-capsule document revealing the mores of ancient India and the transcendence of love across all time and space.

This present collection does not pretend to be a definitive version of the legendary Indian book. It is more of a sampling – illustrated by clever tales in the spirit of both Vatsyayana and

Sir Richard Burton. The positions that follow from the various sections of the *Kama Sutra* will, we hope, give a flavour of the original and convey its robust eroticism, joie de vivre, complexity and universality.

Trisha Telep

Kama Sutra

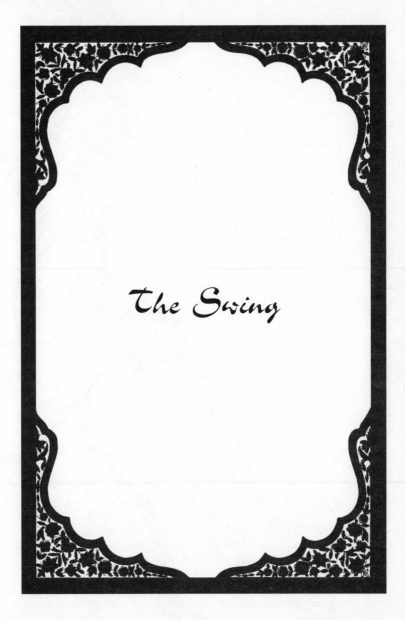

The Swing

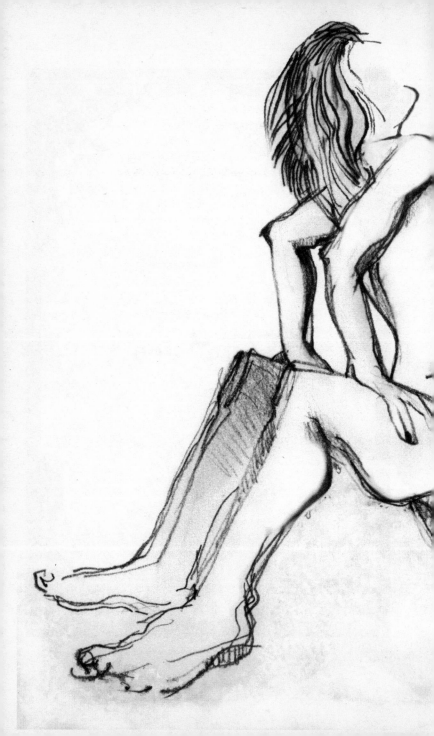

The Swing

Prenkholita
Kama Sutra

Here is a position for the most virile of female partners. As the woman is on top, she is responsible for the quick, intricate movements of this position, without much help from her lover (except the occasional bit of assistance as he elevates his pelvis to plunge further into her). She must move her hips in figure of eights, back and forth, side to side, in fact, in all directions, without her passion or intensity flagging. The swing is a virtuoso performance from the leading lady in a position of dominance and power.

When a courtesan, out of need for money, or freedom from fear, desires to attach herself to a wealthy, educated man, she should show him her considerable skill in the sexual arts, especially in poses such as "the swing". It is by doing this that she might cast a spell over him and make him her benefactor for many years to come.

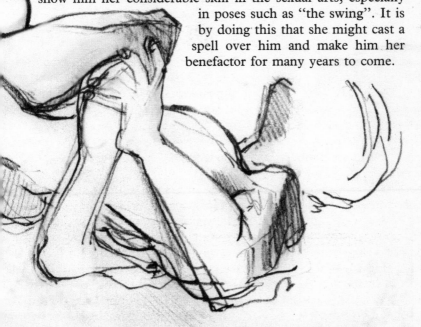

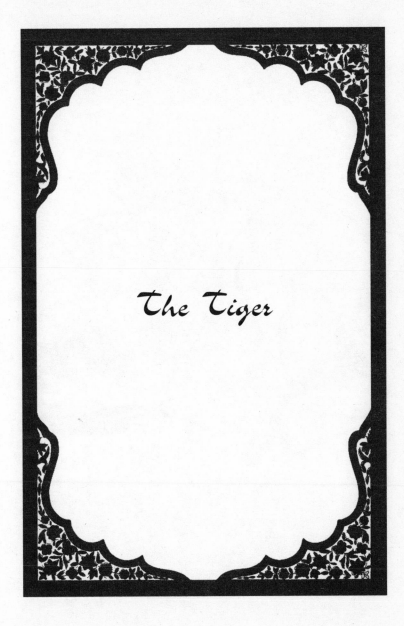

The Tiger

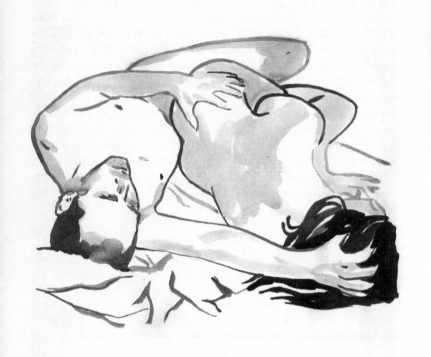

The Tiger

Vyaghera
Kama Sutra

This is a rear-entry position that takes inspiration from one of the most ferocious, deadly beasts of the jungle. It is a position of male domination where the tigress is held down by the male who is atop her. In the wild, male tigers often go so far as to use their teeth to grip the female's neck or head and keep her in position. The male must do everything in his power to foil the female's escape. The aspects of theatre here are evident, for just like other animal positions, the requisite tiger sounds (e.g. fierce growling) are to be produced. The man should also feel free to employ the listed thrusts and strokes to determine exactly what the woman likes. Vatsyayana doesn't prescribe specific strokes for a specific position, but instead lists them on their own, to be used on any occasion. The possible penetration is very deep, however, so some of the more intense strokes will be more than adequate to please your tigress.

The Tale of the Tigress

as told by Andrea Dale

Gather close, my daughters and sons, for I have another tale to tell you, a tale of great courage and great love and yes, great passion, too. You have already heard how the Lotus came into being, and why the Wheelbarrow was so named, and now it is time for you to hear of the Tigress.

Long ago, the gods and goddesses spent more time in the world of men. Some found us amusing; others, an annoyance to be avoided. Still others used us for whatever reasons they chose, or no reason whatsoever except idle whimsy.

Some walked among us in human form and others in their true form, and such was the whim of Budhi Pallien. Yes, you recognize that name: the forest goddess here in the north of India.

Budhi Pallien could be a beautiful woman or a ferocious tiger, and she protected the forest, and of course tigers were close to her heart. So it came to be that a denizen of a small village was out hunting for food. His arrow went wide as he shot at a chital, and it struck a tiger who was also stalking the same deer.

The goddess, as you might imagine – for I see you shuddering with fear – went into a rage. She stalked the young man as he had stalked the chital, and she carried him away into the forest to meet his punishment.

But this is not his story. This story is about Duranjaya, the young man's brother, whose name means "heroic son" and who journeyed deep into the forest to rescue his sibling.

It is said he travelled for thirty days, and it is also said he wandered for a hundred, and it is also said he journeyed for only three, which is the way of these types of stories. The important point is that he found Budhi Pallien before the goddess had killed his brother.

The other, perhaps less important but perhaps more important point, was that when he found them, he was at first struck dumb at the sight of the goddess' beauty.

She was tall, with breasts like ripe mangos and hips as curved and flowing as the Ganges. Her black hair glittered like moonlight and hung to her knees, and smelled like earth and dreams, and her skin was the colour of cardamom.

Duranjaya's *lingam* stirred beneath his *dhoti*. He wanted to bury his face between her breasts, breathe in the fragrance of her hair, caress the silk of her skin and explore the treasures found between her thighs.

It was the goddess herself who broke him from his reverie. Her eyes, golden and slitted like a great cat's, glittered with amusement as she regarded him, and he knew she had seen his excitement. But wasn't such a goddess used to being worshipped? Perhaps that was why she didn't kill him outright.

Instead, she said, "Why have you sought me out, handsome man? I get few devotees at my temple here."

"I have come to take my brother home," Duranjaya said.

His brother lay, bound by vines to a marble column of Budhi Pallien's temple. He shook his head, obviously unable to speak by some spell, but Duranjaya paid him no heed.

Budhi Pallien laughed, and her mouth was as wide as a tiger's when it yawns, and he could see the untamed beast barely contained by her human form. He was fearful even as he was aroused.

"And what makes you think I would just hand over your brother at your request?" she asked. "Surely you know that when you beg a boon from a goddess, you must give her an offering worthy of her, an offering of equal or greater value to the favour you ask."

Duranjaya was not a stupid man, but in his haste to save his brother – and his stunned reaction to Budhi Pallien – he had not even considered the need for an offering.

But being not stupid, and being as astute as he was, he had seen the way her gaze had taken him in, and he had noted that she called him handsome. Although he still assumed his life would be forfeit, he said, "I offer you myself in exchange for my brother." He drew himself up, held himself tight to keep from trembling. "If you let my brother go, I will stay with you

myself, and face whatever fate you would have cast upon him."
For Duranjaya lived up to his name's meaning.

This time, Budhi Pallien did not laugh. Instead, she paced, her silk sari flowing about her and outlining her lush figure. Duranjaya swallowed, unable to stop the throbbing of his *lingam*, even if it meant the death of him. He, a mere mortal, showing his lust for Budhi Pallien could cause the goddess to take deep offence.

If any man had shown such desire and lived, Duranjaya had never heard the tale.

Budhi Pallien circled him slowly, stalking him, and he knew he was prey. When she was in front of him again, she said, "I will consider your offer. If you prove yourself to me, prove you are worthy to take your brother's place, then I will release him unharmed."

"And if I do not prove myself?" Duranjaya asked.

She smiled, and her teeth were as white as ivory and as sharp as fangs. "Then you will both die."

To his surprise, she held out her hand. He took it, and she drew him into the depths of the temple. As they passed his brother, she waved a hand over him, and he fell into a deep sleep.

Duranjaya did not know if a goddess needed to sleep, or whether she sometimes took on her tigress form and stretched on the flagstones before the fire. Perhaps her bed, draped with coloured silks and soft with pillows, was just a place for her to lounge in her human shape.

Or, he realized now as she sliced the *kurta* from his body, a place for her to take pleasure.

The rest of Duranjaya's clothing fell away, and Budhi Pallien paced around him again. This was how he must please her, he knew, how he must prove himself worthy.

His erection grew; arousal shivered through him, hardening him, readying him. Although he had no wife, he was far from inexperienced, and in fact he found himself relishing the challenge of pleasuring a goddess. That she was stunning, that he reacted to her without a touch, would only add to his own pleasure.

It is one thing to be brave – it is another to be overconfident.

She was the goddess of the forest, and thus she had dominion over it. At her unspoken commands, thick vines twined their way in beneath the archways and down along the columns. They reached into the air and wrapped around Duranjaya's wrists, drawing his arms above his head.

Anchoring him in place. Leaving him stretched and vulnerable to the deity's whims.

He had heard of such games before, but never played them, and indeed he had only briefly considered them with the thought that the woman would be at his mercy.

Now he was helpless and, to his surprise, it was not an unwelcome sensation at all, even as he knew Budhi Pallien would not be gentle and was unlikely to be truly merciful.

She stalked him still, sizing up her prey, and yet all he could think of was that even if he died in the end, his last moments would be in ecstasy.

Her hand cupped the fullness of his sac, measuring, considering. She trailed a single nail along the underside of his *lingam*, from base to tip.

He bit back a moan, but the twitching of his member revealed all he felt. Budhi Pallien laughed, low and sultry, almost a tiger's rumbling purr.

"I am glad my *lingam* pleases you," Duranjaya said, although the throbbing of his blood in his veins and the need for relief made it hard for him to speak. "It is but yours to use as you see fit."

He hoped that would be soon.

She laughed again. "Foolish man," she said. "*You* are mine to use as I see fit – all of you. But your *lingam* is indeed proud and well-sized." She encircled the length of him with her fingers. "Long and thick," she said. "You must have given many women great pleasure."

He dipped his head. "It is not only one's *lingam* that gives pleasure," he said. "How one works with the tools one has makes the difference."

"We shall put your tool to good use," Budhi Pallien promised. "But not just yet. I am still taking measure of you."

And as he stood there, helpless, she explored every part of him. Kisses were exchanged with bites, caresses with scratches. Sweat ran down his back, the salt causing the wounds to burn.

But to his surprise, the stinging only added to his arousal.

When she slid a finger between his cheeks, probing, his hips jerked forward. His *lingam* thrust futilely into empty air, weeping fluid, but he knew better than to beg for a touch to bring him relief.

"Shall I find a smooth cylinder of jade to slide in here?" she purred in his ear.

"If that would add to your amusement," he said between gritted teeth.

"Hmm . . ." Her finger flexed within him, and he couldn't help but cry out at the sensation. "Perhaps later," she said. "I never grow weary of tormenting handsome men, but I want pleasure, too, and wish to see what you can provide."

The binding vines rustled away. He had little time to rub his stiff shoulders before Budhi Pallien was drawing him towards the soft, cushioned platform.

How many other men had she brought here? he wondered. He knew he was not her first, and would be far from her last. It wasn't jealousy that made him wonder, but curiosity and again a sense of wanting to gratify her, to be a worthy lover.

He wasn't surprised when she pushed him down into the sea of silk; of course she would take the dominant position. Propped up on his elbows, he watched, mouth dry and *lingam* throbbing, as she let her sari slither down to pool at her feet. As he'd known she would be, she was exquisite.

Sleek muscles rippled beneath her dusky skin, her legs long and powerful. Her breasts were tipped with dark nipples drawn and tight, and when she threw a leg across his lap and leaned forward, he not only knew what she expected, but was eager to comply.

He suckled her, and her hips undulated like a dancing cobra. Her moist heat against him nearly brought him to orgasm, but he dragged himself back from the brink, knowing that if he gave in to his release so soon he would incur her displeasure and perhaps even her wrath.

How long would she test him? How long could he hold out?

When she had reached her fill of his ministrations, breathing heavily, he expected her to simply straddle him. But again Budhi Pallien had other plans, ideas he could not nor ever hope to predict.

She straddled him, yes, but at an angle, with her left leg over his left shoulder as he sat up. To balance her, he slipped his hands beneath her bottom, cupping her round cheeks, and in this way he found he had some control to move her.

When she settled on him, her wet warm *yoni* surrounding and tightening about his *lingam*, every muscle in his body tensed against the astonishing need to release his seed.

No. Not before she had reached her own climax. Not until she allowed him.

He swiftly learned why she had chosen this unusual position, why she was allowing him to move her rather than controlling the motions herself. It left her hands free, and she put her hands to good use once again.

Her nails dug into his shoulders, the pain fierce and bright; he had no doubt bright spots of blood welled up on his skin. But the torment only heightened his arousal. His *lingam* pumped tighter, the skin so sensitive he believed he could feel every inch of her *yoni* gripping him, sliding up and down upon him. He couldn't help a groan of pure lust from escaping his lips.

Then her hands moved, raking his arms, his thighs, urging him to move faster, harder. He was overcome by sensation, pleasure and pain merging and mingling into one greater feeling that transcended anything he'd experienced before.

And as Budhi Pallien's *yoni* clenched and squeezed him, as her body gripped him with her climax, he could no longer hold back. He thrust up into her, and his passion blossomed in the base of his spine, expanding like a lotus until it burst out of him.

The next morning, Budhi Pallien released his brother. The young man, dazed and still half-enchanted, headed into the jungle. The goddess assured Duranjaya that he would find his way home unharmed.

Although Duranjaya was reasonably certain that he had performed adequately throughout the night, he still found he needed to ask her why she had granted his boon and released his brother.

Budhi Pallien trailed a nail down his chest, scraping lightly. He almost flinched, for he was sore from all the harsh caresses of the night. For a moment he thought he saw a tiger's claw, but perhaps it was only a shift of the morning light between the heavy-leafed vines.

"Because you are a pretty human, and you pique my interest," she said. "You are brave but vulnerable, focused on your purpose yet distracted by my beauty.

"And," she added, "you have proved delightfully fun to play with. Yes, I think I will keep you."

It seemed to Duranjaya that this would not be such an awful fate.

There is a certain decadence to living with a goddess. Oh, she demanded much of him when it came to slaking and satisfying her pleasure, but Duranjaya found himself anticipating the bites and scratches and withheld release. He grew to crave her creative and wicked imagination, finding himself bound, whipped, impaled, tortured with peacock feathers, and ultimately soaring on clouds of ecstasy.

When they were not exploring the limits of desire, Budhi Pallien requested he provide her with other amusements. So he told her stories, tales of his people, sharing the joys and tragedies and humour of mortal life. He sang to her, and sometimes she sang too, in a voice that would make koel birds weep.

There was sumptuous food as well: the most succulent of fruits, rice redolent with spices, tart yogurt. There were sizzling meats also, which surprised him at first, but then he was reminded that Budhi Pallien's other form was that of a tiger. The world had a natural cycle, plants and animals and earth and sky and fire and water. The jungle was her domain, and she protected and guided it well.

Duranjaya fell into that ebbing and flowing rhythm, his time with the goddess as fluid as the days and nights themselves. Hours passed, and days and weeks and months, but all was in a haze of pleasure and bliss.

But still there came a time – he knew not how long it took him to come to this moment – when he thought of his brother and his parents and his village. Although he trusted Budhi Pallien's word that his brother had safely returned, Duranjaya longed to see them all again, to see for himself their good health and happiness.

Budhi Pallien did not want him to go. "You will find things very different there," she warned him. "You have changed. Your family and friends have changed. I cannot tell you how, for your world is unfamiliar to me, but I know that you will not be gratified with what you find."

But Duranjaya could not let go of his yearning to return, and in the end Budhi Pallien could not find it in herself to deny him his wish. He would return – of that there was no question. He had no intention of leaving forever and she had no intention of letting him go forever.

Duranjaya had not worn clothes for so long that draping the garments around him seemed foreign, and although he winced as the silks settled on the freshest of his welts, he did not dislike the sensation.

Budhi Pallien gave him water and food for his journey, and after a final kiss he set off into the jungle.

What Duranjaya did not know, and what Budhi Pallien could not in her immortality begin to comprehend, was that time moves differently for the gods than it does for mortals. Although Duranjaya had been with the goddess for a time that did not seem long to him, his village had seen many, many years go by.

The village had grown; there were many more houses than he remembered, with streets he did not know. But stranger still was that he recognized none of the villagers.

Duranjaya was still a strapping young man not yet past his twenty-fifth year, but what he discovered was that his brother, who had been a few years younger when he'd accidentally shot the tiger in the jungle, was now an old man, white haired and gnarled and shrunken.

Their parents were long dead, his brother said, although the fact was plain.

"How could this be?" Duranjaya cried. But even as he asked, he knew the answer, understood how the world of gods and the world of men flow at different speeds as a wide river does not flow the same as a narrow, rocky stream.

His brother had assumed Duranjaya was dead when he didn't return to the village, so their reunion was a joyous one. But although Duranjaya was glad to be with his family again (for he counted his brother's children and grandchildren among them now), he found that he pined for the harsh yet exciting caresses and the supple body of Budhi Pallien, and even the conversations they shared. He also discovered that, as he spent time in his old village, he seemed to age faster than a normal man would.

As a man ages, he often gains a certain, greater desire; thus Duranjaya knew he must return to Budhi Pallien and beg yet another boon from her. He said his farewells to his brother, his family and his friends, and set off again into the jungle.

The journey back to Budhi Pallien seemed to take longer. His joints had begun to ache; his muscles were not as supple as they had been.

Budhi Pallien was overjoyed to see her lover again, but also shocked to see him thus, with his hair growing grey at the temples and the slightest of stoops to his shoulders.

Still he was virile, his *lingam* burgeoning hard and proud in her presence, and he craved her touch. First, though, he had to make his appeal.

"You are immortal," Duranjaya said. "Living ever on, never changing. But I am mortal, and the only way a mortal man can have immortality is to father a child. And I realized the truth of the matter is that I wish to father a child with the woman I have grown to love, goddess though she may be."

He had little hope that Budhi Pallien would agree, but the fact of this tale is, Budhi Pallien had, despite herself, fallen in love with her brave and strong and willing companion. Although the gods and goddesses do not breed as frequently as humans or animals, they do at times feel the desire to create a new life in such a fashion.

Thus Budhi Pallien assented to Duranjaya's request.

She drew him to her bed, and mounted him in the fashion that most pleased her. Although he had aged, Duranjaya still had the strength to lift her upon him, one of her legs across the chest and over his shoulder, leaving her free to brand him with her pearl-tipped nails and sharp teeth.

His passion flared as she did so, and as always it was hard for him to hold himself back. He slipped one hand between them and caressed the hard pearl between her legs, and Budhi Pallien roared like the tiger she could become.

Soon thereafter, though, she was twined with Duranjaya, purring like a cat, and they both knew his seed had taken root within her.

"We will have a daughter," Budhi Pallien said, and together they agreed her name would be Nisha.

But Duranjaya could not stay to watch their precious Nisha grow from a babe to a strong young woman, who he knew would be lithe and fierce like her mother. They both knew he needed to live out the rest of his days – which would not be many – with his people.

His cuts and bruises causing a delicious ache, Duranjaya made one last journey through the jungle. Before he died, he relayed to all in his village the story of his time with Budhi Pallien, leaving out no detail, and he urged them all to keep the tale alive.

The position Budhi Pallien favoured, with her long, catlike limbs wrapped around her partner and her teeth and nails, not quite claws but close enough for memory and belief, marking his skin, thus became known in the *Kama Sutra* as the Tigress position.

While it may be more aggressive than you might have considered in your own lovemaking, my children, do not discount it out of hand. Pain and pleasure twine hand in hand, and if you open yourself to the possibilities, you may find your passion to be as strong as a goddess's.

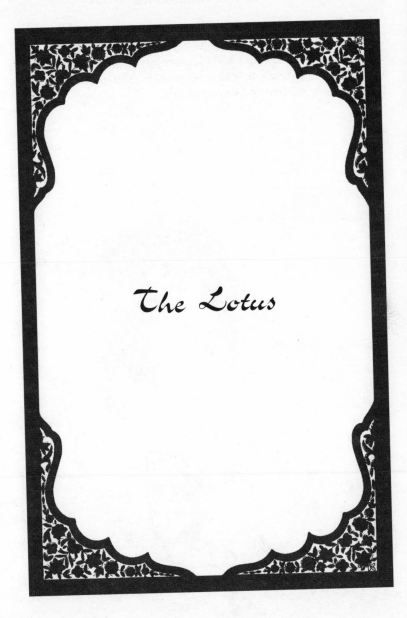

The Lotus

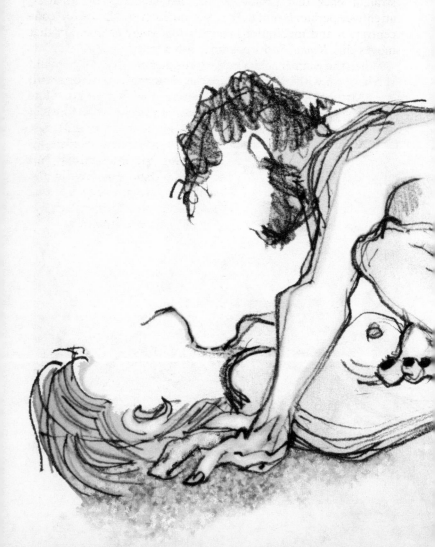

The Lotus

Padmasana
Kama Sutra

In this yoga posture, the legs mimic the look of a blossoming lotus. This is a traditional yoga position with crossed legs and straight back that promotes the characteristics of an alert, attentive, perhaps, mind. It is the position of choice for concentration and meditation, and it's this yogic connection that moves this *Kama Sutra* position into a tantric realm.

When the woman achieves the lotus posture, the lover should rub her *yoni* with his fingers (like an elephant rubs objects with its trunk) to open her and cause a flow of wetness. Slow penetration is best in this position because the foreskin could be injured if the initial stroke is too swift. Sex in this position could not help but conjure up images of worship and the spiritual, but whether the yogic postures in the *Kama Sutra* are a nod to a sexual communication with the Divine is open to interpretation.

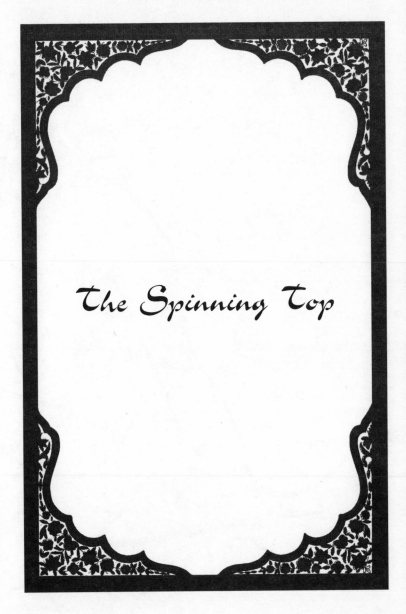

The Spinning Top

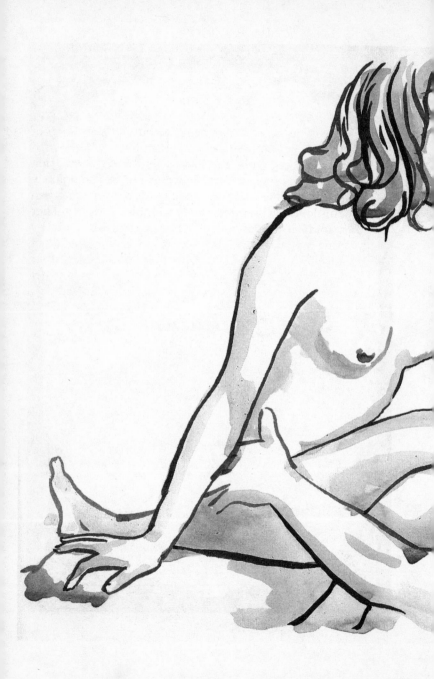

The Spinning Top

Paravrittaka
Kama Sutra

The position is given this name because of the action of the woman spinning in a circle, much like a wheel, without withdrawing from her lover's *lingam*. It seems that some translators believe that the woman moves completely around in a circle while on top of her lover. The man can assist his lover by lifting her body with his hands to aid her in her spin on top of him. The man can also assist by thrusting up his pelvis. This position requires a lot of practice because of the possibility of injury. Also, if either of the partners is of intense passion, they are liable to get so carried away with the sensation involved here that they do the other injury.

The Tale of Mitra and Kumari

as told by Mitch

A time long ago, in the province of Uttar Pradesh on the flood plain of the holy Ganges River, an albino child was born into the Brahman caste. His albinism was seen as a sign from the gods. He was revered not only by his family but by the entire community. He was named Mitra, which means god of the sun, to symbolize his whiteness. His skin and hair were white and his irises pink.

Soon after his birth, myths about his abilities multiplied in the countryside. Reportedly, he could talk and read before he could walk as well as interpret dreams. In addition, it was believed he had magical powers. None of these were true, of course, but perceptions are more important than facts in a fatalistic culture.

It was true he received special treatment. He was breastfed by his mother and a series of wet nurses until he was seven. From an early age he was taught self-discipline. He learned to read and interpret the Hindu classics. He practised tantra yoga, using a mantra he contemplated and meditated in an attempt to achieve oneness with the god Shiva and his wife Parvati, the goddess of love.

The four aims of Hinduism were drilled into him: 1) *Dharma*, satisfy religious, social and moral obligations to those of his caste and to those below; 2) *Artha*, ensure material well-being of self and family; 3) *Kama*, enjoy a life of pleasure and love through sexual proficiency; and 4) *Moksha*, find release from the cycle of rebirth and unity with the universe.

He was seldom seen beyond the walls of the family compound and then only at dawn or dusk because of the danger from the sun to his skin and eyes. Two Sikh bodyguards and members of his family accompanied him on these outings He was always dressed in white, with a visor over his eyes. Even as a youngster his presence was seen as a blessing to the community and his open, casually given blessings, were cherished.

Rumours of his adherence to the priestly practices of his Brahman caste added to the reverence in which he was held. Stories about his intelligence, physical strength and flexibility, the length of his meditative incantations, and his respect for traditional Hindu customs added to the myth.

At the age of ten, in order to prepare him to satisfy his *dharma*, he was given the responsibility of a family that had been unable to pay their appropriate taxes. He listened quietly to the elders of the household, and in consultation with them devised a plan to increase their agricultural production. The scheme worked; the family prospered and was soon able to pay its taxes. Word of Mitra's involvement with the tenant farmers' prosperity added to the myths and to his karma.

Over the next three years he was given the task of managing the entire village. After consulting with the elders and local experts, he saw to the consolidation of fields, to the improvement of the irrigation system and to the use of hybrid seeds. Production of rice, carp, soy and vegetables soared. His efforts provided wealth for his family and improved the standard of living of their tenants. In this way both his *dharma* and *artha* were attained.

At the same time his priestly duties increased. He presided at weddings and feast days with an authority and confidence that far surpassed his elders. His style adhered to classic traditions but added a modicum of unprecedented pleasure and joy. His special abilities, knowledge, skills, winsome personality and heavenly good looks reflected the gifts symbolized by his albinism and made him a legend in his own time. Leaders throughout the province and beyond sought his advice and insight.

As he neared his fourteenth birthday, he had successfully achieved both *dharma* and *artha*. Karma had been realized through his actions, and he had achieved a measure of fame but he had not attained *kama*, the pleasure and love befitting his status. On his birthday his father and mother reminded him of two responsibilities of *kama*: one was that sexual intercourse was a religious duty, and two, in order to fulfil that duty, he had to marry and produce male heirs.

That evening as he reclined on a pallet in his room a door slid open and a female crawled into his room. "My lord, my name is Andhra and it is my honoured privilege to be your first congress. For the next two weeks my associates and I will instruct you in the ways of the *Kama Sutra*."

"Welcome, I've been waiting for the day when my education would be complete. I'll follow your instructions as to the Way of Love, although I am familiar with the process because of my studies."

Andhra disrobed. She stood close to enable him to observe her body because of his poor eyesight. Then she removed his clothes with great ceremony. She gasped when his loincloth dropped. "My lord, you are endowed as the bull. It will give me great pleasure to be your first." She proceeded to take him through the first four stages of lovemaking: the ceremonial slap, the consumption of a small portion of fish, the eating of a bowl of rice and the drinking of wine.

She then took him through the next stages which included: kissing, hugging, scratching, fondling and massaging the skin. He was a good student. He learned to be slow, gentle and caring. She offered her breasts and he nibbled, licked and sucked with unexpected expertise. She stroked his *lingam* until he had a glorious erection, but stopped, allowing his passion to cool. After taking a moment she performed fellatio on his engorged *lingam*. She licked his pre-come. She ran her tongue along the length of his shaft and then took him into her mouth. Her firm lips slid up and down with deliberate slowness and when he showed signs of coming she stopped. She would have gladly sucked him dry, but she had been instructed not to waste royal seed outside the *yoni*.

When his excitement subsided she introduced him to her *yoni*. She took his hand and led him in rubbing her pubic area until her vulva lips began to swell and moisten. Then she taught him how to explore her depths with his fingers and find her most delicate spot. When he did so she said, "My lord, with less experienced women that spot will elicit great pleasure and an orgasm. Even I am experiencing elation."

She moved his finger out of her vagina and to her clitoris. "This small mound, my lord, is the clitoris and is a woman's most sensitive place; take your time and rub it as gently as you can in all directions." She lay on her back and watched his pinkish-white figure, in the shadows of the flickering candles, proceed as a surgeon with care and diligence.

She was becoming aroused when she stopped his probing and instructed him about cunnilingus. She washed and perfumed herself and then, with her guidance, he explored her lotus. First he licked her pubic hair sopping wet, then inserted his tongue between her lips and, after a long time, found her clitoris. Unexpectedly, she had a rush of emotion as his venturesome tongue brought her to an orgasm, "Eeeeeh," she moaned. He pulled away thinking he had hurt her, but she gently pulled him back to her and said breathlessly, "My lord, you have achieved your mission. To bring a woman to orgasm is your solemn duty. Thank you, that was exquisite." She writhed in pleasure as he continued to explore her intimate regions. She had a number of mini orgasms and had to remind herself to return to her lessons.

"My lord, you are a brilliant student, but while these first acts are especially enjoyed by women it is the congress, the joining, that is of most importance to men. The crab position is one of the most common methods of penetration. It can be performed in many positions but the simplest is for me to lie on my back."

He did as he was instructed and was amazed by the satisfaction that swept through him as he penetrated her to his depth.

"Ah, Mitra, you are huge and fill me completely. When you are ready, ride me as though I were a water buffalo," she said as she grabbed him and pulled him deeper into her. She directed him with her hands and was astonished because he didn't climax quickly. Rather, under her urging, he rocked within her for a long time. Finally, she said, "My Lord Mitra, your weight is too much for me. Please rise up on your hands and continue." He did so and resumed. "Faster, my lord."

Mitra increased his speed until he sensed a strange feeling moving through his loins. He stopped and uttered, "Aaaaah."

"Don't stop, my lord, you're close to coming."

Mitra returned to his stroking and within minutes he gave one mighty shove and poured forth continuous gushes of fluid. His body went into spasms and with each jolt he spurted more sperm, until he cried out, "Shiva, Shiva, Shiva," and fell from her body.

Within a short time he said, "That was wonderful, can we do it again?"

"In a minute, my lord, if you're able."

She cleaned both of them and then using both hands she pleasured herself, stroked him lightly, and soon he was ready.

"Now, my lord, we'll use the cow position. I'll kneel on all fours and you enter from behind."

She assumed the position, Mitra placed his hands on her hips and with her guidance he entered her. He held her hips and stroked without instruction; she was amazed because he lasted forever. She had to drop her head to the floor when her arms grew weary, and he stroked her into a continuous state of ecstasy. He stopped when she began to moan. She begged him to continue because her moaning was from pleasure. Finally, his *lingam* swelled, to what seemed twice its size, and he pumped stream after stream of semen into her.

She spent the rest of the evening instructing Mitra about the art of after-play. Early in the morning she crept from his chamber, leaving behind a tired but happy 14-year-old.

Over the next thirteen evenings he was visited by a different courtesan, each of whom furthered his instruction in the Ways of Love. The fundamentals of the *Kama Sutra*, other tantric verses and individual variations were added. Mitra was an enthusiastic and apt student who learned quickly. Comments of the courtesans to his servants were soon circulating throughout the community. They whispered their "secrets" with pride: the size of their master's *lingam*, his endurance and his rapid recovery ability.

The search for a satisfactory wife began. There was no shortage of applicants because rumours of Mitra's worldly and sexual prowess spread far beyond the province of Uttar Pradesh to the whole of India. The process, it was thought, would be short and that the prince would marry and carry out his husbandly and worldly duties in a short time. However, years passed and he had not yet found the one.

The moon was full, the breeze light, Mitra reclined on his pallet waiting for his twenty-first birthday gift. The same present he had received every evening for the past seven years, a female willing to serve him as a sexual instrument, willing to be the one who pleased him, willing to be the one who enabled him to become one with the gods.

In the chamber below another partner was being prepared by a cadre of specially trained servants. They saw to her physical cleanliness. They participated in a purification rite led by Mitra's father, and they uttered for the 2,543rd time, "Shiva, Parvati, Shakti, we humbly ask that Kumari be the one, allow her to lead Lord Mitra to oneness with you. Amen and amen!"

Kumari was led up the stairs to the entrance to Mitra's room. Everything had been prepared for her performance. The door was slid open and she entered on hands and knees.

"My lord, I'm here to serve and give you pleasure."

"And, I you," he responded.

She knelt in front of him dressed in a pink sari. In the candlelit room his nude, white body reflected the flickering flames. They exchanged ceremonial slaps, a sign of commitment. She served both of them a portion of carp, a glass of wine and finally a rice cake. When they finished, she stood and removed her sari so he could see her better. Kumari turned in a tight circle in front of him. Even with his poor eyesight he could see she had skin darker than most, a Dravidian, her body a perfectly proportioned fiddle back with hips as wide as her shoulders, a slightly protruding derriere and breasts larger than most. Mitra noticed a different scent, it wasn't the soap used by his servants but it was a smell that caused his nose to tingle. He was pleased.

They kissed; it was not passionate but sensuous. Mitra noticed the softness of her lips and a zesty taste that complemented her aroma. The ritual kissing, rubbing and scratching was more stimulating than usual. She stroked his *lingam* erect, and loved it with her mouth: kissing, licking and sucking until he neared a climax. Surprised, he pulled her away.

"My lord, have I done something wrong?" she asked looking worried.

He hesitated. "Nothing is wrong," he said, looking at her beautiful face with a spark of wonder. "Lie down please."

Lying side by side in the Crab position they kissed and he enjoyed the warmth and flavour of her lips. He lowered himself to her breasts. They're beautiful, he thought as he suckled one and massaged the other. She tasted sweet, tangy and zesty and saliva sparked in his mouth. She was soon sighing in pleasure. He moved his tongue faster and harder until her body convulsed and she moaned, "Yeeeh, oooah, aaagh." Mitra was delighted with his efforts and her reaction.

He rolled her onto her back and fastened himself to her other breast, and with his hand massaged her silky, pubic hair. When he noticed her moistness and her vulva lips slightly separated, he inserted a finger deep into her vagina searching for her delicate spot. She was warm, she was moist, she was reacting to his probing and his sucking.

"Faster, my lord," she said.

Mitra was surprised for few of his partners with the exception of the courtesans ever gave him directions.

He moved his hand faster and faster. She was writhing in pleasure. He stopped and pressed his finger at the top of her opening, her ecstatic spot, and she cried out, "Oh, oh, oh, my lord, oh, my lord, you've sent me to paradise."

Mitra was thrilled and he stopped, allowing her to recover. He was leaking pre-come profusely. With squinted eyes he explored the face and body of this most unusual partner. When she returned to normal, her breathing had steadied, she had a smile on her face and her eyes were closed. He inserted his finger between her vulva lips searching for her clitoris. It didn't take long for his finger to find her mound of pleasure. Carefully, gently, softly, he moved his finger up and down, from side to side and around and around. At the same time, he reattached himself and drew deeply from her elongated nipple.

Without warning, she had an explosive orgasm. Her body arched, stiffened and gyrated in all directions at the same time. She pulled his hand from her; she was crying tears of joy and repeating, "Shakti, Shakti, Shakti".

Never had one of his partners pleased him as much as she. She had almost brought him to a fellatio climax and he had brought her to three orgasms: one with his mouth and two with his hand. Giving pleasure to his partners was one of the benefits of his sexual education but none had ever responded as this one. As he waited for her to recover, he noticed the profusion of pre-come and the throbbing of his *lingam*.

He directed her to the mallaka position. He had his feet on the pallet and his knees raised. She faced away from him as he directed her to hold his knees and lower herself towards the head of his *lingam*. Together they guided his *lingam* into her *yoni* and her *yoni* around his *lingam*. Penetration was an awesome sensation of pleasure surging through his penis and throughout his body. He held her by the hips as she settled upon him. He was completely encased. Shocked, Mitra could only remember the courtesans and a handful of others who were able to take all of him without pain.

With his hands, he helped her ride up and down his shaft. Pleasure vibrated throughout his body. He saw the faint outline of her fiddle-back body and cascading hair rising and falling upon him. Within minutes, she climaxed again with a scream, and her pulsating movements brought him close to a marvellous orgasm. Instead, he enjoyed her obvious pleasure, and he rubbed his hands over her back until she ceased vibrating.

He lowered his knees; she followed until she was prone upon his legs. She took him by the ankles and moved her *yoni* back and forth pummelling his *lingam*. Soon she was moaning. Mitra could feel the fluids rising in his body. The sensations pushed him beyond the point of no return. "Uuugh, uuugh, *uuugh*." He poured his fluids into her vessel.

Mitra glowed in a satisfaction he had never experienced. Spasms coursed through his body; he felt her vibrations and quiet moans.

As he lay enjoying his unexpected release she said, "My lord, your performance goes beyond the legend of your abilities."

"My lady, you have pleased me beyond my greatest expectations."

Sitting up, he brought her to the same position. He nuzzled her neck and fondled her sensuous breasts. Her velvet hair and warm back pressed against his hairy stomach and chest. He held her close and images of his lessons seeped into his mind.

Releasing her, he lay on his back and said, "Please, my lady, I want you to spin until you're facing me."

"Oh, my lord, I might hurt you."

"Move slowly, turn to your right, this movement is possible, it will hurt neither of us, and time is not important. I want you to spin so I can see you. This move is called the *Paravrittaka*."

"My lord?"

"Do as I ask."

She peered over her shoulder in wonder. "Are you sure?"

He nodded and signalled her to move.

She pushed her right foot in that direction, using her hands for balance as she proceeded to move in small increments.

They stared at each other in wonderment, as the strange yet titillating feeling of her twisting around his spindle coursed through their flesh. His *lingam* was tingling in a way previously unknown and her *yoni* was probed in places experienced by few women. The turn took a long time. The twisting movement was exhilarating; their members were inflamed from this different movement.

As she turned his vision mysteriously improved; he saw her clearly for the first time. A light green aura surrounded her body. Her square, dark face gleamed with a broad smile, her breasts appeared as cinder cones topped with areolae of sliced pineapple and nipples the size and colour of raspberries. At long last, she carefully pulled her right leg and foot over his face and experienced a spine-tingling orgasm as she completed her journey, "Yeeeh, oooah, uuuum."

He smiled as her vibrations continued. When she calmed he said, "You're beautiful. Your eyes are jade-stone green like Shakti, the fertility goddess."

"Thank you, my lord, the spin was as amazing for me as it was for you. You're much more handsome than the myths and your *lingam* is a magic wand."

Taking her by the hands, he urged her to move on him. He lay mesmerized by her beauty, the bounding of her breasts and the stimulation of her flesh around his. He felt himself approaching an orgasm. With his hands he stilled her and devoured the energy she emitted.

Pulling her close, they embraced. As their tongues danced to an unheard jungle drum, he again approached a climax. He pushed her away, waited a moment, then gorged on the sweet, succulent fruit of her flesh while encouraging her to ride him like an elephant. She moaned as he switched from one nipple to another: he sucked, licked, pressed and pulled. All the while she stroked up and down the length of his *lingam*.

She placed her hands on his face, pulling him away while bringing her breasts together with nipples touching, and then she commanded, "My lord, suckle and run your tongue around my nipples."

He inhaled her raspberries; then absorbed and ran figure of eights around them. She moved rhythmically and within moments went into a shuddering orgasm that vibrated both their bodies vigorously. Mitra closed his eyes and arched his body into her. Within minutes he exploded in a grand mal of ecstasy, the most mind-blowing orgasm of his life. For an instant, a vision of the gods appeared and he was one with them.

They continued in perfect rhythm until she fell exhausted and spent. They lay side by side in the afterglow of mutual satisfaction. He stared at the ceiling in astonishment.

Mitra turned and drew her close, his normal white body

basking in the lobster red of spent passion and he asked, "What's your name?"

"Kumari, my lord," she responded breathlessly.

"Kumari, that means princess. Tonight you've enabled me to see a glimpse of the gods and to experience, for an instant, release from the cycle of rebirth. I've found my princess," he said, holding her tight and raining her face with kisses. He turned her on her back in the crab position and once again their flesh became one; she stayed the night.

The servants waited patiently at the bottom of the stairs for Kumari's return. She didn't come. They waited and waited, and still she didn't come as had all the others. When the cock crowed, it was obvious she was not returning; she had stayed the night with their master. They were overcome with joy because Mitra's *kama* had been fulfilled. He had found enlightenment in his princess, Kumari.

The servants celebrated for the young master, the revered one, and ran to tell his family. Both father and mother were ecstatic and began arrangements for the wedding feast.

The next day at dusk, Mitra, dressed in his customary white, was accompanied by Kumari, also in a white robe. They stood on a platform before the village. Raising his hands high the villagers fell silent. He took Kumari by one hand and spun her like a top to his right. The crowd erupted in delight at the symbolism of the ritual, because it signified the beginning of the legend of the *Paravrittaka*.

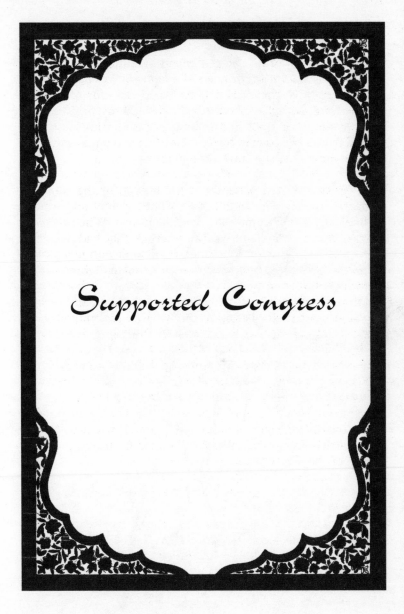

Supported Congress

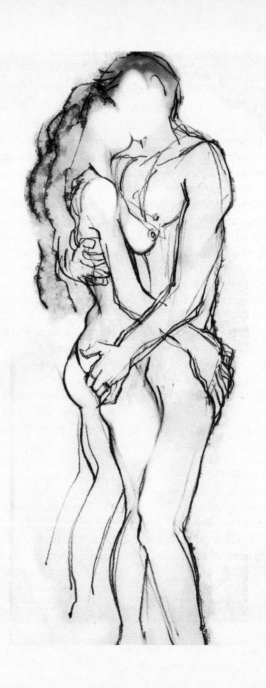

Supported Congress

Sthita
Kama Sutra

In this position, the lovers have to support each other with nothing more than their bodies. It takes tremendous balance and stamina. These are the favoured positions with which sculptors decorate temple walls.

The *Kama Sutra* endorses the need for total reciprocity between partners in sex. Kisses are given and then taken back. In a game where the man grabs the woman's lip gently between his teeth, she then comes back tenfold, determined to catch his lip. When one partner bites the other, it is mandatory that the marked partner comes back to deliver a more intense bite, with greater ferocity and force of mark. When a slap is given, the woman is told to give a slap back to her lover (after a bit of pouting, of course). It is the reciprocity that is the turn-on. Young girls are not to be overpowered and made submissive. Some even say that, where procreation is concerned, if sex is not pleasurable, the baby will be deformed, or that if there is no female orgasm, no baby can be conceived at all. Women are to be made confident, coaxed and seduced, so they can be equal partners in lovemaking. This will make it better for both parties.

So, because a woman and a man depend on each other in sex, there needs to be a methodology set out. In this position, the lovers actually do support each other, providing, in many cases, the only place the other has to gain some purchase. They have to be there for each other in every way. The only way to achieve this type of lovemaking is to remain a steadfast support for your partner, a kind of calm eye-of-the-hurricane solidness and consciousness in the midst of the whirlwind of desire.

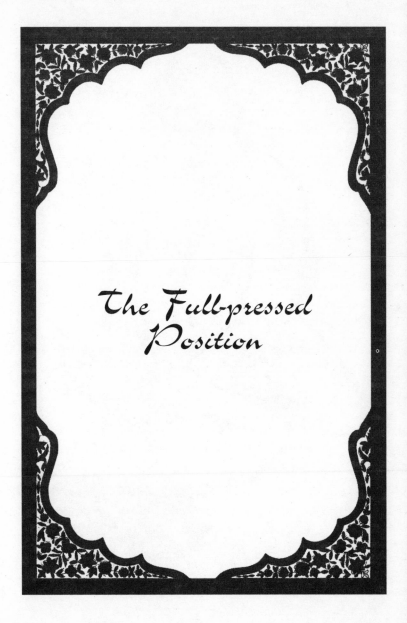

The Full-pressed
Position

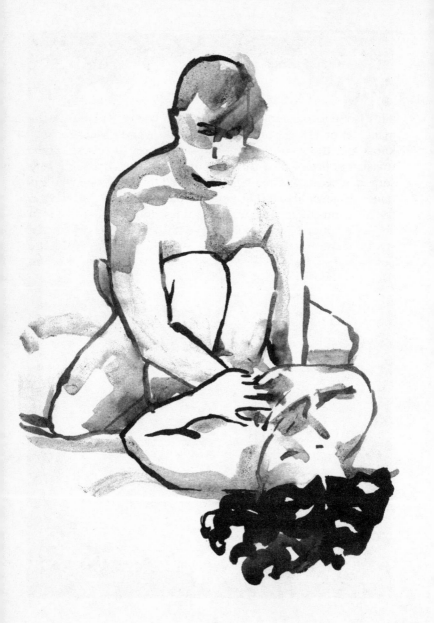

The Full-pressed Position

Utpiditaka
Kama Sutra

This is a possessive position where the woman is beneath the man. Her breasts are pressed into her chest and she can feel her knees and the warmth of her lover also on her chest. Some translators have called the position "high pressure" or "high squeeze" because of the tension created by the contracted legs under the lover above. The penetration is deep and the man can use his hands to grip the woman's sides, and also to pull her in and grind more deeply into her with one of the designated strokes. The man is able to kiss her and bite her lips as he possesses her, but she is not really in any position to bite him back, try as she might.

The Tale of Courting Sumansa

as told by Sephera Giron

Sumansa stood by the blossoming buds of purple and pink flowers. Her back was to me but I recognized the long black braid that swung across her pink and green sari. Her hips swelled out from the cling of soft fabric and I could just glimpse her ruby-stained lips.

It seemed like a lifetime that I had adored this splendid creature. In fact, it had been a lifetime that I had known her.

As children, we had played together in the fields, chasing each other in glee between chores. Even then, her dark dancing eyes and long silky hair inspired a longing in me that echoed from another place.

While I was away advancing my studies, many beautiful women caught my eye. I smelled the sweet perfume of one, listened to the melodic singing of another, wrapped long dark hair in my hands as my mind always extended back to Sumansa.

Every pulse of my body, lips against lips, flesh against flesh, were overtures that would one day lead me back to her. Her eyes, her laughter, her playful tricks, set her apart from any other human maiden. No one could match my Sumansa for vibrancy, for splendour. Impatiently I served my years of study under my strict uncle's hand, and as soon as I could, I returned to my town.

Our reunion was joyful, yet now we were adults. We couldn't run off and play, for now, she was a single woman and expected to follow protocol.

However, my free-spirited flower still had her old defiant ways about her.

"Sumansa," I said to her, extending my hands so that she could greet me. Her slender fingers slipped through mine as she looked up at me with wide dark eyes. Her face glowed as a flower to the sun, and I could barely contain my enthusiasm as I brushed her cheek with mine.

"My affections grow stronger for you by the day. Come with me to hear the musicians in the square. Today is a day of celebration."

"Oh, Bhadrak," she sighed, breaking her grasp and turning away. "You know I can't go with you to town. It isn't right."

"We're only going to hear some music. Nothing more," I reassured her. "You will love the harmonies of my friends. They are eager to meet you."

Sumansa stepped away from me and pretended to inspect the stalks of the tall flowers. "There are bugs in here," she said. "Soon they will destroy my beauty."

I laughed. "Nonsense." I stroked her arm gently. The heat of her flesh was warm against my fingertips as I grazed her lightly with my nails. "Your beauty is magnificent. No flower could ever match it. As these flowers wither and die, your beauty will only deepen."

Sumansa's face grew flushed as she coyly turned her head. "I wasn't fishing for compliments. I was only remarking that I can't go off to town while my flowers are being eaten. They rely on me to nurture them and I have to remove the bugs."

"I'm teasing you. However, what if I help you with the bugs? Will you then take an hour to relax with me at the festival?"

"I see how much you desire my company, Bhadrak. I would love to have help but I don't want to keep you from your own entertainments."

"Sumansa, you are my entertainment. And I yearn to show you so much."

Sumansa picked at the bugs and nodded towards a basket over by a table. I retrieved it and set it at her feet.

"Show me these bugs you detest so much."

Sumansa held one of the despicable creatures between her thumb and forefinger, its vile legs wiggling in the air at me. She squished it quickly and after we both heard the pop, she tossed the body into the basket. I pulled my handkerchief from my pocket and handed it to her.

"Thank you," she said, wiping bug mess from her fingers. It mattered not, for once the hunt began, we didn't worry much about niceties. We set to work picking and killing bugs until it seemed that we had found every last one of them. Bits of bug spatter clung to our clothes but we didn't mind as our chore was finally done.

After we had washed our hands in the fountain that flowed in the centre of the garden, she turned to me, her face flushed with excitement.

"You were so kind to help me. It made a dreary job so much less horrible."

"I still would like you to come to town with me. I'm sure we could still hear some songs."

Sumansa smiled. This time her face was open and relieved. "Yes. I'll come along with you."

As we turned to go, I noticed a fallen stalk of flower lying on the cobblestone. I picked it up and turned it over in my hand. There was a perfect bud just ripening to open. Translucent purple petals seemed to want to burst forth from the green leaves that contained it. I stroked it for a moment then turned to Sumansa. My gaze fell into hers as I gently kissed the soft head of the flower. She smiled.

"A perfect bud," I said as I put it behind her ear. She giggled as she felt it slide along her flesh, and I smiled as I realized that neither sunset nor woman had captured beauty as wonderfully as this virgin bud behind Sumansa's ear.

The streets were crowded as we pushed our way along. The festival had been busy all day. Vendors sold foods and drinks from their carts. Artists displayed urns and paintings and carefully woven fabrics. Oils and incense for enticing lovers were readily available, their gentle fragrances teasing our noses as we passed by. Teas to inspire love and fertility, along with charms and potions to produce long-lasting stallion *lingams* were examined by hopeful lovers. For us, there was no time to stop or browse, our bug-killing had seen that we had missed the busiest part of the festival.

At last we found the musicians. We heard their music before we saw them in their colourful clothes. A small group of people stood in rapture as my friends enticed them with their mysterious wailings. A little monkey on a chain danced beside the small makeshift platform.

In the air, thick clouds of perfumed smoke mingled with the sweat of overheated people and the cloying scent of sweet spices.

Sumansa stood near the front of the gathering and was immediately mesmerized by the dramatic renderings of sitar and *bansi*. Her lithe body swayed and I stood behind her, pressing against her as I wrapped my arms around her waist. The gentle swell of her buttocks rubbed against the silky cloth of my pants and we moved together as the seductive rhythms washed over us.

My enthusiasm for her soft yet firm flesh overwhelmed me and my fingers danced along her arms. She closed her eyes, leaning her head back onto my shoulder. The fullness of her breasts was just a breath away from my fingers. I stroked the softness of her arms and the silkiness of her sari. Too soon the song was over and she broke free of my embrace.

"Bhadrak, we mustn't do this. It's a public place."

"But you drive me to distraction. I can't help but want to hold you in my arms whenever I'm near you."

The musicians broke into a lively dance and I swept her into my arms. Along the cobblestone streets, many couples danced to the gleeful swell of the music. Sumansa was light on her feet and I spun her with confidence. Our legs and arms mimicked each other and, with ease, we danced as we had danced as children. The years we had spent apart dissolved as the music drew us close.

Sumansa laughed and pointed towards the monkey.

"Look at him. He's so cute!" she cried.

I had to agree that the monkey spinning and chattering while slapping his hat up and down was highly amusing.

"Would you like your own monkey?" I asked her as I spun her once more.

"No . . . I love monkeys. I love to see them running free. I don't think I would be happy to keep a monkey on a string."

"My Sumansa, you are so giving. How could I ever be apart from you again?"

"Quiet, Bhadrak. Let's enjoy the music before my father sees me out with you."

"Doesn't your father like me?"

"I don't know what my father likes. But I do know that he wouldn't be pleased that I'm alone with a man."

"I'm not any man. I'm Bhadrak from your childhood. We played together, studied together . . . we did everything together."

"But you went away." She stepped back and dropped her arms. "You went away."

Her eyes were so sad and the sight of them pained me.

"My Sumansa. You missed me?"

"I worried that you would never come back."

"I was only advancing my studies under my uncle. He's a smart and wealthy man. I'm going to have a rich profession after my final initiations."

"But you were gone so long. I thought you found yourself a wife."

I laughed. "Oh my Sumansa. All I dreamed about was you. One day, when I marry, it will be to you and no other."

"Fine words, Bhadrak, but how do I know that you aren't just trying to seduce me?"

"Can you not see my love for you in my eyes? Do you not know how I thought about you every waking moment until my studies were done?"

"But you didn't write."

"I started many poems but none were good enough. I wrote you songs. I carved your name into rocks and sand. I shouted my love to the skies but all meant nothing till I saw your face again. I realized that I had to come back and prove my love to you. Then perhaps, you will come away with me."

"My head is swimming, Bhadrak. Can we talk later?"

My prattling was ruining our wonderful dancing time, so I took her hands and set to work showing her some new steps. Her delicate feet picked up the rhythms quickly. We laughed and danced, the years melting away until we were children once more.

Too soon, the concert was over. As my friends packed away their instruments, I proudly introduced Sumansa. They stared at her with envy, for her beauty was more magical than any sound their instruments could make, more enticing than any garden in the city. They bowed to her, kissed her hands, playfully shoved me and then were gone to their next appearance.

The sun was sinking on the horizon as I led Sumansa back towards her home.

"The music stirs a passion in me that makes me want to sing to you," I said as I started to hum. Sumansa giggled while I sang an old folk song. We were walking alongside a low stone structure that kept the road clear of roaming animals and I impulsively hopped on top. I poured my heart out to my love, waving my hands, staring earnestly into her eyes. Her giggles turned to quiet admiration. My strong bass voice echoed through the air. When I was finished my yearning lament, she clapped.

"Beautiful. I see your uncle trained your voice as well. When I last heard you sing, you squawked like an out of tune reed."

"I wasn't a man then. I was in-between. But now, I am well versed in the 64 *kalas*."

Before she could answer, I raised my voice with a new song. Quickly recognizing it, she sang along with me. Her lovely voice trembled with a rich vibrato as we made our way back through the winding streets. Drunk with happiness, we sang our duets to the setting sun, smiling at the people who passed who saw us giddy in love.

At last, we reached the garden once more.

"Sumansa," I said as I kneeled before her, the perfume of flowers filling my head. "I love you. I've loved you for a long time."

"I know, Bhadrak. I love you too. Our childhood days hold many happy memories for me."

I took her hand and kissed it gently. My lips gently tugged on her flesh and she turned her head away. I kissed her hand again, this time firmly. Pushing back the soft fabric of her sari, my lips gently puckered along her arm until I reached her shoulder.

"Bhadrak," she whispered, her gaze directed towards the drooping head of a sleeping bud.

"Shh . . ." I soothed as I nuzzled into her neck. "Your flowers are safe. They are sleeping now, like you've been asleep. I want to wake you up, spread the petals of your lotus blossom."

Her body leaned back into me, her chin tilting towards the vibrant rays of the setting sun. Musky smells filled my senses, my lips longing to touch hers.

She turned to me, her eyes wide and dark, looking up at me with both longing and fear. My arms reached out and pulled her close. As our lips met with short tentative touches, she lifted her leg to loop it around my thigh. My heart beat with joy as her remaining foot gently covered mine in the "climbing of the tree".

My mouth covered hers and our tongues danced to the memories of the street musicians.

After many minutes of drinking in each other's hunger, Sumansa put her foot down and stepped away.

"Come with me." She took my hand and led me along a stone path that wound through the garden, round and round in a maze until we reached the centre. We stood under a small fruit tree as she held my hands.

"It's more private here," she explained. "I come here often to think."

The tree and flowers were even more fantastic in this secluded spot. Her loving touch was felt here too. The colours in the setting sun vibrantly reflected off the foliage as if a thousand souls were watching our courtship. Beside the tree was a long stone bench.

"It's a beautiful place," I said. "Even a place to sit."

I led her towards the bench.

"Yes." She turned her gaze from mine. "I've never had a man here, Bhadrak. You are the first."

"This makes me treasure you all the more."

"I've been waiting for you. My soulmate. And while I waited, I took my lessons in the 64 *kalas* as well. I think I'm doing well at many of them."

"Your singing and dancing and most certainly your wonderful garden show you've been learning well." I placed my finger on her lower lip and lightly scratched it. Sumansa turned her head.

"I know your seductions. I wonder how you learned them. How many have you practised?"

"I don't know all the seductions and, my love, I only wish to use my knowledge on you."

"Show me what you know."

My *lingam* throbbed with anticipation as my fingers pinched at her nipples, tugging and pulling at them through the soft fabric. She sighed as her nipples grew harder, turning into hard buttons beneath my repeated pinching.

Her head tilted back, her mouth opened as one of my hands reached down to her leg. Lightly I stroked her firm inner thigh through her sari.

The strokes grew longer and harder in length until my fingers made their way up to the warm fires of her *yoni*. She trembled a little beneath my touch, her breath a little faster. My hand pressed fully on the length of her groin with the heel of it bearing down. After a few pulses, her hips instinctively began to follow the rhythm of my hand. I slid the heel down a little more and she spread her legs wider on the bench. In fact, she turned sideways and propped her feet up on the sides.

I lifted her sari and saw with delight, her soft glistening *yoni*. My fingers gently touched the outer folds of her labia as I marvelled at her mystery. Her eyes watched me, expectation growing in her. I opened up that beautiful lotus and stared at the inner bud.

"I need to taste you," I said as I lowered my head. Between her legs, my tongue sought her out, lightly licking and probing her quivering little button. My own pleasure was mounting with every gasp and moan that my dancing tongue inspired in her.

My finger slipped into her vagina while my tongue continued to dance.

"Oh my," she sighed. "I've never felt that before."

"Does it feel good?" I asked as I raised my head to answer her.

"Yes."

I lowered my head again and licked every fold of her lovely lotus.

Her legs quivered as my tongue and fingers danced on her more urgently. Her low moans inspired me to lick at her harder. I hooked my fingers until I found the spot inside that would make her shiver with delight.

It wasn't long before she tensed and released with a climax, her juices flowed down my fingers, her cries matching the pulsing within. When she stopped trembling, I withdrew my hand and mouth and sat up.

"I want to take you," I said. "I want to be inside you."

"Yes. I want to feel you inside me too."

Slowly we undressed, our gazes lowered shyly until we stood naked in front of each other. Her breasts were high and firm, her nipples protruding with the pleasure she had just experienced. I took her hand and led her to the grass under the tree.

"Lie down," I said.

Leaning over her, I stroked my *lingam* until it stood firmly erect. Her eyes stayed focused on it, watching it grow beneath my own hand. I let her touch it and she firmly grasped it. She stroked it, lovingly at first, then harder, mimicking the movement she had seen me perform.

She lay back, her legs spread, and I lay on top of her, placing my *lingam* into her *yoni*. She gasped as my hardness entered her. My hands held her shoulders as I pushed in deeper. As marvellous as she felt, this ordinary position didn't bring the pleasure we both craved. I carefully pulled one of her legs up over my shoulder to re-enact the splitting of the bamboo. My strokes were slow and gentle and she rocked with me. The warmth of her *yoni* felt good around my *lingam* yet I still wasn't happy with the position. I wanted something new and different.

I pulled away from her.

"What is wrong?" she asked.

"I want to try something new. Something that hasn't been done. You are a gentle flower and I want to pluck you. How can we do that?"

"I don't know, my sweet. I have no real experience."

She playfully pulled her legs up to her chest in a hug, exposing her *yoni* to me.

"Oh, my lovely lotus, this is what we need to do." As she stayed with her knees drawn to her breast, I pulled her hips onto my kneeling thighs. Instinctively, she placed her feet against my chest as my *lingam* sought out her *yoni* once more.

"This is it. This is the way to suckle, my lotus," I sighed as the new angle brought me great pleasure. We stared into each other's eyes, one of my hands on her thigh, the other stroking her hair. Her hands clutched at my own thighs as she sighed with every thrust of my *lingam*.

The sun was gone as our pleasure mounted. Our sighs and groans were animal-like as we worked our way towards our climax.

Her *yoni* clenched and released, giving another rhythm to my strokes. My hard *lingam* was eagerly accepted deep within her virginal body. In the darkness, I didn't know if she bled from her first penetration.

I leaned over to touch her lips with my fingers; a glorious rush surged through me. As our juices flowed together, we cried out.

For many weeks, we met in secret in her garden. Her lovely bud was always willing to accept me and we loved our new position. By the time we announced our wedding day, we had named the position: the full-pressed union.

The full-pressed union represented our own life-long union. We had many children and many more positions of pleasure were created. But we never forgot the first position or the first moments where we gave our love to each other in her secret garden.

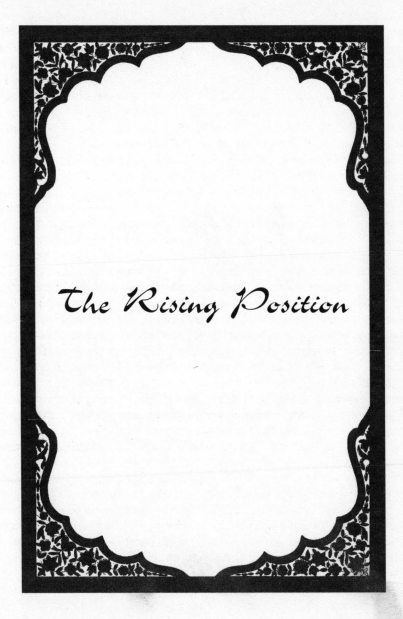

The Rising Position

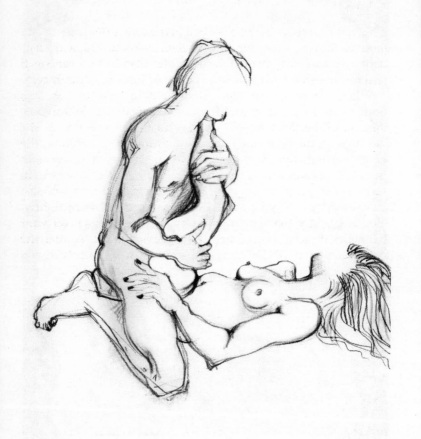

The Rising Position

Bhugnaka
Kama Sutra

The lady lies on her back on the bed in the centre of the room and motions for you to join her. She is naked and beautiful, with large dark eyes and wavy hair to her shoulder blades. You can smell jasmine and wonder if it's her perfume or just her natural scent.

When she raises her legs up straight in front of her, you notice how lovely they are. Perfectly shaped and voluptuous, long and lithe. So you hold her legs in the air like that as she lies back on the bed, enjoying your admiration of her legs. She keeps her legs tightly closed while you drag your finger over her tight, exposed bud, feeling the hairs rise on her skin in response to your touch. In this position, the woman can also clasp her legs in her arms, closing them even more tightly. You might try that later. For now, you sink down on your haunches directly behind her closed, raised thighs so that she can't see you at all. On your haunches with knees raised, you penetrate her and pull her hips towards you while she keeps her legs closed and stretched to the sky.

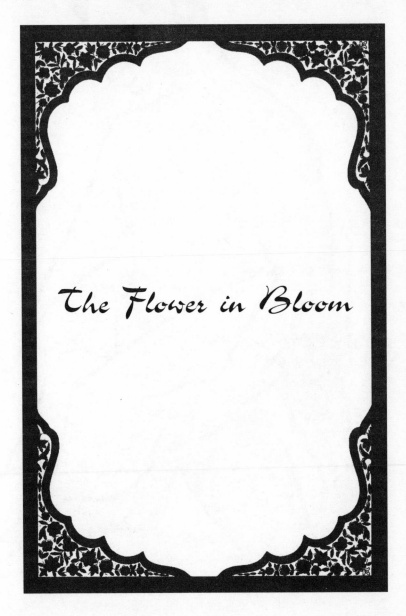

The Flower in Bloom

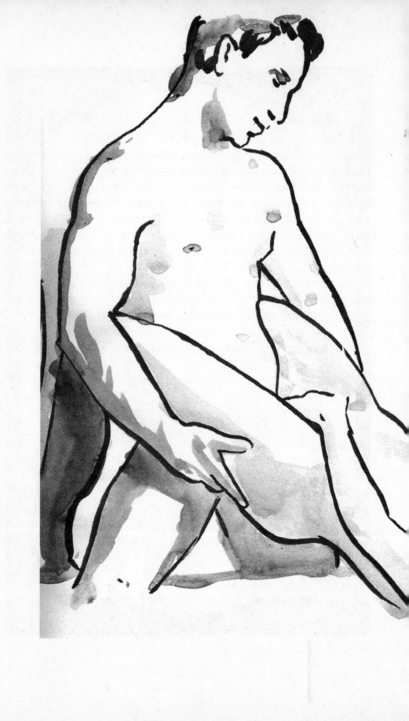

The Flower in Bloom

Utphullaka
Kama Sutra

The *yoni* blossoms open, ready for the *lingam*, when the woman pushes up her hips towards her lover inviting him to penetrate her. He spreads her thighs and she keeps her head low. Vatsyayana recommends applying a lubricant to make the entrance easy. At this time either the woman or the man can place hands on the inside of the thighs to widen her further, or the man can steady himself by grasping her ankles and opening her up to receive him.

A pillow can be placed underneath her buttocks if she is unable to raise and hold her hips in the air for the period of time while intercourse takes place.

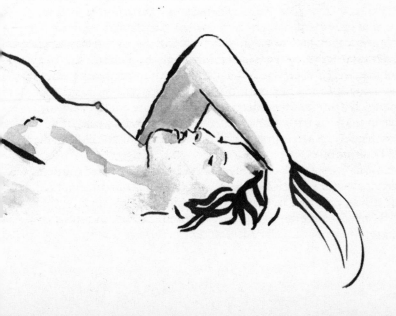

The Tale of the Serpent in the Garden

as told by Jordan Castillo Price

Most of your once-upon-a-time type stories begin with a wide-eyed young maiden who's a blushing flower. Not this story. This story is about a girl named Shirina, and Shirina was as far from blushing flowerdom as a girl can get. No flowers here. Not even plants. Or turtledoves, or butterflies, or anything charming and nice. If anything, Shirina was a serpent.

Shirina was elegant and slim, but she was also cold-blooded and sneaky. She moved with a deadly grace that was breathtaking to behold, and the sting of her venom could paralyse, even kill.

At least, she hoped that someday it would, once she'd grown the proper flowers and herbs and combined them correctly. And once she had found someone to test the poison on besides her mother and her brother, Dharmesh. She never dared to spike their drinks with anything much stronger than a sleeping draught; she figured the two of them came in handy from time to time.

Someday Shirina would be a master poisoner, a deadly enchantress who did nobody's bidding. But, unfortunately, for now she was just a girl in a garden.

Shirina scowled down at the battered, faded surface of a much-read scroll, its presence known only by Dharmesh, who had discovered it on one of his daily forays to the marketplace and bought it for her on a drunken whim. She scanned the ornate characters. She'd need senna before she could brew any poison that was truly fearsome. And it would take weeks, if not months, for the seeds to grow. If those seeds could be had at all.

"Dharmesh!"

Shirina's brother poked his head into the courtyard garden from the window of his bedroom. His hair stuck out on one side, but it was balanced by his crooked smile. "Hey."

"I need something for my garden. Take me to the market."

Dharmesh leaned both elbows on the window sill and considered, which was not a good sign. It meant he was doing something other than getting ready to leave. "I don't think it's safe," he said.

"What?"

"All kinds of rumours are flying around."

Shirina gritted her teeth. As big brothers went, Dharmesh was easy enough to get along with, and he knew how to keep a secret. But he could be such an idiot when it came to spitting out a story. "Could you give me a reason?"

Dharmesh crooked his finger and gestured for Shirina to come closer. "I'll tell you," he said, "but I don't want Mother to hear."

Shirina stepped forward carefully to avoid crushing the rue beneath Dharmesh's window and leaned towards him. "Well?"

He looked one way and then the other, as if checking the courtyard for anyone who could overhear them, and then lowered his voice with dramatic flair. "There's a rapist loose."

Shirina shivered. "What?"

Dharmesh leaned out further still, half in, half out of his bedroom window. "Everyone was whispering about it when I picked up the groceries."

Shirina drew her wrap around her shoulders. "What did they say?"

Dharmesh managed to stick himself out even further. Shirina leaned forward to listen, worried that he'd end up dumping himself in the rue. "That the women he's 'visited' don't seem all that eager to press charges." Dharmesh waggled his eyebrows. "That they've started leaving their windows and doors unlocked in the hope that he'll visit them again."

"That's disgusting," said Shirina. She chafed away the goosebumps that had formed on her arms beneath her wrap.

Dharmesh shrugged and pulled back from the window. "So I'm not parading you around the square to invite trouble into our house. Mother would kill me."

"I need senna," Shirina insisted, voice low and clipped. Her brother never seemed to notice when she was practising her serpent voice. Her brother was a fool.

"Making up more of those secret potions, eh? All right, give it here." He stuck his arm out of the window and Shirina handed him the scroll, pointing.

"Senna."

"Yeah, OK. I suppose I can pick some up this afternoon."

"Why later? You haven't got a job. Go now."

Dharmesh winked as he tucked the scroll into his vest. "That's when the pretty girl at the samosa tent starts work."

Shirina crossed her arms and rolled her eyes, but the evidence of her displeasure was lost on Dharmesh, who'd ducked back into his room. Shirina supposed it was all for the best. Serpents didn't roll their eyes.

Shirina set a cushion down on the ground and began pulling weeds. The sun was high and warm, and bees meandered from flower to flower while she hummed to herself and worked. Her mother always slept through the middle of the day, and Dharmesh would eventually leave for the marketplace where he'd loiter for hours, which left Shirina in peace to enjoy her solitude and her garden.

Shirina lost herself in her work, in the feel of the soil beneath her fingers, and the scent of the plants as she plucked them from the earth. She worked slowly, stretching often, until she'd cleared weeds along the entire west wall. She was rinsing the dirt from her hands when someone spoke.

"Hello?"

Shirina stood and turned towards the door. It was a man's voice, but it hadn't sounded anything like Dharmesh.

She stepped behind a cardamom bush and peered through a tangle of needlelike leaves. The only way into the courtyard was through the house. Her brother was at the market, and her mother was likely to be dozing in her room at the far side of the house. There was only one other person it could be.

The rapist.

Shirina felt her heart pounding in her throat. Footsteps rang on the tiles as the stranger got closer.

"Hello?"

He wasn't very stealthy for a rapist, but maybe it was his unusual method that made him as successful as he was rumoured to be. Shirina glimpsed him in the doorway through the cardamom. He was very tall. His face was mostly hidden by a hanging pot of *manjishta*, but as he moved, turning this way and that, Shirina glimpsed his profile – strong, with a neat moustache and small pointed beard, a proud jaw and shrewd eyes.

She felt a fluttery warmth deep in her belly.

So, this was the man who would finally deflower her, after all of her ploys and manipulations to escape the marriages her family had arranged, so she could spend her time in the only place she'd ever loved: her garden. Maybe it was fitting, that the rapist with the flashing dark eyes would take her here. The garden was, after all, the source of the *ulat kambal* that kept her mother drowsy and docile, and the poppies that ensured Dharmesh would never outsmart her.

The heat of the day leached into Shirina's back from the stones of the courtyard wall. She pulled her wrap tighter and shivered despite the heat.

The intruder dropped a cloth sack onto the paving stones and strode to the centre of the garden, hands on hips, surveying the space.

Shirina cast around for something to hit him with while his back was turned. A stone pitcher full of rosewater sat on a table nearby, close enough to grab and swing. She stretched out one arm, and then hesitated. She couldn't imagine why. It was easy enough to drug her mother's tea. Why should she worry about knocking some stranger on the head?

Unless she didn't want to hurt him.

She decided not to think about that. Instead, she told herself that she could get a better look at the rapist once she'd laid him out.

Shirina grabbed the pitcher and took a few silent steps towards the man in the centre of her garden. The shadow of the upraised pitcher fell across the bed of poppies directly in front of him.

He turned to her and smiled. His teeth were dazzling white. Shirina blinked. She felt like she'd been staring into the sun.

"Thanks," he said. "I'm parched." He took the pitcher from her. She surrendered it with limp hands, staring. No man had a right to look like that, so confident, so self-assured. Especially a rapist who'd just been discovered. He stood, back straight and shoulders squared, and gazed down into her eyes. "Where's the cup?"

Shirina blinked. She went back to the table and returned with her own cup. The rapist took it from her, poured himself some rose-scented water and drank deeply.

"Ah, that really hits the spot. So, where do you want it?"

Shirina crossed her arms. Her wrap slid down into the crooks of her elbows, baring her long, pale, serpent-like throat. "Is that all?" she hissed. "No preliminaries?"

The rapist's eyes widened. As a fellow predator, he obviously saw her for what she was. "My apologies, *yuvatii*. Feel free to inspect the merchandise."

Oh, the arrogance. Shirina would show him. He had her cornered, her brother was away and her mother was dreaming the drugged dreams of *ulat kambal*, but Shirina still had her pride. She stepped right up to the rapist and did as she'd been told.

His eyes went wide.

"*Yuvatii* . . ."

"Don't 'young lady' me. My name is Shirina."

"Shirina . . ."

She cupped him with her hand. There was quite a heft to the goods that dangled between his legs. She squeezed gently, getting the feel of the soft, fleshy, resilient parts. It wasn't that unpleasant. She'd been put off for so long by talk of sticks and staves and battering rams. But this handful of "merchandise" was inoffensive enough.

And the handling of it would stop any man in his tracks, given the reaction of the rapist. The bronze cup clattered against the paving stones and the pitcher thumped into the poppies. But even with his hands free, the rapist did nothing to subdue Shirina. He seemed stunned. She explored further, two-handed now. Ah, there was the staff she'd heard so much about, but it felt more pliable than she'd imagined. She stared into the rapist's eyes and felt herself smile. He might have cornered her like a mongoose, but he hadn't realized she was the cobra who'd enthral him.

The intruder managed a few more words. "What are you . . .?"

"No one's ever bested you at your own game, have they?" And maybe the battering ram was bigger and stiffer than she'd originally thought. But no matter. Shirina wasn't afraid. She wasn't afraid of anything.

Once Shirina had felt her way around, she pulled her wrap from the crook of her elbow and looped it around the rapist's neck, since, strangely enough, he looked like he might collapse. The heat of the day was probably a bit much for him. She pulled his face down to hers and spoke low and sibilant. "If this is going to happen, I demand a kiss. It's the least you can do."

His lips were surprisingly gentle on hers, for a rapist's. His mouth brushed against her, soft and perhaps even shy. His warm breath was perfumed with rosewater, and his moustache felt bristly and strange where it trailed along her upper lip.

Shirina flinched when she felt his fingertips against the side of her face, but they were as gentle as his mouth, tracing the curve of her cheek with delicacy. Her lips parted in surprise, and the rapist took it for an invitation. His rose-scented tongue slid into her mouth, brushed against the edges of her teeth, teased at her tongue. The unfamiliar thrill that had overcome her when she'd first seen the rapist, the warm tingle in the centre of her body, spiked and intensified. It coalesced into a point of sharp, damp heat, right between her legs.

Shirina gasped, breathing in the rapist's breath. He slipped an arm around her waist, pulling her more firmly against him. She held him against her tightly. And there, pressed into her hip, she could feel the stiffness of his "merchandise".

One of the rapist's hands moved lower, cupping Shirina's bottom, while the other slid beneath her long braid at the back of her neck and clasped her to him, skin against skin. Shirina kissed him harder and his pointed beard tickled her chin. Everywhere they touched, he was hard against her softness, and each point of contact sent jolts of arousal straight to her sex.

Shirina's knees felt weak, as if her legs would refuse to keep her upright much longer. She pulled the silk wrap around the neck of the rapist – if she could even think of him like that any longer, since he was obviously something else entirely, a seducer, a lover – and guided him down beside her on a bed of mint.

She let go of the wrap, and instead cupped his face. So strange, the feel of his skin, so different from hers, the stubble where he'd contoured his pointy beard, the strong curve of his jaw. He lay over her, tongue sliding deeper into her mouth, lips pressing harder. He slipped a hand between them and cupped her breast. Shirina cried out, just a tiny gasp, but it caught her by surprise. The sound spurred her lover on. He covered her breast with caresses, stroking it tenderly, each touch bringing him closer and closer to its peak.

When he stroked her hard nipple, Shirina's hips rocked against him as if they had a life of their own. The feelings he sent blazing up and down her spine, sizzling between her legs, might be new to her, but her body knew how to respond.

Shirina's lover turned his face and trailed kisses towards her ear. "You're so beautiful," he said, and his words tickled strangely, more layers of sensation that built and built, still more shocks of pleasure causing surges of wetness between her legs. "Shirina," he said, and the sound, the feeling, the hiss of her name was like a caress on her sex.

Shirina slipped her fingers beneath his tunic. He felt smooth along his side, rippling with muscle and the shape of his ribs, and then hairy as she ventured further between them, bristle scant on his belly and thicker towards his chest. The hard pebble of his nipple startled her when her fingers skittered over it, and he gave a broken sigh beside her ear.

"I want you so badly," he said, his voice hardly a breath. "Please."

How clever of him to ask. No wonder his victims never reported him. They'd consented.

Shirina was too proud to grant permission – with words, at least. But her hips said yes for her, grinding her sex against his hard thigh. The motion allowed him to slide his hand under the small of her back and grasp the back of her *dhoti*. He tugged the end from the waistband and pulled. The silk fell open, baring her to the open air.

His fingers trailed up her inner thigh, moving, exploring, while Shirina guided his mouth to hers again, seeking more kisses to bury the whimpers that kept trying to escape her throat. Their tongues were bold now, having learned each other's mouths. Shirina's hands slid lower, into the waistband of his trousers. He raised his hips, and she slid the trousers down. His thighs felt scorching hot where they pressed into hers. And there, the unmistakable hard length of his shaft.

Shirina did whimper after all.

"Please," he murmured against her lips.

She'd pulled down his trousers: what more invitation did he need? Shirina spread her thighs. Her sex felt drenched as she opened her legs wide, so ready for him that it ached. She pushed her hips against him, wiggling them in an effort to line everything up. But he was on top. He'd need to co-operate.

"I want you," he murmured against her cheek. "I want you so much."

Shirina gritted her teeth. She was a serpent. If he wouldn't give his *lingam* to her, she'd take it. With a cunning effort, she swivelled her hips, spine flexing. His *lingam* fell into position, right between her legs. The smooth tip of it rocked against her opening, slick, hot and blunt.

All he needed to do was lower his hips. But instead he planted his elbow and slipped a hand onto her other breast. He caressed them, one in each hand, and the feathery brush of his fingertips on both her nipples at once made her moan.

Fine. If he wouldn't press into her, she'd impale herself on him from beneath. She bent one knee, then the other, and pulled her heels up high. She dug them into the ground on either side of her hips, then slipped her hands under her bottom, waiting for the perfect moment to strike. He covered her mouth with his and fondled her breasts, teasing the nipples into taut peaks. She kissed him back, flicking her tongue out, and, when he was distracted by her tongue, her hips snapped up.

Both of them went suddenly still, frozen in the sunlit garden. Shirina stared into her lover's dark eyes and dared him to make her beg. He stared back, eyebrows twisted up high; maybe he'd always been able to make his women plead for him. Shirina spread her legs wider still and thrust herself onto his staff again, forcing it inside her even deeper. Her lover's eyelids fluttered shut, and he buried his face in the crook of her neck. Shirina writhed beneath him, helping herself to forget about the pain of his entry by losing herself in the sensations that coursed through her when she ground herself against him.

Soon, his body's moves began to mirror hers, thrusting in counterpoint to her insistent motions. It was clumsy at first, slick and strange and even a bit painful, but they fell into a good rhythm of slow, deep thrusts that ended with a grind that left her shuddering with pleasure. Shirina stopped thinking about where her hands and hips and mouth were, and lost herself in the undulation of their bodies.

Her lover's thrusts grew faster, and his breathing in her ear went ragged. Shirina lost all sense of her garden, herself, and instead became pure pleasure as the burn between her thighs blossomed into a white hot wave of sensation that rolled through her body over and over again, until finally it ebbed and seeped from her bones, leaving her limp, and damp, and utterly spent.

"Shirina," stammered her lover. "I . . . I . . ."

"Don't say anything," she whispered. Serpents had no need of speaking.

Shirina pulled her hands out from beneath her bottom and laid them across the back of her lover's neck. He was damp, his tunic soaked through, and his skin chilled where the late afternoon shade covered it.

Warm in the sun and cool in the shade; maybe he could be a serpent too, if she showed him how. Shirina had never needed to put it into words. But this man seemed to be a quick study.

They lay together on the bed of mint as their breaths slowed, and Shirina allowed her mind to be clear, to enjoy the heaviness of her lover's body on hers, the strange dampness between her legs and the lassitude that pervaded everything. But just as she began to drift between wakefulness and dreams, an awful clatter came from the house.

"Shi-ri-na!"

Shirina pushed her lover into a galangal thatch. "That's my mother!"

Her lover's eyes went wide.

"Shirina! Where are you? Where is Dharmesh? I can never find either of you when I need you."

"Go," said Shirina, jabbing her finger towards the door. "If she finds you, she'll kill you."

He staggered to his feet, cast a glance towards the window, hiked up his trousers and ran to the doorway. With his hand on the latch, he turned to look at her. "Shirina . . ."

"Go," she said, waving him away. "Go the way you came in. Her room's on the other side of the house. Go."

He stared for one more moment, then ducked through the doorway and was gone.

Shirina wrapped her *dhoti* quickly, and tugged her tunic back down around her hips just as her mother, fanning herself, appeared in the window. "Why are you covered with leaves?"

Shirina glanced at the mangled bed of mint. Her wrap was a rumpled ball of silk among the crushed leaves. "I was working in the garden."

"Where is your brother? I have a terrible headache."

"Don't worry about Dharmesh. He went to the market. Go and lie down. I'll make you some tea."

Shirina settled her mother in bed with a strong dose of *ulat kambal*, then made her way back to the garden. It was the same garden it had always been, only it seemed different now, smaller somehow. The mint was ruined, but it would come back in a few weeks as it always did. Shirina stared at the spot where she'd met her fellow serpent. She wondered if the mint knew; if it would taste different now.

The door banged open and Shirina looked up. Dharmesh lounged in the doorway, cheeks flushed with wine. "What was that thing you wanted? Senna? Did Atal have the one you wanted? I guess there's at least a dozen different kinds."

Shirina glared at Dharmesh. She liked him better in his room than in her garden. Dharmesh tended to step on plants when he staggered, and not all of them were as resilient as the mint.

"He showed up, didn't he?" said Dharmesh. He looked puzzled. But then, he usually did when he'd been drinking. "Tall man, pointy beard."

Shirina went very still.

Dharmesh took a few meandering steps into the garden and looked around aimlessly. His eyes fell on the sack Shirina's lover had been carrying. "So, he was here! Why are you being so weird? Was the senna wrong?"

Shirina blinked slowly. "Yes. Entirely wrong. I need to see some more."

Dharmesh squinted at the sack. Shirina wondered how she could explain why she'd kept it if it was "entirely wrong", but thankfully, Dharmesh just shrugged and turned towards the gate. "I'll tell him tomorrow."

"What did you say his name was?"

"Atal."

Shirina mouthed the word. It felt like the jab of a fang. A good serpent name.

"Yes, tomorrow," said Shirina. Dharmesh was busy fumbling with the latch. "And visit Mother before you go to your room. She's been asking for you."

The door finally popped open. "Yes, of course," Dharmesh mumbled as he wandered into the house. He wasn't the smartest brother a girl could hope for, but he always remembered what Shirina wanted from the marketplace. That had to count for something.

Shirina sat cross-legged in the mint and watched the shadows deepen. Her thoughts turned to Atal. He'd seemed so gentle, so tender . . . even reluctant. As he fled, he'd stared at her with such a strange, poignant look on his face, as if he had no idea how to react when he was caught compromising a girl's virtues.

She hardly knew what to make of him.

She decided it was very clever of Atal, very clever indeed, to gain entry to women's homes by posing as an innocent merchant – one known to everyone in the village, even her brother. Not that Dharmesh was all that hard to deceive.

How fortunate for her that there were a dozen types of senna. Dharmesh wouldn't be bothered to puzzle out the proper variety himself. He'd send Atal.

Shirina went to Dharmesh's window and pounded on the sill with the flat of her hand. "Where's my scroll? You'd better not have lost it."

"Calm yourself, here it is." The scroll flew over Shirina's head and landed in the poppies.

Shirina picked it up and scanned down past the various tinctures and poisons. There, at the end, was a section she'd barely skimmed in the past: aphrodisiacs.

She read the formulae and discovered that she already had many of the ingredients right there in her garden. She moved swiftly from plant to plant, gathering flowers and leaves. She had until tomorrow to brew a very special tea.

Because when Atal got here, he'd probably be thirsty.

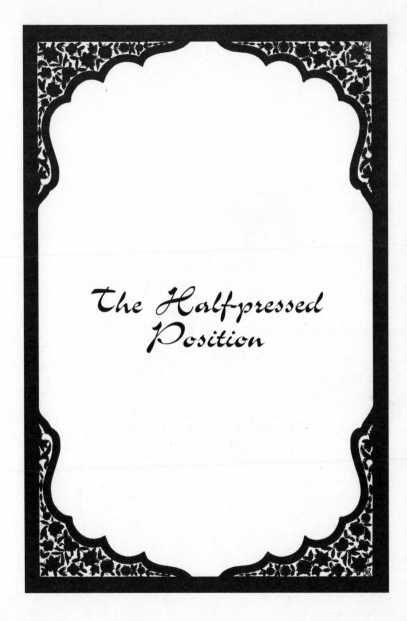

The Half-pressed
Position

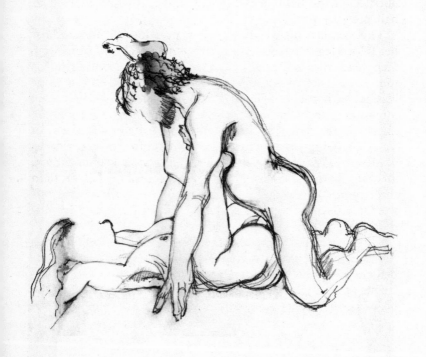

The Halfpressed Position

Ardhapiditaka
Kama Sutra

If a woman's leg is contracted and held before her lover's chest, gently pressing against his heart, while the other leg is stretched out flat on the floor, it is *Ardhapiditaka*, the half-pressed or half-pressure position.

The man lays his weight onto her, pressing his chest against her folded leg. He feels her against him and takes her this way. Her *yoni* is pleasantly constricted in this position and this adds to the man's sensations. The man may lean his face in close for kissing, let her take small nibbles at his lower lip, or touch her forehead or breasts. The man should remember to employ many strokes and thrusts to please his lover. Because, as Vatsyayana says, men and women have different experiences of pleasure. While the man's semen comes at the end of the act, at orgasm, the woman experiences a continual fall of fluid throughout the sexual act. A man thinks, "I am having this woman." While the woman thinks, "I am being had by this man."

In this position, the woman has the option to unfold and refold each leg, stretching the alternate one out flat as the one before. This movement and changing of position can be extremely pleasurable for both. Satisfy her with the "blow of the boar" or the "sporting of a sparrow".

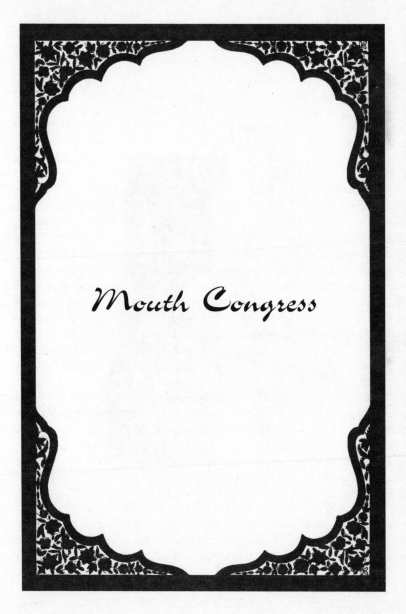

Mouth Congress

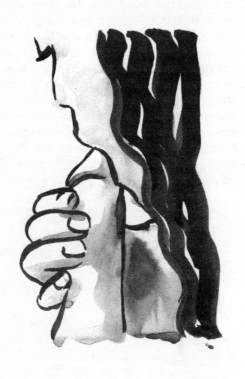

Mouth Congress

Auparishtaka
Kama Sutra

Prevalent in India since ancient times (an ancient Indian work on medicine some 2,000 years old describes a wound being caused by the teeth to the *lingam*), oral sex gets a complicated and slightly ambiguous treatment in the *Kama Sutra*. On the one hand, it is a pleasurable sensation that leads to sexual release and mental health. On the other hand, it says it is not a good thing to have oral sex with your wife, or to kiss the mouths of those who you go to for oral sex if they are unclean. However, the *Kama Sutra* goes on to mention that many of the ancient religious texts say that a cow's udder is unclean except at the time of milking, which means that during loveplay, everything is allowed. Homosexual men were the appropriate givers of oral pleasure in ancient Indian society.

The Tale of the Mouth Congress

as told by Thomas S. Roche

Dharma is better than *Artha*, and *Artha* is better than *Karma*. But *Artha* should always be first practised by the king for the livelihood of men is to be obtained from it only. Again, *Kama* being the occupation of public women, they should prefer it to the other two, and these are exceptions to the general rule."

The Kama Sutra of Vatsysayana (Burton translation)

Many years ago in the land of Alaritramishi in today's Sharashura province, south of the great mountains where the great Lasharka River meets the endless ocean in a fertile river delta, there lived a prince named Alari-Tasharik who, instructed in the teachings of the Thinkers at a young age, sought to live a virtuous life. You might say he had mixed success.

Though he did not want for any material possession while he was growing up, Tasharik was known throughout the court of Alaritramishi as a troubled youth. From an early age, he sought the wisdom of books over the pleasures of the court, and many said he was destined not to be Rāja, or King, but to be a holy man.

Tasharik was very unlike his father, Alari-Lashrim, who placed the pursuit of *kama* over *dharma* and *artha*. Lashrim's indulgence in the rich foods and wines provided by the agricultural wealth of the Lasharka delta was well known throughout the region, as was his love for the tactile enrichments of rich clothes and furnishings, scents, baths, intoxicants and the performing arts.

Speaking of performing arts, Lashrim quite notoriously brought women from many lands to perform for him; their sensual behaviours were on display at his court revels as well as in more private surroundings.

King Lashrim died when Tasharik, or Rik as he was called by those very few in his inner circle, was nineteen. Lashrim's early death, many said, was owed to the king's indulgence in sensual pleasures, and certainly the scene of his passing was a lascivious affair, though it could certainly be said that Lashrim died with a smile on his face.

Despite Lashrim's many rumoured and claimed offspring, Rik ascended to the throne peacefully. This was a testament to the goodwill of the citizens of Alaritramishi, as well as the fact that Alari-Tasharik alone had been the son of Shanri-Al, Lashrim's first and favorite wife. Shanri had died when Tasharik was twelve, many said from her own over-indulgence in *kama*: the queen also died with a smile on her face.

That his father and mother had both died without achieving the fourth goal of life, *moksha*, or liberation, was of great trouble to Rik, and he promised himself that he would not fall prey to their weaknesses. Had not the Great Thinkers, whom Rik admired so profoundly, said that *dharma*, or virtuous living, was superior to *artha*, or material success, and that *kama*, or sensual pleasure, came third? The Great Thinkers had also stressed in their teachings that *artha* was the first duty of a king. In any event, by almost anyone's reckoning but his own, Rik had already achieved the goal of virtuous living. But the unhappy youth could not see it.

He concluded that his only virtue as king could be the enrichment of his people, whom his father had taxed heavily to strengthen the richness of his trade and support his indulgences. He would further *artha* for his people, as the Teachers have said a great king should do.

Rik's first act was to banish from his household all those temptresses who had so tempted his father. Providing moderate quarters for them on the outskirts of the city, Rik staffed his house instead with eunuchs purchased from the Sholal-Shoshara region, famous for their discretion and obedience. More importantly, they would provide no temptation for the new king to stray from his works of public good.

Lashrim's many concubines were unhappy with this, but we'll get to that in a moment.

Rik restructured the payment of taxes and redirected the monies that had previously enriched his father's court into great public works. His people became rich, but the land still richer, as the agricultural wealth of the valley grew into legend. Known throughout the world for producing delicious foodstuffs, the land and its people were greatly enriched by trade and, even with the restructured tax base, the land's king also grew enriched.

But the king's many public works projects had begun to take a toll on his health; he became angry, dyspeptic and volatile. Embarrassed on several occasions by public outbursts of displeasure, he elected to isolate himself more and more, to disappear within his household of eunuchs. Some years later, a historian would comment that the great Rāja probably had the world's worst case of sexual deprivation, but Rik would have furiously rejected this assertion.

Shortly before his death, King Lashrim, having heard rumours of the odd proclivities of Punjabi women, conceived a most inventive way to pursue a little *kama*, and sent for a courtesan named Parvati from his friend the king of Punjab. In Punjab, women are renowned for making congress with each other using their mouths, which makes Punjabi men famously nervous, but they don't mind so much as long as they get to watch.

Parvati was named after the Devi of Love, and she met this calling with great enthusiasm, showing uncommon ardour. Unfortunately for King Lashrim, he never got a chance to try out his hypothesis that the legendary act of Punjabi love could also be performed on a man. Parvati had never met with the king, and was unknown to men. But she was what we, today, would call "popular" among the other courtesans.

Secreted in their modest harem far from the new Rāja's eyes, Parvati had already taught most of the former courtesans the ways of the Punjab women, with the result that none were wanting for pleasures, and few felt embittered by their banishment from the Rāja's household.

Except one. Her name was Salimari and she was a woman who had held the first place in the Rāja's bed since his wife's death. She was a haughty, proud woman, and could not live without luxury, influence and power.

Salimari called Parvati to her one night after the Punjab woman had extracted the dew of creation from a large number of the courtesans. Salimari invited Parvati to extract her dew, and Parvati complied with bored, mechanical efficiency.

"Your skills are truly great, beautiful one," said Salimari with succulent grace.

"Thanks," said Parvati suspiciously. Her tongue was beginning to hurt.

"They would find better appreciation if we dwelt in the house of the Rāja, beautiful one," said Salimari.

Parvati sighed patiently, for Salimari had been working on her for weeks. "But we do not dwell in the house of the Rāja, Most Delicious-Loined Mother," she said.

"Perhaps we could," said Salimari cunningly. "If the king could be tempted to embrace *kama* as did his father, surely he would welcome all of us back into the household and times would be as they were back in '06."

Parvati's eyes narrowed, for she had heard the many tales of the decadent sixth year of the king's reign.

"Aren't you getting a little old for orgies?" asked Parvati.

"One is never too old for orgies," said Salimari innocently.

"Nevertheless," said Parvati, "is it not well known that the Rāja has embraced first *dharma*, living virtuously, and thereafter *artha*, enriching his subjects? Only after he has provided for the material wealth of all his people will the King embrace *kama*."

"But perhaps that would change if he could be tempted by one as beautiful as you," purred Salimari. "And one as skilled."

"My skills do not extend to congress with men; as you know, Great Succulent Mother, I am a virgin."

"But could the congress you enjoy with the woman's dew of creation not also be worked upon a man?"

Except for the late King, this idea had not yet occurred to the people of Alaritramishi, though more than one Punjabi man had thought about it while watching the congress of

Punjabi women. Parvati, however, was innocent of such ways, and she was repelled.

"Are you mad, Mother Whose Delicious Thighs So Tempt Me? It is natural for women to seek such pleasures with each other when a *lingam* is not around, but why should a man submit to such pleasures, when a woman has a perfectly good *yoni* to please him?" Here Parvati betrayed her own preferences, for she'd grown desperately bored of congress with her fellow courtesans and no longer understood what the fuss was all about, especially since no one ever thought to perform such congress upon her, which she really would have appreciated.

Salimari caressed Parvati's face. "Indeed no man would waste time inviting that pretty mouth of yours to perform its magic on his *lingam*," she cooed. "But do not Punjabi eunuchs engage in such practices?"

Parvati made a disgusted sound.

"That, Great Mother With Delicious Dew, is just *weird*."

"Hear me out, Parvati. Could not the king be convinced that such a thing did not violate his vow to forego *kama*?"

Parvati swallowed nervously.

She said weakly, "But there is no Punjabi eunuch in Alaritramishi, O Mother With Creamy—"

"My little Parvati," said Salimari. "Always co-operative."

She pulled out her shears.

Not one day later, Parvati found herself miserably shorn, her lustrous black hair cut close in the manner of the King's eunuch attendants, her ample breasts cinched tight to her body with bandages so that even were she to be mostly undressed, her female beauty was not evident. This was important, for the eunuchs lived communally.

Salimari had bribed the chief steward of the Rāja's house so that Parvati could fill the position of body servant to the Rāja. From the first moment Parvati laid eyes on Rik, she desired him; how could a trained courtesan not desire her King? More importantly, Parvati, well into the prime of her desires, had a fierce case of sexual deprivation herself.

As the Rāja's body servant, Parvati helped him bathe, dress and do many other intimate things, which did not help her swiftly growing attachment to him, nor her desire. Worst of all was the fact that the eunuchs' communal living and bathing made it virtually impossible for the wretched girl to touch herself. She had grown quite accustomed to multiple daily partnerships with her fellow courtesans, and within a few weeks was out of her mind, ravenously desirous of Punjabi congress, or for that matter any other sort of congress, with the Rāja or any other random stranger, eunuch, female or male – she wasn't particular.

Witnessing the frequent erections the Rāja suffered when he bathed was no help, and her own growing tendency to let her hand linger down there while she washed him contributed to stiffening tension between them.

"I could take care of that for you, sir," she said huskily one day when she had elicited such an erection by spending quite a time with saffron oils on those parts of his body inclined towards erection. Upon doing this, she had thought to herself "This is a very, very bad idea," and had done it anyway, unable to resist the draw of taking the King's growing member in her hand.

Inflamed, the Rāja raised his hand to strike her and would have done so had he not recalled suddenly his vow to seek *dharma*. He took a deep breath and firmly removed Parvati's hand from his *lingam*. "Bah! How could a eunuch relieve me?"

"Here," said Parvati, returning her hand to his erection. "I'll show you."

"What are you doing?"

"I am Punjab, great King, and there the eunuchs, we practise . . . a technique that'll take your mind off *kama*. Should help with those headaches you've been having, too."

Rik frowned. "How can the temptations of *kama* be relieved without succumbing to – oh." That was the last word he said for quite a time, for Parvati had begun to move her hand.

Parvati's voice was as rich as the sweets enjoyed in great quantities by Rik's father. "Surely, King, the Great Thinkers who proscribed *kama* until *dharma* and *artha* could be achieved – did they not also say that youth is when *kama* should be enjoyed?"

"That's sacrilege," said the King hoarsely. "Or a great idea . . . I can't decide." He gulped.

"Then don't decide," she whispered, moving her hand more quickly and insistently. "Let me decide for you, great Rājan-Gopa-Samrat." She used the term that means "King-Protector-Supreme Ruler," mostly because she'd been about to say, "You stupid fool."

The king let out a cry of pleasure, and his own dew ejected forcefully into the air and hit the oil lamp hanging far overhead, sizzling as it landed.

Parvati had never really had any interest in furthering Salimari's plot; now she just wanted to lie with the King. She felt tormented, however, for in addition to being hungry for him, she had started to fall in love. She had no wish to tempt the King into compromising his morals for the sake of Salimari's ambition. But she wouldn't have minded a little compromise in the service of her aching sex.

Each night when the King bathed before bed, Parvati used her hand to anoint his member, which in turn anointed her hand (and often the lamp). After months of this, Parvati's mouth watered more and more as she serviced the King; finally, she said breathlessly, "Great Rājan-Gopa-Samrat, if you wouldn't mind getting out of this bath, I could finish this job properly."

The King looked suspicious. "You wouldn't be suggesting I forsake—"

Parvati had quite lost her patience with the King, and interrupted him irritably: "Hand or mouth, what does it matter to you? The only difference is whether I enjoy myself." Testily, she added, "O Great Rājan-Gopa-Samrat," with great emphasis on the plosives.

The king gulped. "Mouth?" "What was your name again?" asked the King nervously.

Parvati had been using a variety of them around the castle,

which didn't help her cover much. Now, she said the first thing that was on her mind: "Auparishtaka," which means "mouth congress," and really isn't a very commonly used name, for obvious reasons.

"Auparishtaka?" blurted the King. "My dear sweet eunuch, that is a very strange name."

"Perhaps, great King, you'll feel differently in ten minutes," snapped Parvati. "Get on the bed."

The King was not accustomed to being spoken to in this manner, but he was quite close to completion and therefore more inclined to be forgiving of the beautiful eunuch about to provide it. The King rose and allowed Parvati to dry him, then to guide him onto the edge of the bed, where he sat with legs parted while she knelt before him. Her lips and tongue suckled wetly up and down his shaft, and the King gasped. She slurped her way onto his tip and coaxed a low moan from the great Rāja's mouth.

"By the Great Teachers," the king murmured. "Auparishtaka, are you sure this doesn't violate my – oh!"

Finally having a shaft in her mouth, Parvati was not in the mood to argue with words, nor would she have been equipped to do so.

She convinced the King the way her followers would convince kings and brigands for thousands of years to follow: she swallowed his shaft.

The king's eyes rolled well back into his head. Parvati withdrew just long enough to sweep the Rāja's legs out from under him and spread him over the edge of his enormous bed. She climbed on top of him and continued to apply her mouth to his shaft hungrily, resisting only with profound effort the urge to hump his leg. The King's hands began to rove on their own, groping for her body; Parvati deftly eluded them and, when they came too close, slapped them away. The King was not accustomed to having his hand slapped.

"Auparishtaka, I must touch you!" growled the maddened King.

Parvati came off the king's shaft with a drooly gasp, thinking fast.

"To do so would be to violate your oath, great King," she murmured, "and you wouldn't want that, would you?"

The King frowned, but Parvati's logic was fairly unassailable. His hands gripped the bed covers as Parvati's mouth returned to his shaft and her head bobbed up and down enthusiastically.

Tricked into surrendering to *kama*, the young King had found his virtuous mind quite out of control. His eyes roved over Parvati's beautiful face as she continued to lavish his shaft with affection.

The thoughts he had then surely reflected his growing madness, for was it not unthinkable for a man to love a eunuch the way one loved a woman?

The King came with a bleat not unlike a dying lamb, and Parvati tasted his dew, previously unshared by mortals. He lay there under her writhing as she eagerly licked his dwindling shaft, then wept softly as Parvati's skilled mouth caressed him. It had been a long three years.

Parvati found the crying more than a little creepy, but she forgave the King; after three years without release, she felt he was entitled to be a little emotional.

After the first dozen or so times, the King was no longer reticent at receiving Parvati's oral attentions; on the contrary, he began to demand them with great frequency. Moreover, Parvati became quite aware of the King's sultry, lustful glances cast towards her whenever they would cross paths. The day came when the King did not allow her to conduct mouth congress with him after she undressed him for bed. Instead, he took her chin in his hand when she sought to do so, bent forward and hungrily pressed his mouth to hers; she melted into his kiss, shuddering with her want for the King.

"Return to your quarters," he said. "Allow the other servants to see you taking to bed. Come back in an hour. Auparishtaka, tonight you are to share my bed."

"My King," said Parvati, "I mustn't. Such a thing will draw you into the web of *kama*, when your vow—"

"I've had enough *dharma* and *artha* for the time being," growled the King demandingly. "I wish to enjoy *kama* with you, in its fullest forms."

"My King," said Parvati, tears in her eyes. "I mustn't."

"You must," said the King, who clearly wasn't taking no for an answer.

Parvati returned to the servants' quarters and removed her outer clothes, remaining in the snug undergarments she always wore to disguise her sex. The other eunuchs always slept nude, but Parvati had been able to explain away her modesty as a strange Punjabi custom. The explanation caused the Alaritramishi eunuchs to nod knowingly as if they'd heard of it.

All night Parvati tossed and turned, deeply desiring to go to the Rāja but unwilling to do so lest he discover her deception. What would he do? By the Great Teachers, she'd better not think about that. She pushed her thighs very tightly together, and tried to think of aged holy women.

Parvati arrived at her master's chambers early the next morning red-eyed and pasty-faced. He, too, had not slept, but where Parvati was merely troubled by that, the Rāja was greatly angered, as evidenced by the armed guards flanking him.

"I waited all night for you," he growled.

"Perhaps a little mouth congress, great King?" said Parvati weakly.

"Seize him," snapped the Rāja, and Parvati was grabbed by the palace guards and taken to the dungeon of the palace, where she was placed in a cell.

A week passed, and with every new day Parvati's despair deepened. She expected every morning to hear of her impending execution, but to her surprise, after a week the door of her cell was opened and the Rāja arrived.

His eyes were red, much redder than on the day he had banished her. She also noticed that he was walking in a funny way.

"Auparishtaka," said the King meekly, "my imprisonment of you violates my oath of virtuous living. I had no right to demand of you what I did. I pray you will accept my apology. I . . . I have no right to know the pleasures you offer. From now on you'll work in the kitchen, Auparishtaka."

"The kitchen, my King?" said Parvati peevishly. She smiled vaguely and licked her lips, which caused King Rik's eyes to widen and his throat to tremble as he gulped nervously.

"Yes," said the proud King, and left her there to find her own way out of the dungeons and back to the servants' quarters.

After a week in the dungeon, Parvati was badly in need of a bath, and her enjoyment of one greatly inflamed her own desires. This, perhaps, guided her imprudent actions that night. After an hour spent tossing and turning in her gender-shrouding garments, she slipped out of bed. "This is a terrible idea," she thought to herself, but did it anyway.

Though the King's bedroom, as always, was guarded by men with spears, Parvati knew the back entrance and silently made her way into it.

She discovered him tossing and turning. He sat up in bed as soon as she entered his chambers.

"Auparishtaka?" he asked.

The room was quite dark, and Parvati did not answer. Instead she approached the bed while the Rāja protested meekly into the darkness.

"You mustn't come to me, Auparishtaka," he said. "I am a wretched, wretched king. I have let myself be tempted, and in tempting me you have received my wrath. I am a bad, bad king, Auparishtaka. You must go."

Parvati pulled back the covers. She found the King erect and began to administer the mouth congress to him. His protests were punctuated with rapturous moans, until Parvati knew that his dew was soon to be hers; after a week's denial, she was hungry for it.

In an instant, as he thundered towards his climax, the Rāja's tone changed. "Come to me," said the King. "Remove your clothes. I want to feel you against me."

Parvati drew back, her mouth slick with spittle and with the King's steadily leaking dew. "No, King – I mustn't! Please, let's just enjoy the mouth congress."

"I must have you, Auparishtaka," cooed the King, seizing Parvati and drawing her insistently onto the bed. She twisted and writhed under him, her craving so great it was agony, but knowing that if she allowed him to undress her then her secret would be revealed.

"No, King," she blurted as she struggled with him. "Your vow! *Dharma* must go before—"

The Rāja's desire, dammed for so long, was not to be denied. He uttered soothing sounds to Parvati, who struggled as he tore at her clothes – until they came free and he realized, suddenly, Parvati's awful secret.

That was just before she saw her opening, and kicked the Rāja in his private parts.

"Vixen!" he choked in the instant before her knee made contact; thereafter, he was not saying much of anything, though if "GGGGGGGggggGGGGGG" was a word in Alaritra-mishi, he would have said it.

Parvati, now revealed as a woman, had nothing to lose. While the naked and injured Rāja moved to get out of bed and run for it, Parvati grabbed him and, displaying exceptional strength for her small frame, dragged him back into bed. Admittedly, the King was not exactly in top form, though the blow to his manhood had failed to reduce his erection.

The Rāja continued to struggle, so Parvati, unable to hold out for long against the King's greater physical strength, used the most convincing argument she could. While the King struggled inadequately to get away from her, she returned her mouth to his shaft and within moments was performing mouth congress upon the King as if her very life depended on it. Soon the blow to the King's private parts was forgotten and he knew nothing but his desire. When the King's back arched and he approached climax, Parvati realized that this might well be the very last time she was allowed anywhere near her beloved King, and she decided to go for it.

Making short work of the torn remnants of her clothes, Parvati climbed naked atop the Rāja, who was still weakly protesting. She spread her legs and caressed his shaft with her hand, drawing it close to her centre. Feeling her hairy body, and particularly her hairy loins, against him, the Rāja felt certain he had indeed encountered some magical form of male, for the women of Alaritramishi groom themselves with meticulous care. As he felt her sex against him, caressing moist at his shaft, he uttered her name rapturously: "Auparishtaka."

She kissed him passionately and said: "The name's Parvati."

Now all seemed clear to the Rāja. Obviously this was an avatar of the great goddess, come to teach him that even at the expense of the two superior goals of life, *kama* must not be denied. His hands came to rest on Parvati's shapely backside, and as her body surged against him she began to press herself onto him.

The king's upward thrust met her downward one, and before she could finish her protest she felt her virginity give way painlessly. Parvati passionately made love to the King, and no more protests were heard.

And so it was that the great and famously celibate Rāja took as his wife a Punjabi woman with whom he had first fallen in love while she was masquerading as his eunuch body servant.

Though the king had learned to accept the pursuit of *kama* in his life, Salimari did not realize her goal to return to the royal household, for she, in fact, was but an avatar of the goddess Parvati; her goal was to bring the two lovers together, for she got the sense that the king needed a good session of mouth congress.

Though he continued to pursue both *dharma* and *artha*, and greatly enriched his people with public works, the Rāja learned a great appreciation for *kama* in the arms of his love Parvati.

In the traditions of *kama*, Auparishtaka is the name for "mouth congress". When properly enacted, it may be performed by men, by women or by eunuchs. To this day, the timeless ritual is enacted in honour of Rik and Parvati throughout the world. When the man is aroused, and the woman proximate to his aroused parts, if he is unwilling she must place her mouth upon him and commit Auparishtaka even while he protests. But if he becomes ardent and insists on her continuing – for instance, with his hand on her head or by gripping her hair – she must protest.

Once he has been cowed, she may return to the congress, but if he becomes demanding again she must refuse to continue. Only when this ritual has driven them both to the delirious heights of pleasure may the man's dew of creation be extracted properly through mouth congress, or another form of mating engaged in.

Thus is the goddess Parvati most pleased, and thus do the lovers reach *moksha* – liberation. And even the Great Teachers can get behind that.

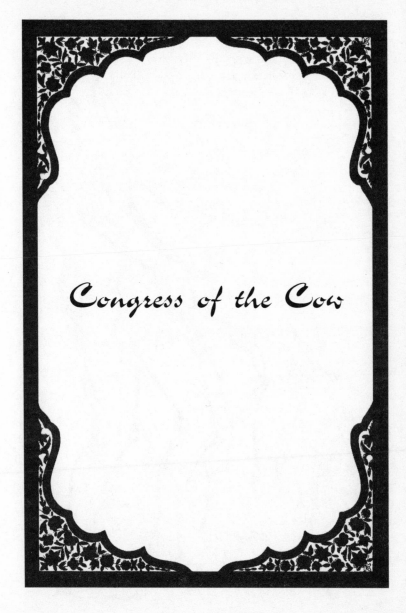

Congress of the Cow

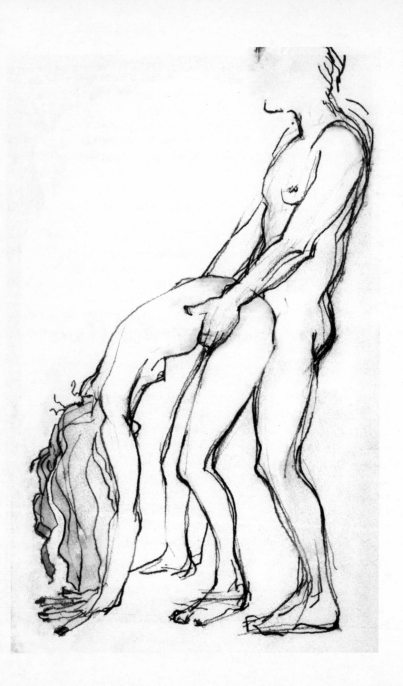

Congress of the Cow

Dhenuka
Kama Sutra

The *Kama Sutra* tells us that a man may choose to take his lover like a cow, like a beast, when the mood takes him. But although lovemaking may be animal in style, it should be elevated and civilized, as sex between humans should be. Animals have sex instinctually and without a methodology like the *Kama Sutra*. After all, aren't humans civilized and superior to animals in every way? Therefore, we look to *kama* for a method that two people, the lovers, will study and participate in, being equal lovers in this civilized sexuality. The man takes his lover as if she were a cow – bellowing and caressing her back roughly. But he is only acting, impersonating a bull and all his base desires. And she will respond to the animal lust at her back, and push against him, mooing in return, spurring him on to orgasm!

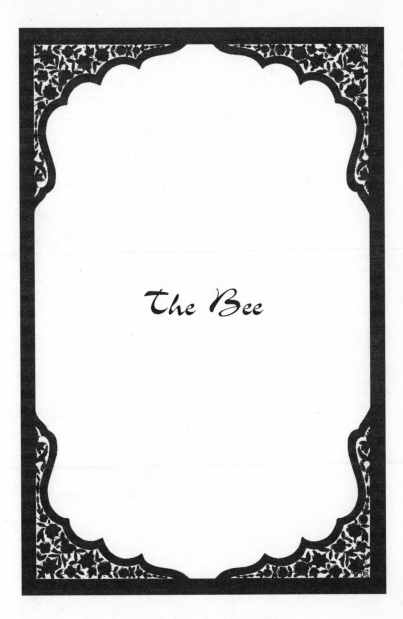

The Bee

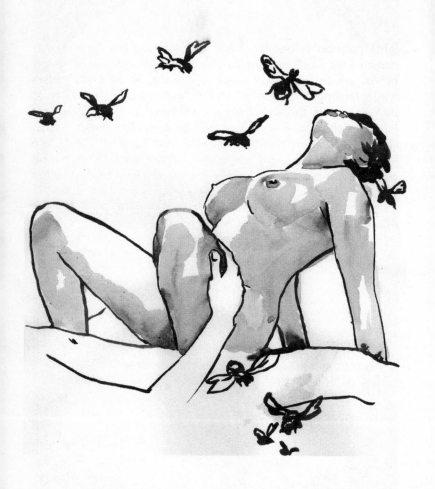

The Bee

Bhramara
Kama Sutra

This position is one of the woman-on-top positions and is named "the bee" because of the movements of the woman's pelvis, which mimic the bee's movement as its body pulses while feeding at a flower. Her pelvis makes rapid, circular movements on the man's *lingam*, rubbing it on the right and left sides of her *yoni* as she sees fit. She draws her feet up so that she is sitting above the man in a squat and uses her feet to help her achieve an ease of movement. Penetration is deep and passions can be intense. This is a position where love scratches can be left easily. The woman is also free in this position to interrupt the frenzy of her movements to give her lover any number of kisses.

The Tale of the Black Bumble Bee

as told by Kweli Walker

Before I saw them, I heard the drum of their horse's hooves beating towards me. The fiery brilliance of the evening sky painted their faces. Brisk winds tossed my Aunt Tejal's silver locks like flames. Cousin Aruna galloped beside her.

"Welcome home, Vatsyayana!" she cried, carving a spiral of red dust into the belly of the earth with her mare's hooves. We dismounted and rocked each other with hugs and tears.

"We've heard that you advise royalty, Vatsya."

"It's true, Auntie, but you're the stone who sharpened me into seeker and sought. Where is cousin Jyoti?"

My youngest cousin, Jyoti, always accompanied them when they rode to meet me.

Tejal's smile evaporated. "Jyoti's the reason I sent for you, Vatsya. He had a nasty fall and hasn't been himself, nephew. Sometimes he leaves before sunrise, and we don't see him until dark. Once, I found him sulking under the Palash tree, where his father is buried. Remember how brave and joyful he was?" She shook her head sadly. "You're our only hope."

We were savouring heavenly morsels of spicy vegetable stew when Jyoti slowly hobbled towards us. His head hung like drenched rag until our eyes met.

"Va-a-aaatsya!" He smiled with pain-filled eyes.

His wide shoulders still filled his woolly wrap but he was much leaner. He picked at his food like a child. Where was Jyoti who ate his first two bowls like a wolf in winter? Who was this sombre young man, whose leg betrayed each step? Aunt Tejal left me to find out.

Cousin Aruna shared a spicy tale of a voluptuous courtesan who polished his sword each day to learn my new positions.

"And you, Jyoti?" I asked. "Surely you've tried some of the lessons I shared?"

"Playing blind to my lameness, Vatsya?" he snarled, "Only public women need me now."

"Taken to self-pity, Jyoti? Where is the boy who dug his father's grave?"

"I ask myself each day, Vatsya."

I examined his leg in the firelight. Clearly, it had been improperly set.

"It must be rebroken and reset. Is there a healer near?"

Aruna said, "Bala is the finest healer in Gupta. We carried him there first, but she was birthing Samudragupta's first child."

"Go back to her, Aruna."

I pressed a gold coin into his palm. He leaped on his Marawi and galloped west. Hours later, Aruna returned with Bala and her granddaughter, Makshi. Bala was a regal matriarch with a long silver braid. She moved slowly but sturdily. Makshi was a carob-coloured goddess with hair so black, it shimmered with sapphire. She was petite but through her flowing sari, one could see, Lakshmi had been generous above and below her slender waist. Her voice was soft and sweet as ripe mangoes. She eagerly absorbed her grandmother's instructions, and moved about working quickly, but with seductive grace. Her name definitely suited her. *Makshi* – a honey bee, indeed.

"Makshi will attend Jyoti after I've sedated him," Bala rasped. "I must leave but trust that she is a highly skilled healer." She began brewing a large pot of tea.

As the tea steeped, the air turned bitter. Bala gave final instructions to her granddaughter and left quickly.

Jyoti valiantly refused honey and gulped down the vile-smelling tea. Suddenly, his face knotted into a giant pucker and he exploded into body-heaving gags. Minutes later, after a drunken tirade about "foul-tasting" tea, he grinned and collapsed into Makshi's lap.

I imagined how beautifully the whites of her kohl-lined eyes would glitter, as the tip of my tongue pillaged through her luxuriant forest to burnish my prize. I thickened with each wicked fantasy of her seduction. Unfortunately, Jyoti held her full attention.

Makshi was small but strong. Alone, she pulled Jyoti's leg apart and wrestled it into position. While she wrapped his leg securely in red clay, bay bark, and cloth, Aruna and I were hypnotized by the tremble of her smooth flesh.

Long before daybreak, I heard Jyoti and Makshi whispering. Lightning blazed between them in the plum-coloured dawn. From a pitch-black corridor, I watched their flirting escalate from a simmer to a boil. Jyoti did everything but circus tricks to keep her attention. He intentionally spoke softly to draw her near. In erotic retaliation, she bent slowly and deeply . . . *to hear* – spreading her wide hips and spilling her full breasts inches from his mouth. She used her long jet-black hair and the silky corners of her sari to torment him.

"Are you hungry?" she asked, coyly.

He burned a hole in the lap of her sari while rhythmically quivering his sharp tongue. She smiled, but soundly scolded his increasing boldness.

"In a house full of people, Jyoti?" she giggled. "And with your freshly broken leg? You'd do all that for me? How exciting." She laughed, seductively stoking the inferno he ignited between her thighs. "Empty the house . . . and *then* let's see how clever you are."

"*Almost empty*," I swore to myself. "*A threat this exciting demands a witness.*"

Makshi prepared a large bowl of barley and yogurt for Jyoti. The spectacle of Makshi, slowly licking an errant drip of yogurt from her two deep brown fingers, caused Jyoti to moan with desire.

"Please join me," Jyoti coaxed. "Surely, you must be hungry and tired."

Makshi filled a small bowl for herself and knelt near his pallet. The attraction was mutual. Their hungry eyes loitered without guard. Jyoti's huge *lingam* made a long rigid curve beneath his *dhoti*. Every time she glanced at it, her nipples carved sharp points into the bright orange silk of her wrap.

Finally, she held his cheeks in the tiny mauve bowl of her hands and asked if he needed anything.

Jyoti slid his *dhoti* aside and whispered, "You know exactly what I need," and then slid his clenched fist from the tip to the root of his long thick member. Jyoti was pulsing, as Makshi took her last bite . . . and so was I. With her gaze locked into his, she calmly slid his cloth aside and spiralled the beaded crown of his burgundy shaft, with his first pearl of lust. When it began to dry, she resorted to a slow storm of her own wet kisses, sweetened with a dab of honey from a bowl nearby. Emboldened now, Jyoti slid his fingers deep into her folds, and discovered feverish warmth and silky wetness. The sound of their breathing filled the room as he stirred her bowl, exploring her depths.

"My grandmother told me to gather several herbs to make a poultice for your leg. I'll be back just after sunrise."

"Everything about you promises pleasure. Your scent is intoxicating," he said with a smile, weaving his fingers through her tiny triangle of black silk. "Can we take up where we left off when you return, Makshi?"

"We'll see how empty the house is when I return from the fields," she sighed, reluctantly pushing herself from the heavenly combination of his touch and tongue.

Jyoti casually reminded Aunt Tejal and Aruna that it was market day. The market was an hour away. Perfect!

Jyoti urged me to join them. I claimed fatigue. My staff was still locked in a knot of anticipation and I was determined to stay . . . and watch.

Upon returning, Makshi gave Jyoti two *dhat* seeds to relax, and then warmed water for his bath. I watched, from the cool shaded hallway, like a starving hawk searching for prey. Anticipating their lust-filled celebration, I bound the root of my *lingam* with a taut collar of carefully knotted satin cord. I was not disappointed.

Jyoti reclined like royalty as Makshi bathed and oiled him. Afterwards, she bathed herself for him, in an amber wedge of dust-stippled light near a window. The water and light adorned her smooth brown skin with radiant garlands of sky blue and gold. After oiling herself, she spread her thighs and nimbly parted the soft hair of her velvety lips, still swollen from his playful bites. Her bangles chimed as she circled her glistening clitoris. With every orbit, her tiny bright red bowl gulped to be filled. She dipped her fingertip in honey and strummed. Soon, she stroked his shaft with her honeyed hands. He sucked each finger clean. On her elbows and knees, rhythmically sucking him to marble hardness, she backed her honeyed treat into his mouth. She gracefully eased onto her back and realigned her clitoris with his talented tongue. As Makshi leisurely climbed to pleasure, Jyoti again sawed into her luscious sex with his giant fingers . . . first one, then two . . . until a cone of three. She lowered herself on him, kissing him deeply. Like a bee, she hovered, vibrating and circulating her hips. Turning slowly and sensuously, she descended repeatedly for filling. When he felt her twitch and tighten, he pummelled her clitoris with his fluttering fingertips. She shuddered with release and Jyoti followed soon. He lightened his touch to extend her shaft-clenching waves of pleasure.

I stealthily retreated to my room. In my haste, I tripped over my aunt's rosewood step stool. Makshi came running to see what had happened. I pretended that I had just awakened and was slightly disoriented.

"Are you OK?" she asked with genuine concern.

"I'm just extremely tired from my journey. I'm going out to relieve myself and then I'm going back to sleep."

"Would you like a cup of sweet blue lotus tea, to relax you?"

I wanted much more but just said, "Yes. Thank you."

It was clear that my cousin Jyoti would be the one to forever enjoy Makshi's skills and beauty. But, I would forever enjoy my stolen memory of their passion.

After attending Jyoti, Makshi brought my tea.

"Would you be kind enough to tie my eyes shut with this?" I asked, holding out the long silk tie to my robe. "The sun is so bright, I'm having trouble sleeping."

I could have easily tied it myself but, before pleasing myself, I wanted to enjoy one last flash of her dark beauty and feel her tender touch, but most of all, to gather her just-taken scent.

How profoundly and rapidly I climbed towards release! I wallowed in the erotic memory of them, as I slowly undid all but the last two knots enslaving my shaft. My first strokes were slow and slippery but my last ones were fast and wild – almost violent. Finally, I erupted powerfully with extraordinary pleasure. Once I regained my strength, I wrote "Black Bumble Bee". It will make the *Kama Sutra* even sweeter.

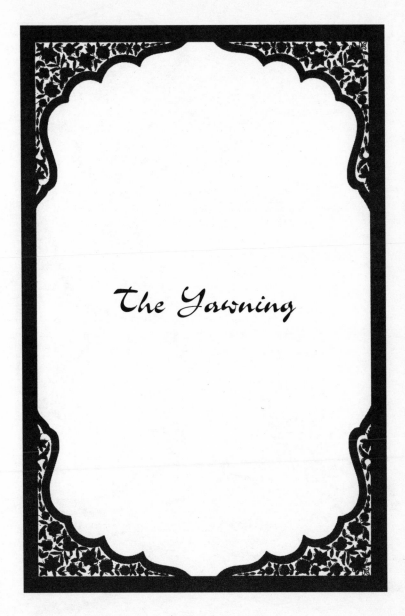

The Yawning

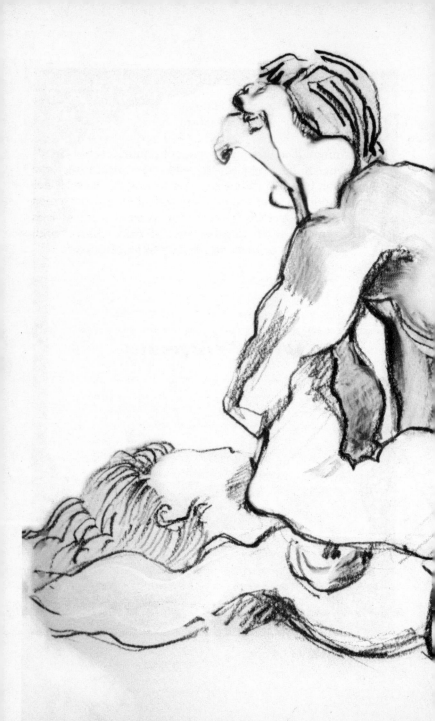

The Yawning

Jrimbhitaka
Kama Sutra

"The yawning" is a loving position, appropriate to the Gand-harva type of marriage (a love marriage) which sees the woman on her back with either her feet or the backs of her knees on her lover's shoulders, with the lower legs then draped over his back. In this position her pelvis is nicely tilted to allow ease of access and enough friction for both partners to reach orgasm.

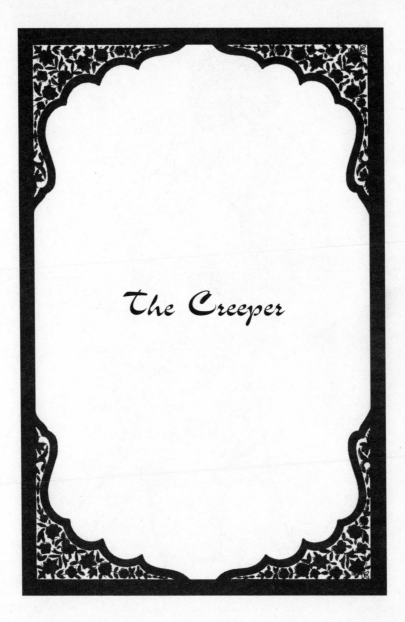

The Creeper

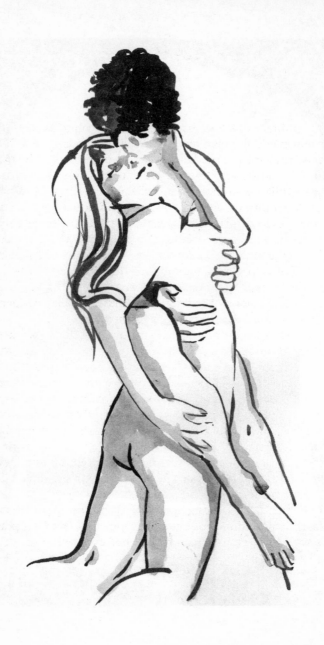

The Creeper

Javaveshtitaka
Kama Sutra

In this embrace that happens before sexual congress takes place, the woman and the man cling together, she gazing up at him as if she were a vine growing up the length of his body. She tries to bend his head down to her in order to kiss him. It is a loving embrace full of adoration from the woman to the man. When he stares down into the eyes of his lover and notices her beautiful shining eyes looking up with great love and affection into his, he is overcome with desire. She begins to wrap herself, in the first of the loving embraces, around him like a vine, like a plant or trailing flower that wraps around the thing it covets. She starts at his ankles, tracing small circles of pleasure on the inside of his foot; he gasps aloud. Looking up at him like this, she parades her beauty and leaves nothing to chance.

Looking down on her, he sees the swell of her heavy breasts spilling out of her sari, and he sees the young, firm leg that is slowly wrapping around his like a trailing creeper, the firm female flesh of his lover combining with his in a pleasure concoction born directly from Kama himself. She groans, breathes quickly against him, pushing her bosom against his so he feels the slight prick of her nipples as they brush and harden against him. She reaches up lithe, doelike, with per-fumed arms to slide around his neck, caressing and causing sensations in his private parts below, a stirring she can no doubt feel as she further wraps herself, like a vine, like everything that is trailing and constricting and natural (like an aphrodisiac tree from which cunning potions are made). She smiles up at his eyes with love, yes, she can feel it, her eyes tell him.

The Tale of the Creeper

as told by Nan Andrews

Her limbs, entwined in yours
like tendrils of fragrant jasmine creeper,
draw taut and slowly relax
in the gentle rhythm of *lingam* and *yoni*;
this is *"Lataveshta"* (The Clinging Creeper)

Long ago, in a far-off time, Rajiv Kumar yearned to take a wife. Sent by his parents to live in the house of his uncle, he soon saw a local girl drawing water at the village well.

"Uncle, who is that vision?" Rajiv set down the jars of oil he was bringing to the market and stared at the dark-haired beauty in the deep yellow sari.

Vikram laughed and clapped him on the back. "That, my nephew, is Arundhati. She is the daughter of the baker."

From that day, Rajiv only had eyes for Arundhati. He volunteered to do any errand that might take him into the village and especially to the bakery.

One day, he met her walking to the river with her wash basket. "May I escort you?" he asked.

"It is no concern of mine if you wish to walk this road, but I have work to attend to and can't delay."

"Oh, I don't wish to take you away from your duties." Rajiv bent to pick a flower growing at the side of the path. "But let me bide the time with you." He offered the flower and she took it, ducking her head so that he only caught a glimpse of the smile on her deep red lips. Such delicious lips. He intended to taste their sweetness before the season was through.

"Nephew," his uncle called out to the field one evening, "come and walk with me." The men followed the path to the river and walked along the bank. Rajiv could see a goat herd on the far bank urging his flock up from the wet stones at the river's edge.

"Rajiv, I have had word from your father. He intends for you to marry soon and return home to assist him."

"Uncle," Rajiv turned to ask, "I have been meaning to speak to you about this very subject."

"Have you?" Vikram chuckled. "I have seen you looking at our fair maids in the village. Would it be Shruti who draws your eye?" Shruti was the oldest unmarried woman in the village. She walked with a limp and Rajiv often saw her out gathering firewood at the edge of the forest.

"No, uncle." Rajiv shuddered. Shruti was the least attractive maiden in the village.

"Ah, then it must be Ritika who lightens your heart." Ritika was a simple girl, daughter of a farmer. She was so shy that most villagers had never heard her speak.

"Oh, uncle, please," Rajiv sighed. "I want to talk to you about Arundhati. She is the one I want."

"The baker's daughter? Will you take stale bread and flour as your dowry?"

Rajiv was stricken. In matters of marriage, the dowry was an important consideration, but his heart and loins were stirred by this girl and he must have her. "Please, uncle, will you speak to her father for me?" He knew he sounded desperate, but he couldn't help himself.

Vikram laughed. "Yes, Rajiv, I will speak to the baker. I'm sure he has a goat or two hidden somewhere for the girl's dowry."

Rajiv and Arundhati were married as soon as the families agreed and the signs were auspicious. When they were alone in his room at his uncle's house, Rajiv lifted her veil and traced the outline of her delicate lips. They were the colour of ripe mango and glistened in the sunshine like sweet morsels of cut fruit. He bent and smelled her fresh scent: warm spring air, freshly baked bread and the heady smell of a maiden. As he touched his lips to hers, he thought he would melt away, she was so sweet.

They lay under the draperies of the marriage bed and he caressed her dusky limbs, uncovering more and more skin as he covered her with kisses.

"I have waited for this pleasure for a long time, my love."

Arundhati smiled at him shyly and returned his kisses with her own new-made passion. Together, they explored the simple pleasure of their first congress.

The next day, he carried her home to his parents' house in a cart, drawn by an ox given to him by his uncle. The cart was filled with household goods provided by the baker and his wife. A single goat was tethered to the back.

Rajiv's parents welcomed the couple into their household for a season and then Rajiv was given a land holding of his father's to farm. There was a tiny house for them to live in. Rajiv moved their things in as soon as the rains allowed and they began their new life together. At first, Rajiv had some success. The land was fertile, the water was strong and clean. The animals flourished and the grain grew tall and golden.

Every night, Rajiv returned home to Arundhati and his own hearth. She met him with a fine meal, a warm smile and the sweetness of her kisses. They were very happy.

But then, all across the land, came a drought. As the summer grew hotter and everything grew drier, Rajiv became increasingly worried about their future. Their crops failed and the stream from which they drew their water was reduced to a muddy trickle. Some of the animals wandered away, in search of better pastures. Others were taken by fierce creatures in the night, desperate for food themselves. The roars of the tigers came from the forest each night as Rajiv barred the door.

After many sleepless nights, Rajiv drew his wife close and kissed her. He told her that he would go in search of a solution to their problem. "I can wait here no longer. There must be some help for us in the wider world."

"But, husband, where will you go?"

"I will go where the Goddess leads me. I'm sure there is an answer to our prayers out there waiting."

Arundhati packed him a small skin of water and some fried breads. Before he left, she cut a long strand of her hair and wove it around his right wrist.

"Let this token of my love keep you safe and remind you of home."

Rajiv kissed her deeply in the early morning light and left, only looking back once to where she stood at the doorway, watching him.

He walked for many days, over high, dry hills and into deep valleys, but everywhere there was only dust and rocks and mud. There was nothing green and no water anywhere.

After many days of walking in the hot sun, Rajiv grew weaker and weaker. He started to think he might die without finding an answer to his prayers. Until one morning, as he was stumbling down a dry river bed, he rounded a bend in the canyon and saw something miraculous. It was a tree of mythic proportion, green and fragrant. Its highest branches reached the top of the canyon walls and beyond. Beneath its delightful shade burbled a tiny spring. And best of all, it bore the most amazing fruit. Shades of rose and pink, as delicate as his wife's *yoni*, the fruit clung to the branches. He hungered for it desperately, but it hung out of his reach.

As spent as he was, he dragged small boulders and smaller rocks together under the edge of the tree in order to climb up and reach the fruit. Trembling and nearly falling, he climbed and reached as far as he could and felt the soft, ripe fruit just at the tip of his fingers. As he was about to pluck it, he was suddenly entwined and held fast with vines. Flowing with the speed of water, they grew out of the tree and clung to his arms, his torso, his legs. He could feel the tendrils between his legs, slipping into his clothes and gripping the root of his *lingam*. He could not move.

A voice thundered in his ears. "How dare you touch my fruit? Despoiler!"

"Please," Rajiv begged, "I am hungry and near death. I hoped to taste the delicate sweetness before I died. If only I could bring it back to my beloved wife, it would save us both. Please help us."

As he was held in the embrace of the vines, huge thorns began to grow around him, imprisoning him. One pierced his side cruelly. Several more encased his manhood, making him quiver in fear. When next the voice spoke, it was the vengeful voice of the Goddess Parvati.

"So, your beloved wife is all that you can think of? You would plead for her before me?" She stood with hands on hips and glared up at him. "If you wish to live, send for your wife. Let her come and pluck you from my grasp. Let her demonstrate this great love. If she loves you enough to do that, she shall rescue you and I will provide for you. But if she does not come, or if she should fail, you will die a terrible death upon my thorns."

With these words, the Goddess broke off a huge thorn against his chest, tearing his flesh and causing his blood to spring from the wound. Pressing a leaf of the tree against the tear, she wiped off some of his blood and threaded the leaf onto the thorn. Another such leaf she pressed into the wound to stop its terrible flow.

Calling a small monkey to her side, Parvati handed it the totem: the thorn-pierced leaf, red with his blood. "Take this to his wife, Arundhati, and beg she come to his aid."

With that, the monkey dashed away.

For many days, Rajiv hung in the tree's embrace and listened to the voice of the Goddess Parvati. She spoke to him of love lost and desire inflamed. She taunted him and praised him until his head spun with her fierce scent.

"You are a handsome man. Is your wife as beautiful as I?" Parvati asked as she walked around the base of her tree. "I have had many lovers but none have been worthy of my love in return."

Rajiv looked down at the Goddess. She had shining black hair that hung like silk to her feet. Her hips moved with the rhythm of the tiger; her breasts swayed and bounced with each step. She reached up, lowering her blouse and cupping her breasts up towards Rajiv. "Are her breasts as fine as mine?" She caressed the nipples with her fingertips. "Would you like to taste them? To compare their sweetness? I'm sure they are finer than hers."

Rajiv struggled in the vines that held him tight. He loved his wife and thought she was very beautiful. But the Goddess was more beautiful than any woman he'd ever seen. She was also more powerful. Who was he to reject her?

The Goddess spread a blanket on the ground beneath the tree. Lying back, she spread her legs and drew back her sari. Rajiv could see the black curls covering her *yoni*. She reached between her legs and stroked her thighs. They were golden and delicate. He imagined the softness of them. He closed his eyes and the vision of his wife reclining on their marriage bed filled his mind. He remembered Arundhati's sweet lips and the slick heat of her as he entered her. Rajiv turned his face away from the Goddess.

The next morning, Rajiv woke within the cradle of his vines to see the Goddess sitting on a branch of the tree within an arm's reach of him. That day, she was dressed in a blue and silver sari that glinted in the rising sun like the wide ocean itself.

"You are a fine man, Rajiv. You would be an excellent consort for me." She touched his arm lightly with the tips of her fingers. A fire spread through him. Rajiv sucked in his breath and held it. He could smell her delicate scent: a combination of flowers and the earth, womanly and rich.

"Tall and dark, with intelligent eyes. I can see that you are a man of wisdom."

"I am but a humble farmer, Goddess." He did not know how to respond to her compliments although the closeness of her body was causing him to feel the growing heat of the day. Sweat dripped down the back of his neck and ran along his spine. He could feel the drops as they fell from the fringe of his hair.

She laughed, leaning close and kissing his brow. The kiss sent a lightning bolt of desire through his body, making his *lingam* stiffen. He feared that he would be pierced by the thorns and so he struggled, but the vines held him fast.

"I have given a vow of marriage to my Arundhati, Goddess. I must keep it."

"Ah, a good man who honours his word." She leaned away, a look of disappointment on her face. His heart fell. He felt terrible about turning her away.

"Perhaps . . ." The word was just a whisper.

The Goddess turned back. "Perhaps? Perhaps what, Rajiv? Would you throw your honour to the ground, to be broken into dust at a mere kiss from me?" Her laugh was taunting now. "Perhaps you are not the man I imagined, not worthy of my attention."

A flash of light blinded Rajiv and when he blinked it away, she was gone. He sighed and hung from his prison, his body wilted and his terrible thirst returning to punish him.

As the heat of the day seemed to melt his body even further, Rajiv remembered the taste of his wife's flesh, the sweet nectar of her womanhood as he plundered it with his tongue and fingers. She would lie beneath his mouth, her legs across his shoulders as he drank her passions.

Just as these thoughts were coursing through his blood like molten lead, the Goddess reappeared. Once again, she sat across from him in the tree, only this time she was higher, her knees at the height of his head. He strained to look up into her face, to see if she was full of wrath or amusement.

"Are you thirsty, Rajiv?" She parted her sari and spread her thighs. Rajiv could see the rose petals of her *yoni* glistening in the afternoon light. "Would you care to drink of my nectar?" The Goddess gently spread herself so that more and more of her delicate centre was revealed.

Rajiv's parched mouth began to feel the barest hint of moisture. He licked his parched lips and imagined how she might taste, of honey and rich fruit. He could barely swallow, but he could only think of the taste of her. He leaned as far towards her as the thorns would allow, mouth open and eyes begging. He reached out a hand to draw her near and just as he was about to touch her, he caught sight of the woven strands of hair around his wrist.

At the reminder of his wife, Rajiv jerked back, stung. He had nearly forgotten her in his thirst for a taste of the Goddess. No, he could not betray her love in such a way.

Parvati watched him, aware of his struggle. She must have been able to read his thoughts, for she covered herself and turned away, making a disparaging sound.

Rajiv watched the sun setting through the leaves of the enormous tree. He was not sure how much longer he could last, but it wasn't clear whether he would succumb to his thirst or to the tests of the Goddess. One way or another, he prayed that Arundhati would come soon and release him.

Meanwhile, the monkey brought the talisman to Arundhati and made signs for her to come. The shock of seeing something green after so long nearly made her swoon, but the sight of her husband's blood, for she knew with certainty this was truly his, filled her with fear and longing. She took the thorn, pricking her palm and mingling her blood with his.

Bowing to the altar in their home, she said a prayer to the Goddess and then went out. Following the monkey, she made her way to the sacred tree. There she found Rajiv entrapped in the vines.

"Dearest Arundhati," he called at the sight of her, tears coursing down his face, "we may only be reunited by the strength of your body and your love of me." He paused as they heard the Goddess laughing. Perhaps she scorned him for denying her and was hoping that they would fail. "You must climb up amongst the vines and the dreadful thorns and embrace me. Only then can you pluck me from the grasp of this tree," Rajiv called. "It will be dangerous and dire, but it is the only way."

Arundhati stared at him for the longest time without speaking and then wound her sari tightly around her body, as some safeguard against the thorns. Climbing amongst the vines, she was scratched and pierced, her blood running down her arms and legs. But still she continued. Rajiv feared for her life in the embrace of the thorns. He realized that she was more important to him than anything.

"Take care, sweet love. I would rather die than see you harmed to save me."

"I'm coming, husband. Be patient."

Eventually, she climbed until she was next to him within the embrace of the vines. Her delicate scent was as dear to him as life and with her near, he was roused from his terror. His member rose to meet her, ringed with its crown of thorns. He opened his arms to her. She seemed to know then what she must do. She reached out with one delicate hand and touched his hardness. He shuddered at the rush of sweet sensation, one he had not felt in so long. His desire for her grew.

Careful of the thorns, she grasped the head of his *lingam* as if cupping a flower and lightly scratched him with her nails. Rajiv groaned and yearned to feel her surrounding him, but he was held fast by the vines.

Wrapping her arms around his neck and twining her legs around his waist, Arundhati slipped herself against him, in between the vines, until her *yoni* opened, pink and moist, at the tip of his *lingam*.

"Fill me, dear husband, and share the fruit of this tree."

"But you will be pierced by the thorns. They will tear your delicate parts to bits."

"It must be done, Husband, to save us both."

With that, he took her at her word and pushed himself into her. Arundhati cried out as the thorns between them drew blood but just as suddenly, they withered away and were gone. Rajiv found himself standing under the beautiful tree, his wife clinging to him as he filled her with his staff. Her arms and legs twined around him, replacing the vines which had held him captive. Fruit began to fall upon them as he moved gently inside her and soon she threw back her head and called out her pleasure. They were saved.

The Goddess' quiet laughter was heard receding up the valley as the fruit rained down upon them.

Rajiv and Arundhati finally broke from their embrace and gathered up as much fruit as they could carry. When they returned home, many days later, they found the stream rushing with new water and their land beginning to turn green. They planted many seeds of the delicate fruit and when the leaves were green and the scent of ripeness hung in the air, Rajiv took his wife in his arms and kissed her.

"You saved us, my love." He caressed her hair and cheek. "Without you, I would have been lost."

"Our love saved us, husband." Arundhati leaned her head against his chest, careful of the scars he carried from the thorns. They would be with him for the rest of his days as a reminder.

The following summer, their fortunes continued to be strong. The drought ended and the fields returned to their previous richness. Each night, the breeze brought the scent of ripening grain and damp earth, for which Rajiv was eternally grateful.

At the height of the summer, he brought Arundhati out under the leafy branches of their trees, the offspring of the great tree which had imprisoned him. He lay a blanket upon the ground and drew her down to lie with him.

"My love, we should remember all that the Goddess has given us." He kissed her and cupped the curve of her breast in his warm palm. "She tested both of us and our love saved us, as you've said."

Arundhati smiled. Rajiv had told her, during the long winter nights, of the tests placed on him by the Goddess. Her skin still bore the marks of the thorns which she had braved to pluck him from the Goddess' grasp.

She leaned her head down and bit his chest lightly to remind him of being pierced. Rajiv groaned in her arms, with pleasure this time, rather than pain. He bent her across his lap and set his teeth into her back and shoulders, along the path of the thorns.

Arundhati moved alongside him and twined her arms and legs in his, rubbing her mound against his hardness. She moved until she was once again positioned above his *lingam*. He entered her in one swift movement and, for a brief second, felt the thorns which had pierced them both on that day long ago. But the pain was never there. They held each other tightly and then began to draw taut and relax in the gentle rhythm of the vines, of *lingam* and *yoni*, of the Gentle Creeper.

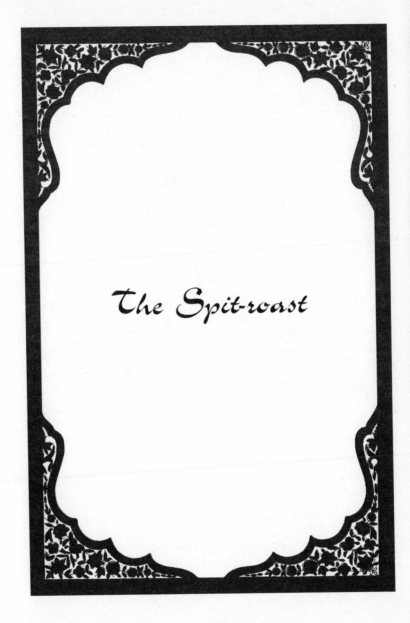

The Spit-roast

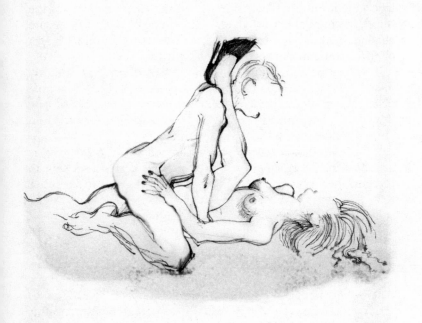

The Spit-roast

Shulachita
Kama Sutra

The *Kama Sutra* is all about practice and study. These are the things to be done and pursued in order to raise sex to a higher level, the level of civilized humanity, the exact opposite of the blind, instinctual mating of animals. Some of the positions are challenging but part of the pleasure of sex is in the achievement of these sometimes pretzel-like couplings.

This is a position that requires great flexibility. It is highly pleasurable but means that the girl has to be incredibly supple because her legs are stretched out in completely opposite directions. Performing the love act with her foot placed on your forehead, balanced there, while her leg is stretched out along the floor, completely straight beneath the two of you, is quite a feat. While you go about enjoying her and seeking to pleasure her with your thrusts, she must attempt to keep her foot to your forehead in an unbreaking connection. Some translators call this position "the spit-roast": who is the spit and who is the roast? Other translators have named it, appropriately, "impaled on a stake" or "fixing a nail": the man thrusting into his beloved in this position must resemble this.

As an additional variation, the girl can alternate her legs, placing the other foot on his forehead and changing as often as she likes. The couple will eventually get into a rhythm and this position will become familiar and easy. The connection between the foot and the forehead is important. The sense of touch is always present in the positions as well as in the embraces, kisses and scratches.

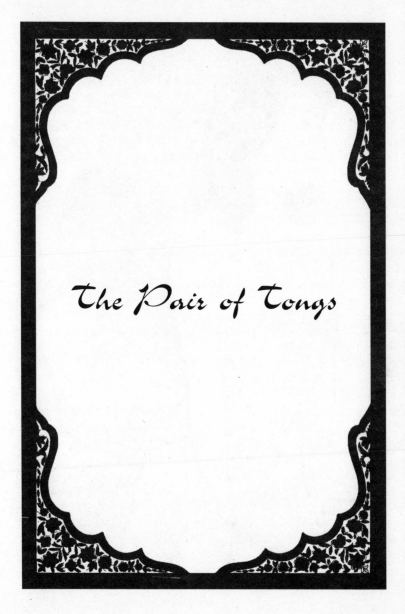

The Pair of Tongs

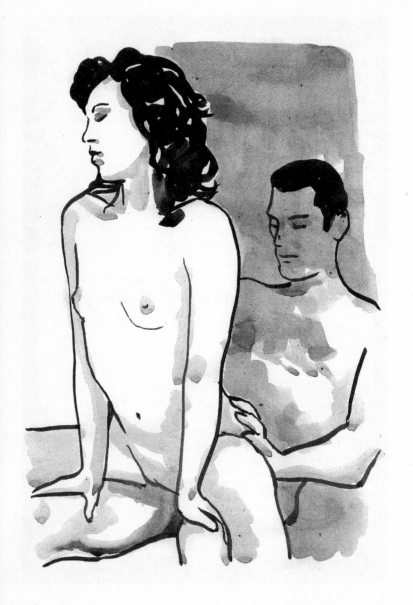

The Pair of Tongs

Samdamsha
Kama Sutra

The mare's trick is achieved when a woman contracts the muscles in her vagina, providing a tighter sensation to the man inside her as he becomes gripped by her muscles. She practises this trick by contracting and relaxing the muscles which form part of her pelvic floor. The "tongs" or the "pair of tongs" is basically a woman-on-top position where the woman uses the mare's trick while in a dominating position astride the man, but for a prolonged, designated period of time. Here, she holds her lover's *lingam* inside her in the grip of her vaginal muscles for 100 heartbeats. There is a dominating aspect to this position. Not only is the man being held tightly by the woman's *yoni*, but she is in a delicate position on top of him, staring down at him, totally in control as she grips him.

as told by Anna Black

The old woman's light brown face was seamed with lines and the whites of her eyes were the colour of rust. Her hair, though long and thick, was as grey as ashes. But she sat with a straight back and her red and gold sari hugged her slim figure.

"But why do they call it the "Pair of Tongs"? It's such an odd name."

The old woman looked over at the young woman who had asked the question, one of among many young and beautiful women in the King's harem.

"Yes," the old woman agreed. "It is an odd name for that position."

She pointed to where two of the harem women were, under her direction, demonstrating it. One woman lay on her back on the floor, silken pillows heaped under her head. She was trying not to giggle. The other woman straddled her, her slim thighs on either side of the supine woman's hips. She was also trying not to laugh.

The old woman shook her head at her charges' refusal to take her lessons seriously. But they were young. As she had once been young.

"Notice," she went on, "how her legs lie on either side of her partner. Do they not remind you of a pair of tongs?"

The young women shook their heads, their collective puzzlement evident on their dark pretty faces.

The old woman sighed. "Well, would you like to hear the story as to how the position came to be called that?"

The women nodded eagerly. They loved stories. The old woman gestured for the two young women who had been demonstrating the position to rise and join them. Which they did, squeezing in among the others who had gathered around the old woman.

"The story begins as most stories do," the old woman began, "with a journey. Long ago a young maiden was taken from her village to the capital city of the kingdom where she became the newest and youngest member of the King's harem."

Fulmala pinched Chandi's arm. "Blacksmith's daughter. Tell us how the people in your village make love." A sly smile twisted Fulmala's face. "I would imagine they all rut like beasts in the field. With all the delicacy and refinement of a bull in heat."

Anger, along with humiliation, surged through Chandi. As she looked into Fulmala's large dark eyes, she wanted nothing more than to scratch them out.

Fulmala tried to pinch her again.

Chandi pushed her hand away. "My father may have been a blacksmith. But at least he wasn't a criminal."

The other women in the harem gasped although it was certainly no secret that Fulmala's father was awaiting trial. A minor official in the King's administration, he had been accused of fraud regarding the conducting of censuses for tax purposes. It was whispered among the women – out of Fulmala's hearing, of course – that his disgrace even threatened Fulmala's current position in the harem as the King's favourite.

Fulmala's face hardened. She leaned over and slapped Chandi across the face.

Everyone gasped again, although most of the women also smiled, pleased with anything that would divert them from their boredom.

"You are nothing, blacksmith's daughter," Fulmala sneered. "And you will be nothing. The King will never take you to his bed. He would not sully himself with such a one as you."

Chandi's face stung from the slap and the desire to fling herself at Fulmala was like a drumbeat in her blood. But fighting among the women in the harem was severely punished. And, despite her determination not to let Fulmala get under her skin, anxiety now rose within her.

What if Fulmala was right? All of the women in the harem were not only beautiful but more experienced sexually. How could Chandi hope to compete with them for the King's attention? All she had to set her apart was her newness to the harem. But even if she were called to his bed, would she be able to please him?

Fulmala thrust her face close to Chandi, drawing her out of her anxious thoughts.

"It was a waste of time bringing you to the palace. I am the King's favourite. I have been for nearly a year. Longer than anyone. You will never take my place with him. I will see to that."

"For nearly a year?" Chandi repeated. "That is a long time for a man to plough the same furrow. Perhaps he will relish a change."

A flash of doubt flared in Fulmala's dark eyes. Then it disappeared and was replaced by her usual scorn. "You will see, blacksmith's daughter. When the King returns from the south. Then you will see."

Chandi was tempted to repeat the slander about Fulmala's father but before she could do so Ishat entered the harem. Ishat was the guardian of the harem. At his entrance all the women turned their attention away from Chandi and Fulmala and focused on the bald, elderly eunuch.

Ishat walked slowly into the harem, leaning heavily on his staff. He stopped in the centre of the room. The women all clustered around him.

"I have news," he announced. "The King has returned. His campaign in the south was a success."

The women all started talking at once. Ishat waved for silence. "He plans to go hunting this afternoon. Then he will host a feast this evening to celebrate his victory. After that there will be entertainment. But, yes, he has requested a bed companion for the night."

Excitement raced through Chandi. But it was quickly replaced by dismay. There was no chance she would be chosen. And then how many days and nights would she languish here, with nothing to occupy her but eating and bathing and sleeping?

But, she also knew, that if she did nothing to further her chances, no one would do it for her. She pushed her way through the women gathered about Ishat. All of them were still chattering excitedly but Fulmala only stood apart, a smug smile on her face.

Ishat looked down at Chandi as she moved in front of him. A frown furrowed his high forehead. "Chandi. That is your name, correct?"

Chandi nodded. Out of the corner of her eye she saw Fulmala give her a dark look. The rest of the women grew silent.

"You were brought to the harem while the King was away in the south?"

"Yes," Chandi replied.

Ishat studied her, his frown deepening, his yellow-rimmed eyes assessing.

For a moment, a flare of hope flickered in Chandi's heart. It died, however, when Ishat firmly shook his head.

"You are not experienced enough," he finally said. "The King will be tired after his long day. He will not want to waste time instructing someone on how to pleasure him."

Ishat turned and looked over at Fulmala. "You will go."

Triumph blazed in Fulmala's face. She glanced around at the other women, her head high.

There was nothing Chandi could do but watch as the slaves scurried to do Fulmala's hair and make-up and dress her in her finest sari and jewels. And, when Ishat returned later that night in order to escort Fulmala to the King's bedchamber, Chandi could also only stand and watch, along with the other women, wishing that it was she who was being taken to the King's bed.

Now that all the excitement was over the women soon found other things to occupy them. But Chandi could not bring herself to join them in their gossip or amuse herself with her pet parrot or take part in the games they were playing.

She could only sit and wonder how long it would be before she was escorted to the King's bedchamber. Weeks? Months? Years? Would she be able to stand it? Could she live out the rest of life without the pleasure of being with a man?

Chandi was not a virgin but her only experience sexually had been a hurried penetration in the back of her father's smithy with a young man of her village. He had entered her body, taken her virginity, and then, after a few hurried thrusts, spent himself inside her.

It had been disappointing to say the least.

Chandi had listened to the gossip of the women of the harem during her short time here and, although she had yet to see the King, they all described him as tall, handsome and virile.

She walked past a group of women who were playing chess. She watched them for a moment, trying to grasp the strategy of their play. Just as she was starting to understand it, a commotion at the entrance to the harem drew away her attention.

Ishat came in, Fulmala trailing behind him. Her face was a dark cloud of anger and humiliation. Before anyone could say a word, Ishat looked over to where Chandi was standing.

He pointed. "You. Come here."

Chandi turned around, assuming Ishat was speaking to someone else.

"You, Chandi," the old man screeched. "Come here. Quickly."

Chandi hurried over, conscious that Fulmala was staring at her with bitter, tear-filled eyes.

Ishat quickly looked her up and down. "You'll have to do as you are. We don't have time. Come."

"Come? But where?" Chandi asked.

"To his bedchamber, of course."

"His bedchamber? You mean, the King's?"

"Yes, of course," Ishat snapped. "Who else would I be speaking of? What are you? An idiot?"

"But . . . shouldn't I . . .?" Chandi began.

Ishat shook his head and hustled her out of the harem. "No time. He's already infuriated. We don't want to anger him further by making him wait."

Ishat walked swiftly down the corridor that led to the section of the palace where the King's bedchamber was located. Normally the old eunuch walked at the pace of a tortoise, leaning wearily on his staff, complaining persistently of his various infirmities.

Now, however, he moved with the vigour of a much younger man, his legs moving swiftly, his staff banging against the floor.

Chandi struggled to keep up with him, her anklets ringing with every step. "What is he angry about?"

"That is no concern of yours."

"But shouldn't I know? So that I don't anger him too?"

Ishat gave her a shrewd look as they hurried along the passageway. "Perhaps you aren't such an idiot after all. It was Fulmala."

"Fulmala? But isn't she his favourite?"

"Was his favourite."

"What happened?"

"Fulmala's father. He was found guilty today. He is utterly disgraced. As a result, the King wants nothing further to do with him or his daughter."

"But why did you choose me?"

Ishat shrugged. "Before he left for the south, other than Fulmala, the King had not requested any of the women in the harem for months. She seemed to have a gift for pleasing him." He shrugged again. "I had no idea who to pick. At least you're new and therefore a novelty. In his current mood you seemed as good a choice as any."

But was she as good a choice as any? Chandi wondered. That eager but clumsy boy from the village was the only man she had ever been with. She knew nothing about how to please a man. Especially someone like the King. What if she was also sent back in disgrace?

They soon arrived at the King's bedchamber. Ishat looked over at Chandi and brusquely gestured towards the hangings that covered the entrance.

"Well, go on in."

Chandi's eyes widened. "You want me to go in alone?"

"Of course. The King does not wish to see me. I angered him by bringing him Fulmala."

Chandi hesitated. She was afraid for she had also heard about the King's legendary temper.

"Hurry," Ishat whispered fiercely." And you'd better please him or . . ." And he left the rest of his sentence to hang ominously.

Chandi's throat tightened. She had no idea what sort of punishment Ishat was threatening her with if she failed to please the King but she had no desire to find out. She parted the hangings to the bedchamber and stepped inside. Ishat quickly closed them behind her, the swishing noise causing her to jump.

As Chandi moved further into the room she saw that it was very large and ornately furnished. Huge windows, framed by silken hangings, looked out over the gardens, pools and fountains. Weapons hung on the walls: spears, swords and ornately designed daggers. Near the centre of the room was a large bed surmounted by a richly decorated canopy.

On it lay the King.

He was staring at her, silently watching as she moved slowly towards the bed. He was partially clothed. His wide chest was bare, smooth and thickly muscled. His shoulders were broad and his dark hair, which was loosened from its customary style, flowed over them.

Her heart beating fast, Chandi stopped at the foot of the bed.

"What is your name?"

"Chandi, Your Majesty."

"I have never seen you before. Are you the girl from the village?"

"Yes, Your Majesty."

"Are you a virgin?"

Chandi licked her lips. "No, Your Majesty. I am not a virgin."

One of his dark brows arched sharply. "Who was it?"

"A boy. From my village. We . . . thought we were going to be married."

The King sat up and, as he did, Chandi saw his penis. It was firmly erect. She quickly glanced away.

"How many times did he pleasure you?"

Chandi looked back at him. "Only once, Your Majesty."

She did not like where this conversation was going. Would he send her back to the harem as too inexperienced to please him? He had slept with hundreds of women. What could a blacksmith's daughter who'd only made love once give him except the novelty of her newness? She doubted that would be enough to please one such as he.

"Have any of the harem women pleasured you?"

Chandi gasped and her eyes widened. "What?"

The King laughed. "Judging by your reaction, they haven't." He waved his hand. "Come closer. Onto the bed."

Chandi climbed onto the bed, her anklets tinkling as she did so. She saw that he had been reading when she came in. He brushed aside the documents to make room for her.

Now that she was closer she saw that the women in the harem had not exaggerated. He was very handsome but there was something in his face that sent a chill down her spine. This was not a man to trifle with. She noted, however, that there were dark circles under his eyes. He looked as if he had not slept in days.

"What you have learned in the harem?" he asked.

"Learned, Your Majesty?"

Impatience hardened his expression "About how to please me."

Chandi looked down at her lap. "I have learned nothing, Your Majesty."

He reached over and touched her arm. His hand, which was large and calloused, slid over to her breasts. He moved his hand slowly across them.

"Your breasts are very big. But you are very small. I can see why you were taken from that dunghill of a village and brought to the palace."

The King continued to caress her. Her nipples hardened under his touch.

He lowered her onto the bed. Chandi trembled but she continued to look up into his eyes. He removed her clothing, revealing her naked body. His hard hands moved possessively over her soft curves.

"I went hunting today," he murmured." I killed a wild boar. The hunt was long. This day has been long."

He moved over her. His thick penis slid between her thighs. Chandi opened her legs wider. She felt the round tip of his penis edging between the lips of her sex. She lifted her hips to pull him inside. He moved deeper.

Chandi's breath caught in her throat. The King was now completely sheathed inside her. And it felt good. Very good.

But he did not move. His breath came long and slow, hot and moist against her ear. Chandi tried to lift her hips but he was so large and heavy. She was trapped beneath him.

Then the King finally moved. Once, twice, his penis poked inside her. But his movements were half-hearted. Then Chandi felt him growing soft within her.

"Is there something wrong, Your Majesty?"

"It has been a long day. And I am tired."

Oh, no, Chandi thought. He was going to send her back to the harem. She might not get another chance. He might even blame her for his inability to perform.

He pulled out of her. His penis was now flaccid. He rolled onto his back. She looked over at him. His head was turned away from her.

"Go back to the harem. And tell Ishat I am to be disturbed no more tonight. I will speak with him in the morning."

Tears stung Chandi's eyes. She had failed. What did she know of men and of pleasure? Her only experience with sex had been the feverish fumbling of a boy no older than she. He had taken her maidenhead and, soon after, had shuddered against her, his seed trickling down her thighs along with her virgin blood.

This could be her only chance. She had to do something.

The King had been hard when she came into his bedchamber. Therefore he had the desire. He was simply tired and unable to ride her. But what if she were to ride him? Then he would not have to move. Did the man always have to be on top? she wondered.

Chandi tried to recall if she had heard any of the women in the harem speak of such a thing. As far as she knew the man was always on top during sex. The few times she had chanced to see her father and mother having sex that was the position they had been in. Her father on top, his thick buttocks quivering as he drove himself into her mother's prone body.

She looked over at the King. He was staring at her, the expression on his face clearly that of puzzlement. She knew he was wondering why she had not yet obeyed him. Before he could speak, she slid over and moved her body on top of his.

"What are you doing?" he asked.

Chandi adjusted her hips so that her sex lay against his penis. She bent her legs at the knees, her thighs straddling his hips. The King put his hands on her hips as if he meant to push her off him.

Chandi quickly rubbed the soft, moist lips of her sex along his penis. She felt it hardening. The King slowly moved his hands onto her buttocks. He caressed their smooth roundness as Chandi continued to slither her soft, wet sex over him.

The King's penis was once again thick and hard. Chandi adjusted her hips and, slowly, eased him inside her, the tender lips of her sex parting to welcome him. The King moaned. Enjoying the feel of him inside her so deeply, Chandi tightened the muscles of her sex around his penis.

The King gripped her hips. "Do that again."

She did, but this time she rhythmically fluttered her sex about his penis.

The King groaned deep in his chest.

Encouraged by this Chandi began to move her hips and buttocks. She rocked against the King's body even as she continued to pulse her sex around his penis.

The King lay motionless beneath her. He looked up at her, his face tightening with his rising pleasure. He moved his hands around her slim waist and then up her body until he had both of her large breasts firmly in them. He squeezed them, his fingers tugging at her swollen nipples.

"Faster," he commanded.

Chandi moved her body faster, her breath coming quickly. Deep inside her sex she felt a fluttering like the wings of a butterfly. Then the fluttering grew into a steady beat like that of a crow. Then it was eagle's wings: harder, faster, stronger.

Chandi threw back her head and cried out as her body violently shuddered from the dark pleasure that melted her loins. The King squeezed her breasts as she climaxed but the pain only added to the ecstasy that swelled within her.

She cried out again, her voice high and sweet.

The King jerked hard beneath her, the muscles in his throat taut, and he let loose a sound that was both a sob and a shout. Chandi felt a slick moistness pooling down her thighs.

She slowed her movements. I've done it, she thought. She looked down at the King's face.

He was staring up at her. "What is it called?"

"What is what called, Your Majesty?"

A frown creased his forehead. "What you just did? This position."

Chandi had no idea what he was talking about.

"Surely it has a name. It is quite pleasurable."

Chandi looked down at their conjoined bodies. Her legs were straddled over his hips and an image of her father standing at his forge, his hand clasping a pair of tongs, appeared in her mind.

" 'The Pair of Tongs', your majesty," she replied. "That is what it is called."

"Indeed," he said.

He grasped her buttocks and rubbed them. She realized he was once again hard within her. She smiled and, adjusting her hips, pleasured him again.

"And did Chandi become the King's favourite?"

The old woman smiled at the woman who had asked the question. "She did. And the position that she called the 'Pair of Tongs' also became one of his favourites."

"So it is a good position to use," someone asked, "when the King is weary?"

The old woman nodded. "But not just when he is tired. The position also brings great pleasure to the woman. Although—"

and she raised a slender finger "—if a man is very large or very long it can also be painful for the penetration is deep."

Another woman leaned forward. "But the King was very large and very long. And Chandi felt no pain."

The old woman smiled and slowly nodded. "Yes, he was. Very large and very long." She quickly clapped her hands. "Now, back to the lesson."

She pointed to two of the girls and instructed them to once again assume the position for "The Pair of Tongs". As they did, she noted that the young woman who had enquired about the King's penis was looking intently at her.

"Is there something wrong?" the older woman asked.

"Has your name always been Narmada?"

The old woman stared at the young woman. "No, not always. Now, go and learn. For someday you may be called upon to pleasure the King."

The younger woman smiled and turned away.

Narmada, who once had been called Chandi and had been the favourite of the current King's grandfather, went over to where the two young women were once again giggling as they demonstrated "The Pair of Tongs" position.

"Remember," she began, "that when you are astride the King and his *lingam* is inside you, squeeze it repeatedly, fluttering your *yoni* about his *lingam* like the wings of a butterfly. Then, not only will he feel pleasure, but you also."

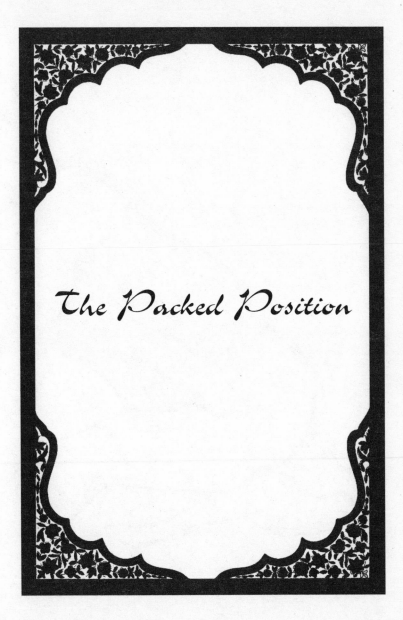

The Packed Position

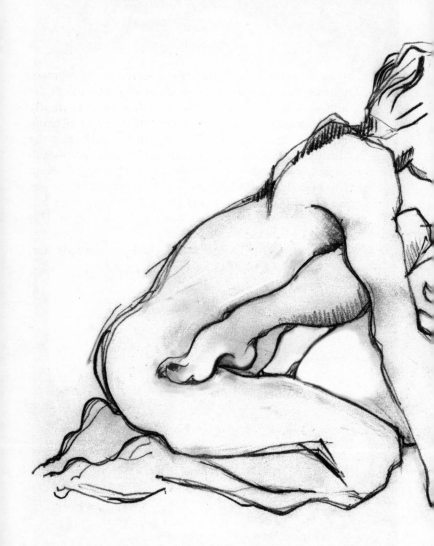

The Packed Position

Piditaka
Kama Sutra

This is a position for a hare man and a larger woman. When she raises her legs up, as if she wants to touch the ceiling with her toes, her *yoni* is on full display, tightly pressed between her closed, raised thighs, and peeking out at you. The woman, her hair flowing out behind her on the bed on which you've laid her, peers around her upraised legs to see your reaction. And then, when she crosses her legs, one on top of the other, still raised, that's when you penetrate her (some translators have named this position "tight") and her *yoni* grips your *lingam* as if in the cruel mare's grip. Use your hands to steady her crossed, uplifted legs. Pull them against your chest, now push them back towards her, restricting her vulva further.

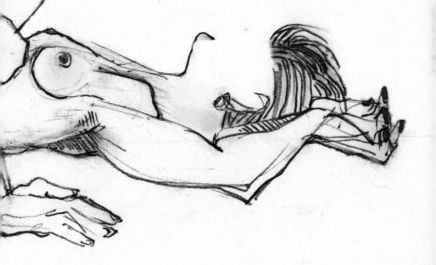

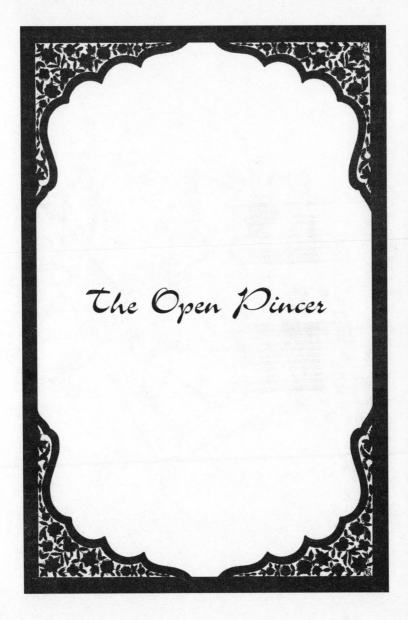

The Open Pincer

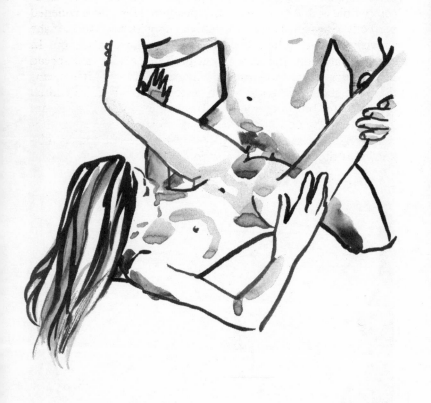

The Open Pincer

Vijrimbhitaka
Kama Sutra

With her thighs spread wide and her legs held in the air with determination and strength, even the small deer woman is compatible with larger men in this position. Her *yoni* is widened perfectly. She can also hold her thighs up with her hands, if she so wishes, offering herself up to her lover for penetration. In another variation, the man might grab her ankles and spread them wider of his own accord. The angle of her pelvis means that care should be taken when penetrating (no quick, initial thrusts here) but once congress has begun, the sensations are intense and the entrance is easy and effortless. In yet another variation, the man can enter her *yoni* from the side (this is then known as the "expanding" position).

The Tale of the Open Pincer

as told by Anya Wassenberg

In the velvet coolness of the evening in the mango grove, their eyes met for the first time; his from the tree branch above and hers, luminous and wide open from where she glistened in the water below . . .

There was a princess who lived with her father the King and seven sisters, along with their gardeners, housekeepers, attendants, cooks and guards in a lovely white palace with arched doorways and many rooms, and a wall that was as tall as two of the burliest guards that encircled the entire compound. Princess Priya had large, dark, almond-shaped eyes, and long hair as dark as the night sky, so lustrous that it shone like the sun when it glistens on the water. And she was neither the oldest nor the youngest, the tallest nor the shortest, but Priya had a certain straightness to her spine, a bright mind that sparkled in her eyes and a sweet, well-spoken manner that made her a leader among the eight girls.

The King had a wide smile, and while he was rich beyond fantasy, he made sure the citizens shared in the kingdom's good fortunes and he was much beloved in return. The Queen had sadly passed away years ago, just after the youngest daughter was born, and their father insisted on a full retinue of twelve guards and eight attendants – one for each princess – to accompany them wherever they went. But, as it happens, eight pretty girls can often persuade even the fiercest of guards to bend their ways now and then, and in the summer, when the heat was overwhelming and crept into every little corner of the palace and the grounds, when the hunting dogs lay in their kennels all day on their sides, tongues panting long and loose, and even the peacocks, whose imperious cries could normally be heard throughout the palace grounds, were stilled by it, Princess Priya went to Narendra, head of their retinue of guards, and in the sweetest of voices she said: "Narendra, so big and brave, it's so hot, my sisters and I can do nothing during the day but take turns to fan each other with palm fronds. Come take us to the pond by the mango grove to swim by night, so that we may at least cool down to sleep."

"But, Princess, what would your father say?" argued Narendra, afraid of the King's wrath.

"But what could happen with my brave Narendra and all his guards to watch over us? Neeta and the other attendants will come right down to the water, they can bring lanterns for light . . . my father is so busy, he need never know!"

"Princess!"

And so it went, but her gentle voice persisted and persisted, and eventually it softened his gruff, deep tones, as it always did, and so it came that Princess Priya and her seven sisters, with their attendants and twelve burly guards, left the palace one hot summer evening and went out to the gardens as the honeyed scent of night-blooming jasmine hung in the air, past the last of the tended bushes and flower beds and into the mango grove. Through the trees, a large, calm pond shone with the light of the moon, and beckoned them with its exotic coolness.

As they passed, their footsteps and voices drifted through the night air to Ravinder, a young man who had crept into the palace grounds to steal mangoes for his elderly mother, who was not well, the sweet fruit from the King's orchards having the reputation for healing properties. He was up in a tree near the pond, as it happened, listening with growing horror as the princesses and their retinue approached, scrambling up to the highest branch that would support his weight as they appeared below him.

He tried to quell his fearful trembling when some of the guards appeared. Ravi only took a few mangoes at a time for his mother, but he knew well that if he was caught in the palace grounds, he'd be jailed at the very least. But, after the first of the guards came the princesses and their attendants, the soft moonlight shining on their long hair. Ravi had heard of the King's enchanting daughters, but never seen them before except from afar. He felt the danger of his position keenly, but his curiosity grew and got the better of him, and in any case, as he reasoned, the watchful guards would surely catch him if he tried to make his escape now, so he slid down a branch or two to see them better. The group followed the banks of the pond to a flat, grassy area around the side. The guards backed away, each taking up a position around the women, backs turned for modesty's sake, and the princesses slipped out of their robes and gratefully into the water.

Ravi watched in fascination as the lovely princesses laughed and played. But then one princess separated herself from the others to swim, the ripples of her easy movements tugging at the water's face. She swam strongly, first across and back, then all the way around the pond along the shore as her sisters stayed in the shallows. He stared, entranced, his eyes lingering on her smooth limbs and the curve of her back, her dark tresses trailing gracefully behind her. A cloud of pink lotus grew in the shallow waters by the banks at the tree where he hid, and he could feel his excitement grow as she swam closer and closer, and, no longer heeding the danger, he crept still further down to a branch that hung just over the flowers, so close he could smell their heady perfume as it wafted upwards.

Priya swam joyfully, her skin blessedly cooled. She loved to stretch her limbs, and swam easily and well. The raft of pink lotus flowers, their heads rising haughtily just above the water, caught her eye and she made her way towards them eagerly. As she reached them, the water became more shallow, and she was careful to do no damage to the roots as she sat to look at a few of the rosy blooms more closely in the light of a moonbeam. She smiled with pleasure as she stroked the soft petals delicately with her fingers. Perhaps there was a slight ripple in the water, or perhaps she saw a movement, but in an instant the thought came to her to look up, suddenly, into the tree. To her surprise, from up in the branches, she could see a pair of eyes that stared back.

Priya was a brave young woman, and felt no fear, so she stared unblinking in surprise for a few moments. She saw no menace in the eyes, and wondered who they might belong to, but just as she thought whether to call out, or otherwise address the intriguing stranger, Neeta called from across the pond.

"Priya!" she called. "Priya! Stay closer to your sisters!"

Priya sighed. "I'm coming!" she called back. She looked up into the tree for a moment longer before slipping through the lotus flowers to swim back.

Up in the tree, Ravi stared, still open mouthed, for some time as the water rippled from her passing, the pink lotus flowers bouncing up and down. His mind was filled with her lovely face and rounded breasts, her perfectly shaped limbs as they shone wetly; so much more beautiful, he thought, than even the flowers themselves.

"Priya," he whispered to himself, and couldn't tear himself away from watching her from across the pond as she returned to her sisters' play. He climbed back up into the higher branches when eventually the princesses, their attendants and guards passed by again on their way back to the palace. He heard the soft whisper of their voices below, and was sure he could pick out her musical tones from amongst them, and it seemed to him that once or twice, she looked back in his direction too.

Once they'd gone Ravinder stuffed the remaining mangoes he'd picked into his pockets and jumped quickly down from branch to branch until he reached the ground. He ran as swiftly as he could through the trees, nearly tripping over their roots in his excitement and haste. Soon he was at the palace wall, where two trees grew close enough that he could work his way up, climbing from one branch on one tree to the other just a little bit higher up. Then, about three-quarters of the way up, a crack in the stonework made a toehold, and from there he lifted himself up to the top, where he could make it down to the trees on the other side – a way into the King's healing orchards that the citizens had passed down from generation to generation. Once at the bottom, Ravi kept running all the way back to his mother's hut, fuelled by his wonder and excitement.

For three days, Ravinder followed his usual routine of rising early to walk down the dusty road as the first fingers of warm sunlight pointed the way into the busy city, to the market with its brightly painted stalls. There, he worked for a tea merchant, selling fine, fragrant teas as the sun beat down during the day. In the evenings, he returned home to make dinner for himself and his mother, reading and studying as he did for the classes he took at the end of the week, on the one day the market was closed. But all the hard work, the endless tasks and responsibilities now seemed hardly an effort. With a light heart, he sailed through the days until night fell, and he could slip over the wall to the mango grove.

For three nights, he sat in the arms of the same mango tree, waiting for Princess Priya to come back, three nights where the only sound or movement to disturb the silence was the occasional rustling of bats as they flew about. Ravi grew disappointed, a little more each night, yet he could not erase her image from his thoughts. His eyes were darkly shadowed with lack of sleep, and he'd collected more mangoes than his mother could eat in a week, but still he resolved to go again the fourth night.

Princess Priya's thoughts kept drifting back many times during those three days to the soulful eyes she'd seen up in the tree. She tried to work at some of her usual tasks to distract herself, in spite of the heat, but not even her loom, where she normally grew absorbed in watching the fine silks take shape under her nimble fingers, could erase them from her thoughts. At night, she would dream about them watching her, and Priya grew warm with a desire she'd never felt before. By the fourth night, her curiosity overcame her and she asked Narendra to take them back to the pond.

Ravi listened in rapt wonder in his treetop perch as the sound of voices became clearer, the flickering lights of their lanterns finally appearing. Just as she passed underneath, the last of the young ladies, Priya looked straight up for a quick moment, and Ravi's heart leapt.

Priya dared not look for very long with three of the guards directly behind her. So, she kept walking, her heart pounding in her ears, following Neeta and her sisters. She tried to contain her excitement as she let her sari drop to the ground, feeling the eyes on her even from across the pond. Her sisters went back to the shallows, and she joined their playing for a time, but she simply couldn't keep herself from beginning her swim, making her way over to the pink lotus flowers as soon as everyone else seemed settled in.

The stems and roots of the lotus flowers tangled in her limbs as she reached the tree, and she smiled as she pulled them gently from her, certain that the eyes would be there when she finally looked up – and sure enough, they were.

"Who are you?" she demanded in a whisper. "Why do you come here? Do you watch everyone who comes by?"

"No!" Ravinder blurted out at this last question. "Only you."

And for a moment the words hung in the air between them. Priya felt that newfound warmth again, from her throat down to her middle. "Who are you?" she asked again, more slowly.

"My name is Ravinder," he began. "I live not far from the palace walls with my mother. I come to this grove sometimes to get fruit for her when she's ill. I saw you, three nights ago, and . . ."

"And you wanted to see me swimming naked again?" she demanded, with a boldness that surprised even her.

"Yes," Ravi confessed simply, "I've been thinking of little but you ever since."

Priya smiled again, pleased at his answer, and felt herself glowing under his gaze. She stood up in the shallows, the lotus fronds clinging to her legs, her skin glistening and her long hair trailing down her back and over her firm breasts. "Do you like what you see?" she asked before sinking back into the water with a watchful glance back at the others.

Ravi could barely speak. "I adore what I see, Princess," he finally whispered back.

Her smile grew wider, peering up at him. "I can't quite see *you*," she said.

"I'll come down!" he whispered.

"No!" she said quickly. "Narendra will surely kill you before I can even beg him not to! He was a fierce warrior on the battlefield – that's why my father would trust only him with protecting his daughters."

Ravi stopped his descent, and sighed. "My father was such a warrior," he said.

It seemed to Priya that his voice had become sad all of a sudden, and she opened her mouth to ask him more when they both heard: "Priya! I tell you, stay closer to your sisters!"

"I must go," Priya whispered up at him. She hesitated a moment, then continued, "Come back in three nights."

Ravi watched her graceful back and the perfect twin mounds of her bottom swim away from him filled with a growing happiness he couldn't quite explain.

And so it went all that summer. Priya would tell him when they'd be back, and Ravi would be there without fail, in the exact same spot. She begged him to stay in the shadows, for his own safety, and for the most part he did, but now and then she would glimpse his aquiline profile against the moon, an image that burned itself into her memory. Nonetheless, it was mostly through his voice that she came to know him. She would remember little things that happened during the day as small treasures she would save up to tell him about. In return, he spoke of his life with his mother, his work and his studies, and his dreams of following in his father's footsteps by entering the cavalry. She came to know every tone in Ravi's voice – when he was happy, when he was sad that his mother seemed to languish or when he was anxious, preparing for his exams.

And she made sure that he saw just as much of her smooth skin as he wanted.

Then one night, towards the summer's end, when the harsher edge of the heat began to soften into the rainy season, Priya swam up to the pink lotus flowers and called softly into the tree, as she always did.

"Ravi, I am here."

"Princess," he began, and Priya frowned at the tone of his voice. "Priya, I must come down, to hold you and speak to you. I must come down from this tree, or I cannot bear it!"

"No!" she whispered back, with as much urgency as she could muster. "I beg you!" She looked anxiously over at Narendra.

"I must!"

Priya could hear his distress, and thought quickly. "We'll be going into the city the day after tomorrow. Neeta lets me slip away for a little while. I've been doing it since I was a child. I can meet you. Can you wait till then?"

He paused, hesitating, still up in the tree, and Priya heard a great sigh come out of him. "Yes," he said finally, "I will wait till then."

After an anxious wait, the day came that the princesses and their retinue made their way out of the palace gates and down the road into the heart of the city for their semi-annual excursion. They turned down a wide street lined with shops of different kinds, brightly coloured silks competing with the sheen of gold jewellery, and all the ladies split up excitedly to begin their shopping. Amidst the bustle, Priya smiled and winked at Neeta, who nodded curtly in return (she always pretended to disapprove). It was their customary signal, and Priya drew the plain sari she'd chosen over her head, hiding behind Neeta for a moment till two of the guards, just nearby, turned the other way, and then raced through the streets to the market to meet Ravi.

As they had arranged, she went to one of the stands and pretended to look at the fruit. Within seconds, she heard a familiar whisper just behind her right ear.

"My Princess," it said, and she turned slowly to take him in with her eyes, from the broad forehead to the dark eyes she knew so well already, all the way down his trim and elegant figure. She found herself blushing as a wide smile grew on her face – just as wide as that which she saw on his. Their fingers reached for each other as if by instinct, hands entwined across the space between them. She looked to the left and saw an alley.

"This way," she said, and, hand in hand, they ran to the alley, giggling like small children.

Once away from public view, he pulled her towards him and they met in a wet kiss. Priya thought she must surely have found heaven in the way she felt herself melt in his strong arms, and Ravinder, as he pressed her soft body to him, knew she'd be imprinted on his soul to the end of his days. After what seemed an eternity, their lips parted again.

Ravi smiled, but then the smile fell as did his gaze to the ground. "Oh Priya, I must be cursed." He sighed. "To have met and now held the most beautiful woman in the world, and then to have to leave her," he finished sadly.

"Leave?" Priya was surprised, and felt her heart sinking. "Why must you leave? When?"

"It should be good news." Ravinder's full lips smiled a little ruefully as he held her close to him still. "I got a notice, they've sent for me to come to training camp for the King's cavalry. I leave tomorrow, for training, then directly into battle."

"Battle!" Priya knew her father's kingdom was at war with a neighbouring state, a conflict that had simmered since she was a child over who controlled the riches of the ocean at a shared border. "Oh no!"

"I'm sad at leaving you –" his arms pulled her closer in his distress "– and now that the time is here, Priya, I wonder too, if I'm really brave enough to be a great warrior like my father."

Priya looked into his troubled eyes. She had heard the fire in his voice whenever he talked of his dreams, all summer long, and in summoning her strength, she became possessed of a womanly wisdom, and she knew what she must do. Priya wrapped her arms around his neck and kissed him, speaking softly into his ear.

"Can you meet me at the mango grove tonight?" she asked.

"Yes, of course I will."

That night, Ravinder sat in his usual spot high in the mango tree, and waited for the usual sounds, but instead, he heard nothing, or perhaps just a very small sound, just a soft whisper over the grasses, then his beloved's voice.

"Ravinder, I am here," she said.

"Princess! But where are the others?"

"It is just me," she said quietly. "I begged Neeta to tell everyone I was ill and went to sleep early. You can come down now."

His heart in his mouth, Ravinder flew down the branches to the ground, finally standing there in front of her where so often he could only look down from above. With trembling hands, he reached for her, and she came to him. Their lips met in another long kiss, one that sent the earth spinning around them in delicious anticipation.

"Come swim with me a while," she said when their lips finally parted again, and quickly, playfully, she stepped back and slipped out of her robes, turning to step into the water.

With a happy laugh, Ravi followed suit and, for a time, they swam and laughed together, forgetting the future, their bodies sleek and wet, sliding against each other like otters. They kissed and caressed each other, feeding on each other's flesh with lips, tongue and fingers.

Priya swam back to the pink lotus flowers under the tree and went up the bank to where the water and the blooms met solid ground. She lay down on the soft, damp earth and said simply: "I am yours, my love."

Full of emotion – for her, for his future and all the questions that remained unanswered – Ravi knelt on the grass and, just as the lotus flower opens in the sun, Priya opened herself to him. He stroked her graceful legs, opening them wider, her back arched towards him, and felt her sweet and utter surrender as he entered her with his stiff member.

They both cried out at the ecstasy, at the liquid fire that grew and grew between them with each thrust inside her own wet and welcoming flower. Underneath him, Priya felt his hands caressing her, stroking her to new heights of intense pleasure. She felt the eternal and feminine ecstasy of strength in surrender and the power in vulnerability as he thrust faster and slower, deeper or more shallow, at will.

Ravi lost himself in their seamless movement. He heard Priya's breaths come more and more quickly, and felt the beginning of a pulsing inside her, so he leaned towards her, and thrust deep, then again, then deeper, until he felt like he must be very far inside her belly. As he reached way up inside her, it unleashed a shivering wave of ecstasy, a strong pulse of *kundalini* energy that seemed to well up from the earth itself, so strong was it, and Priya gasped and moaned his name, "*O Ravi . . .*"

The energy coursed through them both, and he felt the warm gush of her orgasm, and was beside himself with desire, inflamed with a passion that pushed him faster and faster, his rod swelling bigger and bigger. With a cry, he came and, as he emptied himself into her, he felt a surge of powerful strength in return.

All night, they slept little and loved much, until the first blush of dawn began to creep into the sky to the east. Wrapped in each other's arms, their limbs tangled together, they knew it was time to go, and kissed one last time.

"My precious Priya," Ravi said, "I will carry the memory of this night – of you – with me forever. Each day I will think of this and know what a lucky man I am."

"I will wait for you," she whispered back. "I will always remember."

The strength and the feeling she had given him was so powerful it remained with him, and gave him confidence, and with his bravery and natural agility, he excelled in his training, and then shone on the battlefield, rising quickly through the ranks. He became a favourite of the people, who would cheer his home-coming in large crowds, such a favoured son that it became quite natural for him to ask for the hand of a princess in marriage – a request to which Priya, and her father, most joyfully agreed.

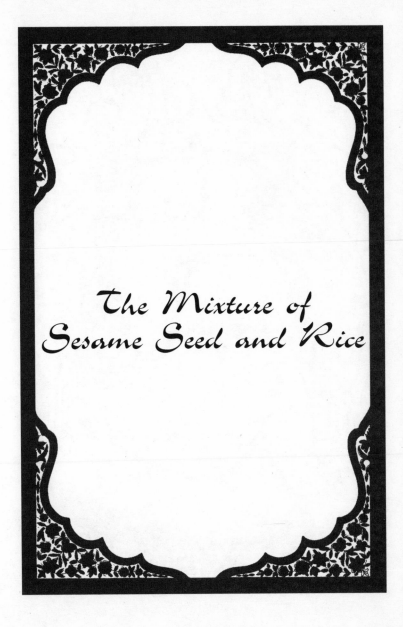

The Mixture of
Sesame Seed and Rice

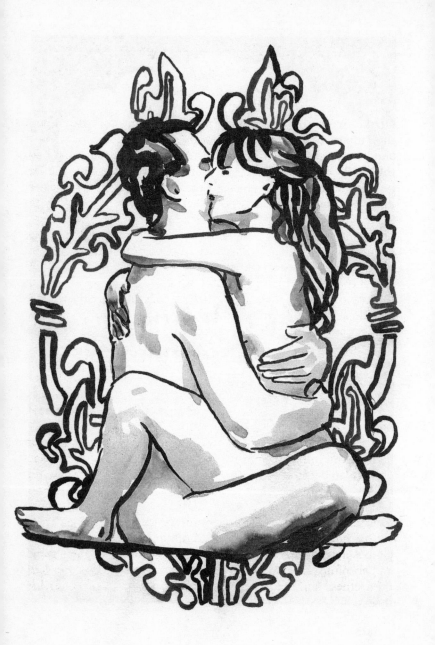

The Mixture of Sesame Seed and Rice

Tila-landulaka
Kama Sutra

Of the two embraces to be performed during the sexual act, the "mixture of sesame seed and rice" is perhaps the sweetest and leads then onwards to further passion and intensity in the "milk and water" embrace. These two embraces should be considered to be performed one after the other, as desire dictates. This heated but still sweet embrace is a good way to begin creating confidence in the desired woman. Women, being of a tender nature, want tender beginnings. First the male should embrace her with the upper part of his body, in darkness first, later in the light. He touches her breasts and if she allows that, then he embraces her.

Once confident, they lie on the bed together, tightly wound round each other's limbs. Their coupling is a jumble of arms and legs and fevered kisses and quiet sighs and pantings. Thighs are touching then have slipped between each other, loins pressed together as if to swallow the other whole. It's like a quarrel this grappling – tightly pressed together as if they never have to come up for air. He might turn her over, attempt to cast her off his body, but she is also strong, and crushes him against her with equal force. And, in truth, the man never actually wanted to get away, and he can feel his private parts joining with hers in this mixing embrace like sesame seed and rice. The desire is to become one with your lover, and so the man presses his lover's breasts against him and crushes her lips to his. And as they move within each other's clasping grasp, rubbing occurs over both bodies. They might embrace this way with all their clothes on, feeling the excitement building, slowly stripping the clothes away from bodies as the desire become indecipherable and absolute. He can feel his hardness pressing against her and the wetness and readiness of her body, waiting, aching for his thrust.

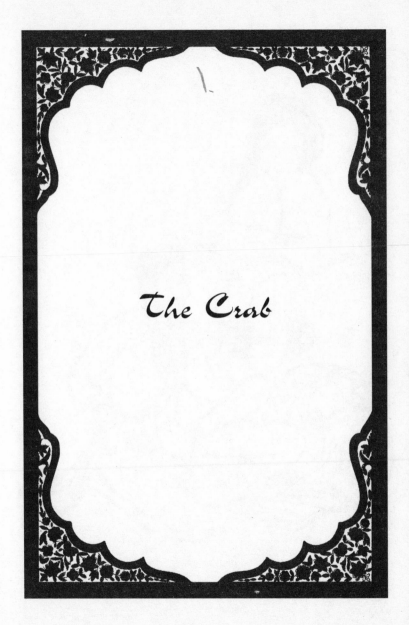

The Crab

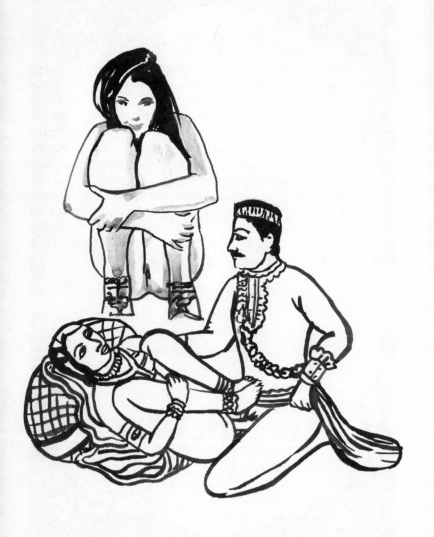

The Crab

Karkata
Kama Sutra

When both the legs of the woman are contracted, and placed on her stomach, it is called the "crab's position" because the contraction of her legs mimics the look of a crab's contracted claws. Her bent legs partially hide her vulnerable sex, but the man presses his midsection down on her pressed legs and buries his *lingam* deeply within her. Some translators have said that this position calls for the woman's feet to be placed at her navel by her lover and pressed together there while he penetrates her. He would then hold the soles of the feet together as he thrust, using her feet to push against and gain purchase. She will have to shift beneath him to get comfortable, because most of his weight will be pushing down on her. The penetration is deep and the sensations are great.

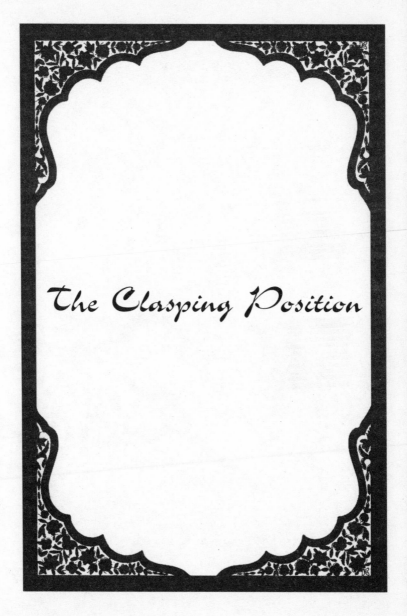

The Clasping Position

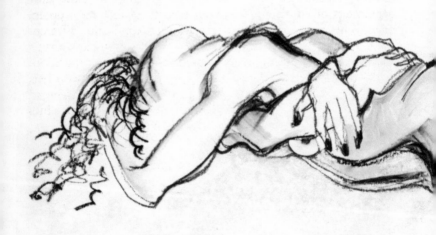

The Clasping Position

Samputa
Kama Sutra

For grasping the *lingam* tightly between the lips of the *yoni*, this is the position to make the elephant woman and her devoted hare man come together and rejoice in sensation: the deepness of her *yoni* is cleverly halved in this position. The smaller man is clasped tightly when the legs of both the male and the female are stretched straight out over each other. The position is of two kinds: the side position and the supine position, according to the way in which the lovers lie down. The woman's legs are straight and constricting her *yoni*, and the lover's *lingam* peacefully gripped inside, they lie and stare into each other's eyes, enjoying the myriad sensations, sometimes not moving for a time until the pleasure reaches a height and forces a groaning and the slow beginnings of churning. The man thrusts against the woman, playing his part, educated in the ways of *kama*, the different thrusts and blows, the ways of gaining a woman's affections. He possesses her in this position; stretched along her length, he overpowers her, and the two laugh at this, him gazing down on her, and her clasping him lovingly inside her.

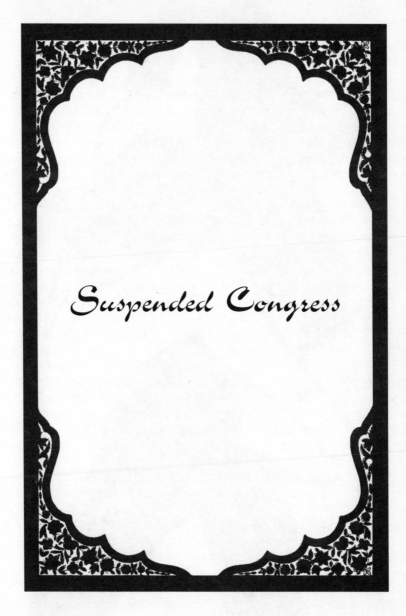

Suspended Congress

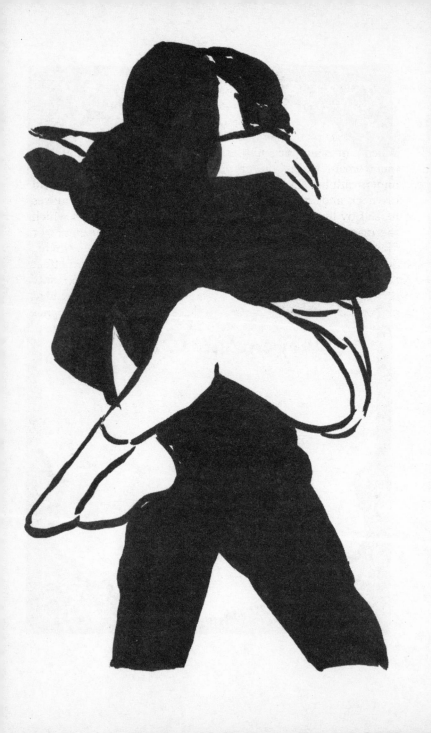

Suspended Congress

Avalambitaka
Kama Sutra

When a man supports himself against a wall or a column, and the woman, sitting on his hands joined together and held underneath her (like a seat, if possible), throws her arms round his neck and, putting her thighs alongside his waist, moves herself by her feet, which are touching the wall against which the man is leaning, it is called the "suspended congress" or "hanging position". The woman squeezes him with her thighs. This is an unfamiliar position that leads to humour and affection between the lovers as they try to negotiate their way through it successfully. The woman ends up being pounded on the end of the man's *lingam* as if on a stake, and easily reaches orgasm.

The Tale of Dvitala

as told by Michael Crawley

Ailaho A'alam!

It came to pass, in the great city of Basra, in days of yore, there lived a moneylender, called Adham bin Ali. This usurer was so ill-favoured that it was said he was begat by a troll upon a midden-heap toad.

Adham possessed but four humours: hate, avarice, lust and the desire to sire an heir. He was obsequious before all who had more power than he but he vented his venom on every unfortunate who fell into his clutches. It was his delight to corrupt the chaste and defile the pure.

Adham had such an instinct for feminine charms that if he but glimpsed the tip of a woman's finger, he could instantly gauge the elegance of her ankles, the roundness of her rump, the configuration of her *yoni*, the depth of her navel, the circumference of her waist and the proportions of her bosom.

His greed demanded that he collect on every debt, even to the tenth part of the tenth part of a copper piece, and that he exact interest, compounded, for every blink of an eye that he was owed.

Adham's lust was never fully quenched. He had lain with women, but only those he had bought as slaves, for even the most depraved whores rejected him. His pride forbade that his heir could be the offspring of a slave, so before all things, he hungered for a wife.

Adham had a servant, a young man who was as handsome as his master was repulsive. The youth's given name had been Yusef, for his father had yearned for many sons and the name means "he that shall have brothers", but his father's loins were cursed so that was not to be.

It happened that Adham's *Mazir*, or Chief Steward, chanced upon Yusef when he was at his ablutions, and was amazed. From that day forth, the *Mazir* called Yusef "Fihr" – a name that means "stone pestle". When the *Mazir*'s wife heard him call Yusef by that name she demanded to know why. The explanation, that the youth was mightily endowed and priapic to boot, inspired the woman's prime passion, to gossip. Before the moon waxed full again, word of Fihr's extraordinary endowment spread from harem to harem, throughout the city.

Wives, concubines and daughters began to pester their menfolk, asking that Adham be invited to visit, as he never strayed out without young Fihr by his side, for it pleased the usurer to keep his servant busy even when there was nothing for him to do. Why feed him if he isn't kept scurrying here and there from dawn to dusk and beyond?

Womenfolk could not be present at these visits, but it's a rare harem that isn't provided with some means for its population to peek out through secret spyholes or from between the bars of intricately formed grills. Each wife, concubine, slave girl or spinster aunt fell besmitten at her first sight of young Fihr and enjoined her master to bring Adham back for further visits. And so it came to pass that Adham the Usurer was feted despite his repulsive appearance and vile manner.

It happened that in Basra there lived a rug merchant, Dilshad Amin, who, as his name implies, was happy hearted and honest, qualities that are rare in merchants and were the cause of his being less successful than most of his contemporaries. Nevertheless, Dilshad's life was joyous, for he had been blessed with a daughter, Niki, the beautiful and elegant, the light of Dilshad's life.

Niki heard tales of the Usurer's handsome servant. No girl, no matter how virtuous, can fail to be curious when told of handsome young men, particularly when the stories are accompanied by giggles and blushes and obscene gestures. And the purest of maidens is not without guile, as many foolish young men have learned.

Niki went to her father and beseeched him, saying, "Father, why have you never sold a rug to the man whose wealth rivals that of the Caliph, and whose floors, no doubt, are in dire need of your fine merchandise?"

Dilshad blinked. "My darling daughter, apple of mine eye, delight of my soul, who is this Croesus of whom you speak?"

"Why, Adham the moneylender, of course."

"He's better known as the Usurer," her father told her. "He is not known to be pleasant company. It is said that he lacks charity." That was the worst Dilshad would say of anyone.

"Even so, is an unpleasant man's silver without value? Is his gold dross? Is it not fitting that an honourable merchant take his profit from a man who lacks virtue? I've read that the brightness of a coin is enhanced when it passes from uncharitable hands, such as his, into charitable ones, such as yours."

These were wise words, Dilshad thought. He asked, "O, sage daughter, how might one such as I entice one such as Adham the Usurer into his humble emporium?"

"I know not, father, but it is said that this man is easily lured into private homes. He is a miser. Every meal he consumes in another's house is one fewer he provides for himself."

Dilshad pondered Niki's words for a day and a night before he dispatched a servant to invite Adham to a feast to be given in the Usurer's honour. A newborn lamb was boiled with saffron and cinnamon. Six types of rice were prepared. Bowls of fiery sumac were set beside gilded apples and sugared dates. Dishes of smoked whitefish and decorated eggs were garnished with spinach and beans.

Adham had not taken five steps into Dilshad's banquette room when his sixth sense directed his gaze towards an ivory grille, behind which Niki and her attendants were concealed. The girl's desire to see Fihr had made her careless. She stood too close. The tips of two rosebud toes showed beneath the scrollwork.

At once, Adham discerned that the toes' owner had high-arched feet; ankles his hands could encircle; dimpled knees from which rose thighs that tapered from almost too slender to just the right side of plump. Her mound would be a silken cushion, divided by a delicate crease. Her *yoni*, he was sure, would have the grip of a blacksmith's fist and yet would be lined by skin with the texture of oiled rose petals. A plover's egg would have fitted into her navel. She'd have the undulant spine of an eel and a waist to suit. Her breasts would be shaped like bells but be yielding and resilient.

No doubt her face would be pretty.

In that moment, three of Adham's humours united. He *would* possess her. He *would* defile her. He *would* get her with child – his son.

But how? As he partook of Dilshad's bounty, Adham plotted. He was too ugly to court the girl. Dilshad wouldn't likely sell her. That left trickery and deceit. By the time the lamb had been consumed, Adham had conceived a scheme.

"I see that you own many fine rugs," he complimented his host.

Dilshad preened. "If you see any here that would not disgrace the lowliest chamber in your fine house," he said, "please accept them as gifts."

Adham wagged his head. "Once, I would have been overwhelmed by your largesse, Dilshad, my friend. Since then, however, I have acquired a – it should not be called such, but I lack another word – a 'rug' that was woven on the Isle of D'Karak. Since I obtained it, I have sworn to neither hang nor lay on any its inferior."

"From D'Karak, you say? I've never heard of such a place."

"It's a guarded secret. Even *I* do not know its location, but the tale is that the weavers there have an insatiable appetite for salt and will sell their finest rugs for no more than a cupful. Can you imagine – they weave the silk of gigantic poisonous spiders. It is said that for every rug they make a man dies in agony. Little wonder their merchandise fetches incredible prices from those lucky enough to acquire it."

"Incredible . . .?"

"The least is valued at a talent of gold."

Dilshad's eyes rolled. "Um – they can be bought for a cup of salt but sold for a talent of gold?"

Adham nodded. "Some profit, eh, my friend? Would that we knew the whereabouts of this fabled island."

The next day, Dilshad heard the cries of an itinerant mapmaker, extolling his wares in the courtyard before his house. It couldn't be, of course, but what harm in enquiring? His servant called the peddler into Dilshad's audience room.

"Mapmaker, tell me, is it possible that you have for sale a map of a distant island I've heard tell of, a place called D'Karak?"

The mapmaker did, for he had drawn it himself, the night before, at the behest of Adham, to whom he was indebted.

Dilshad and the mapmaker settled on a price that was many times the value of any map yet made. Dilshad was convinced that a fortune awaited him if he could mount an expedition to D'Karak, which the map showed as being many *farsangs* to the southeast. If he sold all he owned, he might realize half the cost. Perhaps Adham would partner him?

"I'm no merchant," Adham protested. "A cobbler should keep to his last. *But*, I have every faith in you as a trader in rugs. I'll loan you all the funds you need and charge you but a token interest."

"Wonderful," Dilshad allowed, "but what might a 'token' amount to?"

"Oh, say, a copper penny?"

Dilshad's heart sang.

"A day," Adham continued, "compounded geometrically."

"Compounded geometrically?"

"A penny for the first day, two pennies for the second, four for the third and so on. It'll amount to but a trifle."

Dilshad hired a captain and a ship and filled its hold with salt, and sent it off with the forged map and his sincere prayers.

With his plot in motion, all Adham had to do was wait.

"Wait" has a brother, "Worry".

Worry came to Adham in the still of the night and whispered into the Usurer's hairy ear. "What if Dilshad's daughter has a suitor? What if she *doesn't* but one comes tomorrow? Your trap will take many moons to spring. What if, when it closes, Dilshad's daughter has already escaped and already lies in the arms of her husband, be he a young merchant prince, or a fierce desert sheik, or . . ."

Come the dawn, Adham summoned Fihr. "Go thou to the house of Dilshad the rug merchant," he commanded. "See, but be not seen. Watch for any suitor for the hand of his daughter, Niki, any man, young or old, who comes bearing gifts. Do this every day until I bid thee cease. Return each night and report to me. Perform this task well and I will reward thee."

Fihr patrolled the courtyard before Dilshad's house for half a day before it occurred to him that there might be other entrances. He found an alley that ran beside the house's wall. It twisted before it led to a narrow way that curved and hence to a tiny courtyard that had to be behind Dilshad's house. Set into the wall was a curious wrought-iron gate. On inspection, it proved to be not one, but two gates, one so close behind the other that they touched. The gate on Fihr's side had been shaped into a trellis. The one beyond was formed in semblance of vines. No doubt, at one time the one gate had been painted black and the other green, for a pleasant illusion, but now both were plain from neglect. By the condition of the hinges, Fihr judged that neither gate had been opened for decades.

A sweet soft song sounded from beyond the gates. Drawn, Fihr made a yet closer inspection. Dots of light showed through in many places. In others, there was space enough to admit the blade of a knife. In one place, and in one only, in the centre and at a level with Fihr's chest, the intricate patterns of iron had left a gap through which a hen's egg could have passed.

Fihr put his eye to the hole. In that instant, he was smitten.

Niki was an ardent gardener. The roses on the other side of the gates were her joy. Because it was within her father's harem, it was her practice to work wearing nothing but a *choli* of gauzy cotton that was open to her navel. Further, her self-given task that day was to water her blooms. She had been careless. Dampness had rendered her *choli* transparent.

Fihr sighed a deep soft sigh.

As a mother will hear the gurgle of her babe from two rooms away, so a girl who is budding can discern a young man's sigh from an equal distance, and Fihr was much closer than that. Being a coquette, Niki affected not to have heard and went about her chores, twisting at her waist, swaying at her hips, arching her back. It was a bloom of the rose that grew closest to the gates that she chose to kiss, chastely at first, then boldly, her tongue acting the role of a bee.

Fihr was consumed. Unaware that his presence was known, he clutched himself through his robes in a sweet agony of lust. Niki heard the rustling and Fihr's repressed groans. It was a combination of sounds that she'd never heard before but her fervid imagination deciphered them perfectly.

What to do? If she spoke, her unknown admirer would surely flee. There were two pleasures that obsessed Niki, though she'd experienced neither yet. One was to lie with a handsome youth, preferably Adham's servant, who she'd gazed upon just the once. The other was to have a stalwart lad gaze upon her with love and lust in his eyes, again, preferably Fihr.

How to keep her hidden admirer at his post without frightening him away? Such conundrums are easily solved by a concupiscent nymph. Accompanied only by her own lilting voice, Niki danced. Her swaying and turning, the tiny stamps of her bare feet, her undulations, all revealed and then concealed, giving her observer glimpses of treasures that should have been reserved for her groom on the night of her wedding.

The rustling and groaning became louder and faster until they climaxed in a deep grunt. Then there was silence. Niki went to the gate and bent to the hole. There was no one to be seen but the air was redolent with a musk that she recognized from her father's concubines' rooms.

The next morning, Niki started gardening early, wearing an old *choli* that'd grown tight two years before. She plucked the prettiest pink bud she could find and poked it through the gates. The sun was a hand's breadth above the horizon when the rose's stem disappeared.

Fihr's voice asked, "Niki?"

"Who are you?" Niki asked, not daring to hope.

"I am called Fihr. I am servant to the Usurer, Adham."

"What do you do here?"

"I was sent by my master to spy on you, but now . . ."

"But now?"

"Now I am here by my own choice, or perhaps not, for I ache to be as close to you as I can. You have enchanted me, sweet Niki."

"You have secretly watched me," Niki accused.

"As . . ." And Fihr dried up, for the comparison that came to him was "as a mongoose watches a cobra". His love would hardly find that flattering.

Niki continued in her best pouty voice, "You have seen me – a lot of me – but all I have seen of thee is a glimpse, when you visited my father's house. That isn't fair."

"I'm sorry."

"Then show thyself to me."

"There is a hole . . ."

"I know." Niki bent to the hole. "You are handsome, Fihr, in thy face. I would see more. I would see as much of thee as you have of me. Disrobe, I pray thee."

Fihr glanced about. "What if someone comes?"

"If they do?"

"My master would beat me severely and render me a eunuch."

"Oh!" That was a telling argument. Niki might have been able to bear Fihr being beaten, even severely, but castration, that was another matter.

"Then we shall just converse," Niki decided.

They crouched beside the hole and conversed. By noon, each had hooked a finger into the hole and their fingertips had touched. By mid-afternoon, they had pressed their faces against the cruel iron and had stretched forth their tongues. And the tips of their tongues had touched.

The following day, Niki crushed her own breast between her two hands and forced her delicate flesh as deeply into the hole as she could bear. Two of Fihr's outstretched fingertips touched her tender nipple and caressed it. That day passed in almost-kisses and unsatisfying caresses until the young lovers parted, each aching for more.

On the third day, Niki, the bolder of the two, said, "Part your robes, dear Fihr, and climb the gate. No one would be able to see that your manly sceptre . . ."

Shivering with lust, Fihr parted his robe, pulled one garment up, pushed another down, and did as he was bade. The iron gates were cruel but he persevered despite the bruising. Eventually, the dome of his *lingam* emerged from the other side, like a boss on a shield.

"More?" Niki asked.

Fihr pressed his belly hard against the gate, but to no avail.

"Then be still," Niki told him. She scaled the iron vines until her *yoni* was level with Fihr's *lingam*. She pressed. She contorted. She raised up one leg, pointing her toes at the sky, but no matter how she twisted, the most she achieved was to nestle half of Fihr's damson between her eager petals. In her striving, Niki found that when her pink seed rubbed on Fihr's hard flesh, the sensation was divine. And so she worked, moving her hips no more than the width of her smallest finger, but with avid intensity. Fihr's groans urged her on until finally she achieved a great spasmodic joy.

Overcome with gratitude, Niki dropped down and planted a sweet kiss on that portion of Fihr that had so pleased her. A kiss led to a lick, and a suck, and an open-mouthed gobble, until Fihr bleated like a goat in a slaughterhouse and bestowed his benison onto his lover's outstretched tongue.

"Part of you is inside me now," she told him. "Now we can never be separated."

From that day forward, Niki pleasured herself on the dome of Fihr's *lingam* until ecstasy consumed her, and then returned the gift with the attentions of her lips and tongue. Being young, they performed that exchange four or sometimes five times each day.

Days passed, and months. Dilshad's ship returned with tattered sails, a spoiled cargo, and a report that if the Isle of D'Karak existed, it wasn't where the map showed it to be.

The Usurer demanded that his loan be repaid. By then the interest, "compounded geometrically", came to a sum greater than all the gold in the world. Adham offered Dilshad two choices. He could surrender his all, his daughter included as a body slave, and he himself be sold for dogs' meat, or he could keep his all, if Niki agreed to wed Adham bin Ali.

The wedding was solemn. That night, Niki told her new husband, "I will share your bed, my master. I will not resist you. You may use me as you will, but I will never respond to you, nor grant you the pleasures of my mouth, nor will I ever bear your son."

Adham was incensed. For a watch and a half, he paced his chambers, asking himself why his bride would treat him so. By midnight, he had decided that she must be enamoured of another and that other could be no one but his own servant, Fihr!

He had the lad stripped and dragged down to the vault in which he kept his treasure, which was enclosed by a wall of bars that locked from inside and out, for Adham delighted in spending nights down there, counting his gold and gloating over his gems. There was a mighty pillar in the middle of the chamber. Adham secured the lad to it, wrapping him in chains from his shoulders to his elbows and from his ankles to his knees. He fastened the chains with padlocks and sent for Niki.

"You will perform every act of love that's known, for me, and feign joy in so doing, and you will bear me a man-child. For every night you refuse me, Fihr's torment will increase. To-morrow, I will beat him with nettles from knee to chest. The next night, I will whip him with thorns. If you still refuse me, I'll strike him with a barbed whip. After that, I will cut a piece off him each day, and you may guess which piece I will start with. Think on it."

Adham returned to his chamber and called for strong drink, which he consumed in vast quantities, until he swooned. Niki crept to her loathsome husband and found the key to the vault and the key to its inner chamber about his person but she could not find the keys to the padlocks.

She would spend at least a little while with the man she loved.

In the vault, Niki passed beyond the iron bars and bolted their door from the inside. In her despair, she determined that she would remain within, making love to Fihr, until Adham brought a blacksmith to gain entry, after which she would devise some way to die.

Despite his peril, Fihr greeted Niki with his *lingam* erect. She dropped to her knees to worship the "stone pestle". With no gates to hinder her, she was able to take his full dome and half his shaft into her mouth. Her delight made her eyes weep, her mouth water and her tongue dance.

Fihr cried, "Cease, my love, for I would take your maiden-head and make you truly mine before we are discovered."

Niki scaled the chains that bound her darling. Their mouths met. The tips of their tongues touched and more than touched, slithered and slid and delved and savoured and delighted. Fihr's arms, free from their elbows to his hands, cupped his sweetheart's buttocks and pulled her close, so that his *lingam* pressed on her mound and found its way between her lips but no further, for neither could draw back for a thrust. Niki, inventive as ever, lifted up her feet and set her soles against the pillar that Fihr was chained to. Her legs straightened to push herself away. She paused . . .

"No!" It was Adham, awakened and enraged. The Usurer rattled the bars but could not gain entry.

Niki looked back over her shoulder. "Foul beast! Watch as my true love enjoys pleasures that will never be yours, you monster! I have but one hymen to sacrifice, and surrender it with joy, thus!"

So saying, Niki wriggled to work the crown of Fihr's *lingam* into her vestibule. Her feet left the pillar, leaving her supported by her arms around Fihr's neck, his hands beneath her bottom's cheeks and the sweet hard flesh that impaled her. So tightly did Fihr's member fill her that she sank slowly, taking a dozen heartbeats before her soft mound kissed her lover's muscular pubes.

Sounds that were not words spewed from the Usurer's lips. His face became purple. Veins stood out at his temples. He beat on the bars until his knuckles bled.

Niki drew up her legs. She set her soles against the pillar once more, and pushed with deliberate slowness, drawing her cling-ing flesh up the full length of Fihr's shaft.

Blood dribbled from Adham's left nostril. He clutched at his own head and fell to his knees.

Niki lowered herself again. "I die from joy!" she screamed. Again, she pushed away, but faster, and let herself drop so that her belly slapped Fihr's.

Adham bit through his own tongue.

Niki rose and fell, thrusting and squirming, gyrating her lovely hips.

The Usurer toppled to his side, dead of an apoplexy.

And so it came to pass that the erotic act, *Avalambitaka*, was devised, and that Niki inherited Adham bin Ali's wealth, for the magistrate's doctor confirmed that she had, indeed, lost her virginity on her wedding night and so the marriage had been consummated.

Churning

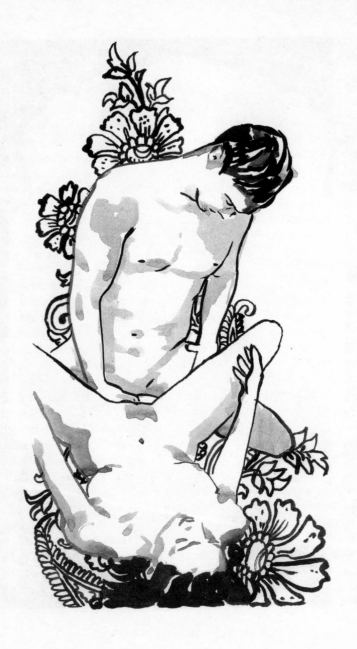

Churning

Manthana
Kama Sutra

Churning is a sex stroke performed by the man in order to satisfy his lover. It is one of nine strokes for which a man is responsible. The *lingam* is held with the hand, and turned all round in the *yoni* without stopping or taking a break, as if churning butter. As well as moving it round the vagina, some translators say it is also moved every which way, according to the man's desires. Vatsyayana would agree: throughout the *Kama Sutra* he mentions that all these rules pale in the face of great passion, and become nullified. Passion is its own teacher and desire will act according to its own rules. The most important stipulation is the constant churning motion that stimulates the woman's *yoni* and readies her for penetration. If a woman is slow to excitement, this type of stroke should be employed for a longer amount of time. When she starts to breathe heavily and a slight sweat breaks out between her breasts, and when she begins to murmur soft sentiments of love and begs you to continue, she is ready for further congress.

Churning is also one of the strokes to be used by the female when she temporarily takes over the male's role. It is then her job to use the man's *lingam* as a dildo and guide it into herself, turning it as fast and in whatever direction pleases her most. When acting the man's role, she should let her passion be her guide. The man has no choice but to allow her access to his vulnerable parts, as he is lying on his back and as helpless as was the woman previously. She should look deeply into his eyes as she uses him, letting him know that she has taken over his job. She is able to please herself now, using him to satisfy herself and reach orgasm. If the man attempts to help her in her task in any way, she should scold him playfully and wag her finger at him. As she approaches orgasm, he will be unable to help himself and will seek to grab hold of her, but she must be steadfast.

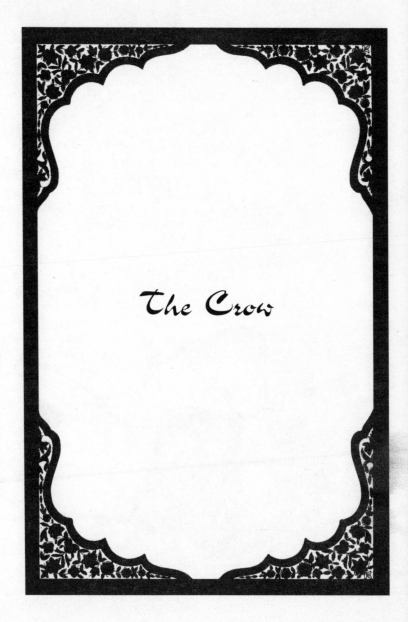

The Crow

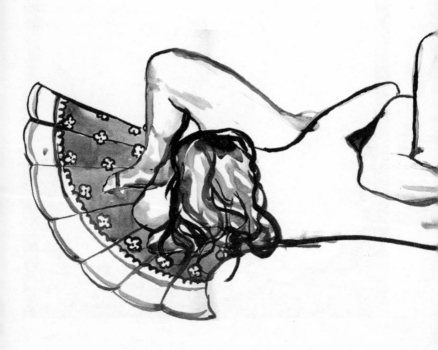

The Crow

Kakila
Kama Sutra

When a man and a woman use their mouths to give pleasure to each other by placing them on the tender love parts of each other – a practice sometimes seen as not holy – and they then proceed to use the techniques and skills inherent in kissing practices yet transferred now onto the lower parts of their lover, it causes great sensation and pleasure, moans and sighs and all the words of love that we've transcribed so far. This position spurs each lover on to greater please the other, to whom in *kama* they are a partner in this act of pleasure. This position is called "the crow". This is because the pecking at the tender love parts by the man and by the woman is like the pecking of crows, nibbling here and there, causing excruciating pleasure, and the release of sounds of delight, such as crows sometimes make circling in the sky.

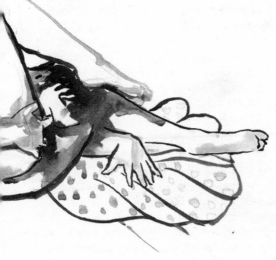

The Tale of of the Crow

as told by Zoanne Allen

This story is told of a time and place many years removed from our own. It was a time of peace and prosperity, when there were no wars upon the land. It was a time when love flowered and was honoured, and there were many ceremonies to Kama and Rati, who granted the gifts of love and passion to their followers.

And in that time, near the city of Peshwahar, there dwelt a comely young maiden, whose name was Amartiah. She was, of course, as slender as a willow branch, with hips of pleasing fullness, and breasts like ripe mangoes, both of which promised much pleasure in the aspects of love. Her hair was long and black as the night of no moon, with a sheen like the coat of a panther. Amartiah was of an age to be married, but her father treated her as his most precious jewel, the only daughter among five blessings from the Brahma. A wealthy trader and a widower, he had no desire to marry off his only daughter merely to increase his own wealth. And so he had long refused to discuss a marriage for her. That is, until he was pressed by his eldest son to consider a young man named Rumindajar.

The young man was as handsome and favoured by the gods as the lovely Amartiah. Like the date palms that grew in the gardens, he was tall and sturdy. His hair fell in dark, shining ringlets around his face. Dark eyes held the promise of passion within and his smile enticed many a local maiden to look boldly upon him. Coming from a family of landowners, Rumindajar had much to recommend him as a prospective bridegroom.

Rumindajar had met Amartiah only briefly when he had come to visit his good friend, her elder brother, Djarlisam. Their eyes had met across the shaded atrium of the house, and Rumindajar had known immediately that she was destined to be the mate of his heart. Fortune smiled upon him, for Amartiah felt the same, and shortly thereafter, secret messages were sent back and forth to determine the depth of feeling which had been stirred by that meeting. Pledges of love were given and so it was that they began to meet secretly in the city gardens or in the groves by the riverbank.

As their love grew and deepened, Rumindajar begged Djarlisam to speak to his father so that he might court Amartiah openly. The voice of an eldest son carries much weight and the father listened. Agreeing that it was time for a selection to be made, and that the young man in question was of good character and good family, Amartiah's father met with the father of Rumindajar and a decision was reached that the two would wed. But no date was set for the blessing of the union, as her father was still unwilling to part entirely with his beloved daughter.

As was the custom of the time, shortly after the celebration to announce the betrothal, the pair joined in that happy congress of her cavern of pleasure with his spear of joy. And, although they continued to meet and practise the joining of their bodies and sharing tender words of passion, Rumindajar began to wish for more.

Lovely as Amartiah was, and beautiful as her body was to touch, and happy as she was to open herself to his eager rod, she was unversed in the many ways of love and the many ways that a woman may please herself and her lover. A young woman of Peshwahar was not encouraged to learn about the amorous arts until she was betrothed and Amartiah had no woman in her family to give her instruction. Rumindajar had tried to encourage her to kiss him and stroke him in different ways, but she was shy and reticent to attempt those caresses that she had not heard the other women speak of. Lacking the patience of maturity, the young man began to consider other methods that might gain him what he desired. And so, like many males before him and after him, Rumindajar turned to trickery.

One evening, when he knew that Amartiah would be alone in her private chambers in a shaded corner of the courtyard, Rumindajar put his plan into effect. Making sure that no one was about to observe him, he threw himself on the ground a few feet from her doorway and began crawling towards the door, softly calling her name.

A lover's ears are constantly tuned to the voice of the beloved and Amartiah heard him even through the door and the sounds of the evening birds and water flowing in the fountain. She threw the door open, ready to greet him with open arms, but drew back in horror when she saw him upon the ground. Again, he softly called her name and reached towards her, with despair written upon his face

Crying out, Amartiah ran to his side and wrapped her arms around his neck, attempting to pull him up. "Oh, my heart, what has happened? How do you come to me like this?"

Rumindajar allowed her to pull him up and leaned against her breasts, secretly enjoying the softness of the lovely pillows. "Most beautiful and beloved mistress, I have come to take one last look upon your divine face and taste one last time the sweetness of your lips." So saying, he pressed his palm against her cheek and lifted his face towards hers.

"No, no," Amartiah cried, pulling back to her knees and grabbing his shoulders. "It cannot be that you are to be taken from me. Tell me what has happened!"

"Heart of my heart," he replied, "while coming to visit you, I stopped to pick some flowers growing by the path. I was only thinking of how they would pale beside your beauty but yet you would take pleasure in having them to brighten your room. I did not see, as I knelt to pick them, that there was an asp hiding in the undergrowth, and before I could act, he stung me upon those parts which have brought such joy to us in the past. Realizing that I had little time left to me, I made my way, as you see, so that I might look upon you and let your beauty be the last sight I see before I leave the earth, and go to join Vishnu in paradise. In his wisdom, we may meet in another life." He reached up and tenderly stroked her cheek which now showed the trickles of tears, the evidence of how deeply she had taken the story to heart. In her agitation, the young woman began pulling at his clothes, seeking the source of the wound.

"This must not be, for how can I live without you, you who are my joy and my strength. You are the creator of my passion and the flowing river that calms my fever. How can I exist without you? I will send my servants for the wisest healer that can be found. I will not let you leave me." Amartiah started to turn to call for help, but he stopped her, holding her hands lest she reveal his unmarked person to the evening light.

"Alas, my own divine Lakshmi, there is no time to send for help. But only assist me to your bed and I will die in happiness that I am in your loving arms." He began to rise, pretending to be too weak to carry his own weight, and so Amartiah put her strength beneath his arm and led him to her bed. Falling into the softness of the cushions, Rumindajar sighed as if in pain and drew her down beside him.

"Please, tell me what can be done to save you, for I swear before all the gods that I will hold nothing back if it will spare your life." Amartiah was crying fiercely now, and he felt the slightest prick of guilt at the deception he was playing upon her. But it did not stop him from allowing his hands to rove about her soft body, caressing her neck and shoulders and sliding his fingers across the tips of her breasts in their covering of thin cloth. All guilt fled as he felt the nipples begin to rise to greet him.

"Oh, most loving of women, there is only one thing that can stave off the hand of death that reaches for me even now. But it is a hard thing for such a young woman as you are, and I fear it is too much to ask, even for my life."

She bent over him and held his face between her hands. "I have sworn. Tell me what it is I must do." Her breasts pressed against his chest, nipples sliding against his skin, and Rumindajar felt his rod swelling as if indeed it had been bitten.

"It requires great courage, for you must draw out the poison yourself. If you are indeed willing, I will guide you in what must be done." Almost before he finished speaking, the girl had begun to remove his outer garments and release the eager shaft contained within. When he was uncovered, she gently stroked him, then paused when he drew in his breath sharply.

"I have hurt you," she said.

"It is nothing," the trickster replied. "I may make many sounds of pain, while you are working, but do not stop. I promise that I will only wish for you to continue your ministrations upon me."

Amartiah nodded and waited for his next instruction.

"You must form your ripe lips into a circle, and then push them lightly against the tip. Then move in tiny circles around it. This will start to bring the poison back from my body."

She did so, lowering her mouth to his *lingam*. As instructed, she slid her lips lightly down over the tip and then began moving them in little circles. The warmth of her mouth and the moistness of her lips caused him to swell even further. Rumindajar pushed himself up against the cushions so that he might see the captivating sight of her lips caressing him, leaving shining, wet trails upon him as she moved her mouth as he had directed.

"Now, my sweetness, grasp my sturdy branch and place your mouth tightly upon the shaft, first on one side, then on the other. In this way, you will encourage the poison to leave me." He gasped as she firmly gripped him in her delicate hand, but again, following his instructions, she did not pause.

First she placed her mouth tightly upon the side of his penis, creating a light suction. Then she began to nip it lightly with her teeth. In this manner, she continued around the length of him, drawing the flesh tightly into her mouth, and then nibbling gently on the tender flesh. Soon her tiny hand could hardly encompass the girth of him, and he struggled to lie still under her ministrations.

"Ahhh," he gasped, as she nipped him again. "I can feel the poison starting to move. Take the head only between your lips and kiss it and pull it as though you were kissing me upon my own lips."

Amartiah now began to show some enthusiasm for the task he had set her. Perhaps she was feeling that her actions were having a positive effect and that her lover might be saved. In her relief, it might be that she began to let just the littlest bit of pleasure take its hold upon her.

Whatever she was thinking, she eagerly pressed her lips around the tip of his maleness, and began pushing down upon it, as if she were almost drawing it into her mouth once again. Then she would let her lips slide together as in a deep kiss, followed by pulling at the edges with her lips. The tip glowed up at her, cherry red from the blood within and shiny with the continuous laving she had given it. Indeed, it did resemble some luscious fruit waiting to be consumed. For his part, Rumindajar was forced to grasp the cushions tightly, that he might not lose control altogether.

Without waiting for his next direction, Amartiah suddenly dived upon the sturdy morsel, taking it completely into her mouth and pressing the shaft between her lips. The unexpected insertion of his organ caused Rumindajar to cry out and his hips pushed himself against her warm lips and tongue, but she pulled back as he pushed forward. Chiding himself for being too eager, he forced himself to lie back upon the cushions, and Amartiah returned to the pleasurable feasting upon him, but again she pulled away. Several more times she did this, each time driving Rumindajar almost to madness as he tried to restrain himself.

Now she took him into her hands and pressed hard, sucking kisses upon the length of him. The noises he made excited her deeply, and his spear no longer resembled a weapon, but instead a long succulent papaya, ripe and running with juices. As Amartiah continued to feast upon him, she unconsciously began to rub her thighs together, feeling her own juices beginning to seep from her hidden grotto. As she moved, her skirt rose even higher, revealing the lovely moons above her thighs.

Rumindajar could smell the scent of her excitement, and he began to think that it was time for the game to end, or indeed he would die from lack of release. But she had found a new trick now and was using her tongue to flick across the sides of his penis as she held him tightly. She would flick it on one side, then the other, then upon the very tip, and had she not held him tightly, he would have sent his seed spurting to the heavens. Unable to release, Rumindajar slid his fingers under her rounded buttocks where she knelt next to him. Almost immediately, he felt a trickle of moisture running down the inside of her thighs. With a soft, circular motion, he massaged the dampness into her skin. Amartiah, for her part, released a soft sigh of pleasure against the red bulb of his shaft. The caress of her breath was followed by her lips closing once again around the ripe tip and her tongue circling as she sucked even harder upon him.

Certain now that his lover was also sharing his passion, Rumindajar knew that he could hold back no longer. He thrust his fingers deeply into her moistness, and felt her push back against him for deeper penetration. "Oh, my beloved! The poison is fleeing from my body. I cannot . . ."

But before he could finish speaking, Amartiah slid his length into her mouth, moaning against the hardness as she sucked more fervently and threw her hips again and again against his penetrating fingers. The clever trickster finally had all that he could ever desire and, with a cry that drove the starlings from the trees outside the doorway, his seed fountained into her waiting mouth.

Even as the spasms shook him, he knew that he must not ignore the fever of passion that he had created within his lovemate. Breathing deeply to restore energy to his now-sated body, he rolled over, gently pushing her onto her side so that he faced her heated *yoni*. The faithful Amartiah still held his glistening stalk within her mouth, still sucking gently to draw out the last dregs of the poison.

"My life is yours, for you have brought me back from the edge of death," he whispered huskily. "But I must be sure that you shall have no ill effects from what you have taken from me, so I in turn must draw the remainder from your body." So saying, he gently pinched together the succulent outer lips of her path to pleasure, and began kissing them as though he were kissing the soft lips of her mouth. As he drew the soft skin into his own mouth, Amartiah moaned against the flesh between her own lips and spread her legs wider to allow him all access to her secret grove.

His own passion beginning to stir once again, Rumindajar pushed his nose between the pulsing lips, burying himself in her womanly scent. He sent his tongue to search the furthest reaches of her warm channel and pressed his face tightly against the open flower of her sex. As he moved in slow circles, Amartiah began the cries that signalled her own climax was near.

Rumindajar pulled himself away from the warm haven of his lover's mouth, and positioned himself between her legs, setting her feet upon his shoulders. The ripe nectar was flowing from her and the little jewel shown and sparkled between the full lips. Like a bird darting to catch the shiny morsel, he pounced against the small pearl within. Now flicking it hard with his tongue, now sucking upon the ripe flesh, he continued until she could withhold no longer. Grabbing his head and pressing it even more tightly against her, Amartiah released her passion, hips bucking in rhythm to the delightful quakes that flooded her body, her legs straightening in the rigour of the waves. As the pleasure receded, she slid around to bury her face once more in the loins of her lover.

Peace now descended upon the silky bed of pleasure. Cushions and sheets ran off the bed and onto the floor. Clothing lay scattered about the alcove. The fountain played softly in the courtyard and the nightbirds began their calls. Amartiah now lay with her lover's softly curling stem against her cheek. Rumindajar lay with his head nestled against the warm dampness of her inner thigh. Both luxuriated for many moments in the lethargy that comes from truly ecstatic lovemaking. As the evening ended, the cunning and now very satisfied young man professed his deepest love for the lady, and swore yet again that she had brought him back from the very brink of death. His tenderest endearments and vows of eternal devotion were matched by her own promises of enduring love and her deepest joy in the gift of his life. And she did not forget to mention his own efforts to protect her from any suffering upon his behalf.

Ah, but some days later, the worm of guilt began to wriggle about. Rumindajar, who was really a good man at heart, was now wondering if he had done a terrible thing in his desire for pleasure. He argued with himself, sometimes believing that he had done no harm, for he had only taught his beloved a new form of pleasure for them both. At other times, he felt he had done wrong in not speaking frankly with the woman with whom he would spend his life. For several days, he wrestled with his conscience, although he found that it was no impediment to sharing the newfound joys of love with Amartiah.

At last, when he could not remove the guilt by any of his arguments, he went to the temple to pray for guidance. Stepping into the cool quiet of the marble sanctuary, he felt his emotions begin to quiet. Devoutly, he walked the length of the temple, with his arms outstretched and his head bowed, praying that his path to atonement would be made clear to him. And his prayers were answered, for no sooner had he lit the incense before the statue of Vishnu, than, with a rustle of robes, the high priest himself came to stand at his side.

"My son, your pain colours the very air around you. There is great confusion and unhappiness within you. Come, let us sit in the temple garden and perhaps you may relieve yourself of the great burden that you carry." The priest laid a kindly hand upon Rumindajar's shoulder and guided him outside to a stone bench.

Seated under a great shade tree, Rumindajar looked into the kindly eyes of the priest, his elderly countenance shining with an aura of warmth and understanding. As if a dam had given way and a great flood had been released, Rumindajar told his story. At the end, he sat with his head bowed in shame, and waited for the priest to berate him for his selfishness. And so he was surprised to hear a deep chuckle come from the holy man seated next to him.

"Oh, my son, you should not look to punish yourself so hard for an act that was not conceived out of maliciousness. Even the gods would not judge you harshly for what you have done. Although—" and here the priest seemed to struggle to find a more serious face "—you have indeed done wrong in using trickery instead of the truth. We are taught that love requires the desire to please your lover as well as yourself. By your actions, you have placed your own desire first. And you did not give your betrothed a chance to show that she might place your pleasure before her own. She seems a properly shy young woman, waiting to be taught the great secrets of love by her husband. It is by patience that you teach these lessons, not by deceit."

"You are right, holiness. I burn with shame for my actions." Rumindajar raised his hands in supplication to the priest. "But it has now become my greatest joy to give her pleasure. And I believe that even though she was acting out of a desire to save my life—" and here a small blush touched his cheek "—she, too, took much pleasure from the act. Indeed, I have had proof since that she greatly enjoys savouring my manhood as if it were some sparkling sweetmeat. And she shows much pleasure when I seek out her shiny pearl in exchange."

The priest rose and placed his hand upon the head of the chastened Rumindajar. "It is taught to us that we should follow the example of the Dog, who is loyal and faithful. And to follow the example of the Elephant, who is strong and wise. And the Crane who is honest and just. You have followed the ways of the Crow, for you have relied upon deceit to obtain what you might have gained honestly. And like the Crow, you seek the bright and shiny treasures placed before you. Go into the temple now and vow before the gods that you will devote yourself to what is true. And with their blessings, you and your wife will have many years of searching and finding those treasures and your pleasures will always be a thousandfold."

And he did . . . and they were.

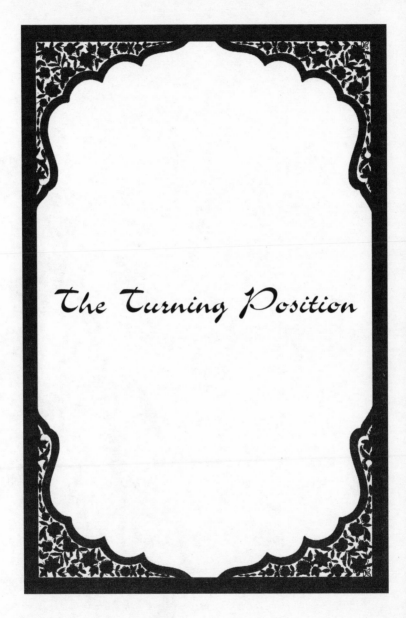

The Turning Position

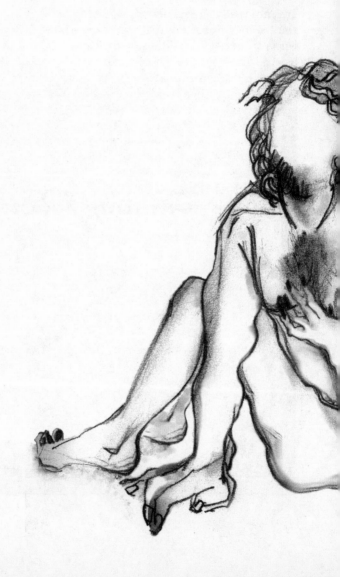

The Turning Position

Paravrittaka
Kama Sutra

It is not really agreed upon how to do the "turning position" or the "spin". Some say that the man, while having intercourse, turns around while still inside the woman, while she grasps him around the back the whole time. In this variation of the position, the woman provides a bit of help as the man effects his spin. She uses her hands on his back and waist to keep him stable and keep the turn easy and smooth.

Others say that the man is seated and grasping the woman from behind, so that while with her back to him, she turns around from back to front so that she is facing him. This position then changes again to a rear-entry position with the woman in control. This is, again, done without the man withdrawing. Penetration is constant while these spins are occurring.

Either way, the turning position is one that requires practice and consideration for the partner. Because it relies on absolute trust, this can be one of the most intimate poses. It is not a position you would attempt with a new sexual partner. Perhaps this is a position best accomplished when there is great love for the other person. Any kind of aggression, even just unchecked passion, could injure the other person.

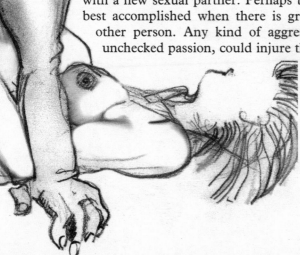

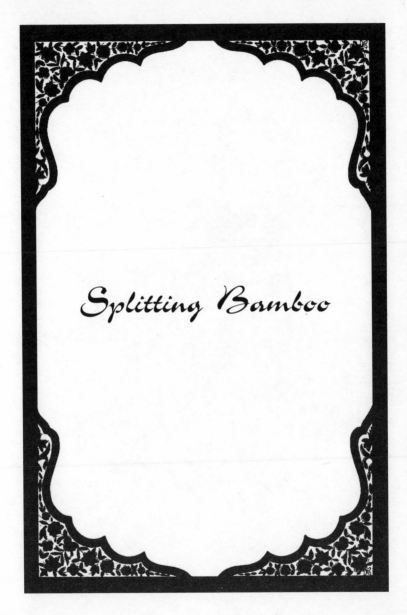

Splitting Bamboo

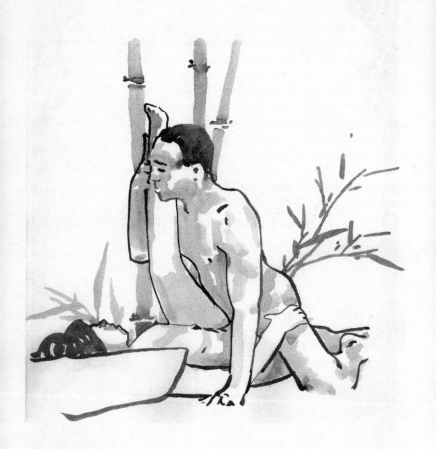

Splitting Bamboo

Venudaritaka
Kama Sutra

When a woman places one of her legs on her lover's shoulder, and stretches the other out, and then places the latter on his shoulder, and stretches out the other, and continues to do so alternately, it is called the "splitting of a bamboo" or "the broken flute". The act of removing the leg from the shoulder and alternating it with the other leg is called "breaking the flute". This is another position which requires intense flexibility on the woman's part, as she is stretched in opposite directions, and all the while, sexual congress is taking place. If she is not flexible enough, this could cause her injury. Penetration is deep and kisses and nibbling are possible, and encouraged, in this position.

The Tale of Music in Silence

as told by Craig Sorensen

The sun had just ascended over the rooftops of the houses that sat safely out of reach across the great river of the Goddess Ganga, the Ganges. Preeti was grateful that she lived so close to the sacred river, and she hoped her husband's famous deep sleep would sustain him in the world of dreams until she could accomplish her task and return to his side.

Few were at the riverbank this morning. Perhaps not many needed to cleanse their bodies and their souls in the sacred river. Preeti's body was certainly clean.

Greatest God Shiva was sure to forgive his precious consort Parvati should she cleanse her soul here. But Parvati would not have transgressed in this way. Preeti closed her hands about her wide cinnamon cheeks and let fresh tears roll from her amber eyes. They gushed so fast that they pooled at Preeti's feet to form a stream to the sacred river.

On a rock near the river, an old man of leather skin sat cross-legged with only a sash about his hips. He played a sacred tune on the most beautiful carved flute Preeti had ever seen. His eyes gleamed with the reflections of the dawn. Preeti denied further tears like a greedy cloud and returned to her objective.

The sun now sparkled in the waves of the river, casting an orange so rich it could only spell the presence of the gods. The smoothness of Preeti's skin and the brightness of her pearly teeth remained hidden under a plain sari, which wrapped around the length of her lithe body, terminating as a cover for her head. The white colour of the sari hinted that she was in mourning. Its tattered plainness inferred she was poor. She even walked hunched over to hide her distinctive height.

The flute player continued his song as Preeti edged to the riverbank. She turned back and watched him. She loved music so, and his was divine. But the musician remained focused on the distant sunrise as he played. He did not return her long gaze.

The song grew more mournful, as if it were speaking the pain within Preeti's soul.

She knelt before Ganga and splashed the sacred waters in her face beneath the protection of the sari. "Please cleanse me, sacred goddess. Do not forsake me." She walked deeper into the water.

Before this day when Preeti walked to the river alone, Chanda had become Preeti's dearest friend. As if conjured by the greatest magician, Chanda had appeared in Preeti's life, and had listened to her secret woes. She led Preeti to what made the young bride's heart feel hollow. Preeti was lonely. Though her husband was learned in many arts, he spoke very little and Preeti cherished the sounds of voices as music. The many sounds she knew in the house of her father had been replaced with the enveloping silence of the house of her husband.

Chanda listened to each detail, and returned sympathy in a soft, sweet voice like music. Chanda penetrated this silence that bedevilled Preeti, but that was not all Chanda brought as a gift to her new friend. She brought a man who knew the music in the spoken word. And he was very wise. He was a young man, younger even than Preeti, but he seemed to understand so much of her secrets: secrets Preeti herself never knew.

Preeti felt the pulse of the Ganges tug her legs while she cleansed. She prayed Ganga would have enough purifying waters to cleanse the deep sins. Again Preeti succumbed to tears, and allowed her voice to chop with the soft rhythm of the river.

In the background, the old man played his flute with an intensity that now bordered on ferocity. Though Preeti was learned in music, she had scarcely heard such a song. It was sad, but it repeated itself in an odd way. It was a different sort of music, beautiful and mournful but harsh. It was so powerful, so mournful that it stole the very tears from her eyes.

Then the player stopped altogether. He said something loudly, but Preeti did not understand. The music rose again from the beginning. The man's voice became accusing, and Preeti wondered who he was talking to. She looked back to see him simply hold the flute in front of his face. He frowned as he stared at it. Not another soul was near.

He resumed playing only to abruptly stop, then there was a horrible snap. Preeti wheeled around quickly to see the broken halves of the flute in the old man's knurled hands.

Preeti felt a sobbing sadness so deep that tears would not quench them. He had as suddenly stolen her woeful song as he had given it. She raced from the water to the musician who had now dropped the halves of the flute to the ground. As he patted his hands, she approached him. "Sir, why do you destroy so beautiful a flute?"

He paused and studied her face. For a moment the expressive lines on his face showed a surprise that seemed to mirror Preeti's feeling when she saw the flute snapped. "Young woman, it is not your concern."

Preeti felt exalted and sacred somehow despite the freshly washed sin that swelled in the river behind her. While it was true that it was not her concern, she felt suddenly that it was. "I must understand."

The old man's eyes narrowed to midday sunlight slits in the soft, pleasant dawn. Preeti knew he was willing her to shrink from him, but she did not. She dared not. She stood as firm as she had when she had fought with her older brother as a girl. The old man drew a deep breath. The impatience in his eyes eased to a quiet patronage. "You truly do not know why?"

"I do not. The music was beautiful."

"Perhaps to your ear, but this music comes to me from the gods. They tell me how it should sound."

"And?"

"This flute would not play it properly. I have endured it so many times trying. I could endure it no more. I have been most patient."

Preeti was bold. "How do you know it was the fault of the flute?"

The old man's eyes widened to deep anger, then he smiled softly, wryly. "You say it was my playing that was bad, girl?"

"I do not. I only wish to understand."

"I see you dress plainly. Your garment implies you are older and poorer than you are. I thought you a widow, though now I can tell you are not."

Preeti folded the top of her sari down towards her eyes. "I am just a poor woman, I have suffered—"

"I am certain you have suffered, but no poor woman speaks or acts as you do."

"I have my reasons to appear poor. I am poor in heart today."

"I understand this. You see," he said as he pointed to the two pieces of flute on the ground, "this was a flute, as beautifully carved as any I have seen and, dear girl, I have seen many. And yet, it would not play the sacred music. It might have been worthy of redemption, though."

"What makes you sure it was not?"

The old man grinned as if he had coaxed a stubborn elephant across a raging river. "Were it worthy of redemption, it would not have allowed me to break it. I have a much simpler flute that plays beautifully, and I will see if it has the will to play this sacred song." He was gone so quickly that she could not utter another word.

She first wondered if this man was real, then she looked down at the broken flute. She picked it up and held it together at the frays along the break. Indeed, were it worthy of redemption, it would not break.

The walk back to the home of her husband seemed eternally longer than the walk she had so recently taken from the home to the river. The old man's music, so perfect in her mind, was flawed. The perfectly beautiful carved flute was flawed. It now lay in two pieces on the ground, fit only to coax a fire. What sense did that make?

Dipaka was a young man, very handsome in the face. He had the gift of words – he was a fine poet, worthy of the royal court – and his warm words cut through the silence of Preeti's life. From the moment Chanda introduced Dipaka to Preeti, she was mesmerized by the power of his soft, lyrical voice. She did not mind that he was such a small, frail man, because his words and music were huge.

Preeti resisted Dipaka's charms fervently. She was a married woman, and Chanda had said he wanted only to be Preeti's dear friend. But his kisses were like his words. Though he did not embody even a fraction of the worldly strength of Preeti's husband Anil, Dipaka filled the void in her heart that he had so meticulously revealed. Dipaka gave Preeti many gifts.

Chanda knew Anil's flaws and reminded Preeti that she deserved to have her soul warmed in a way that only Dipaka could find. Preeti remained at a proper distance from her new man friend, but there came a day, just one day before the morning she went to the river and met the flute player, when Dipaka recounted a poem of passion. The words stirred her deeply, and coaxed the sort of moisture in her *yoni* that her husband would have to work mightily with his hands to create. Such magic, stirring a woman's inner desire with only the benefit of spoken words!

The poet continued his words and slowly began to smooth Preeti's leg beneath her fine, brightly coloured silk sari. His fingers caressed ever higher up her thigh, but it was the words that made her moisture flow like the sacred river Ganges whose song played just outside the window to Dipaka's elegant, secret chamber.

Dipaka's fingers found her *yoni* and played in the soft fur that adorned it. His small fingers plied softly at the magic nub and led her body to feel the strange fear in her core extend out to all her limbs. She felt her will try to fight, but her body went as limp as a dead woman. His hand was cool and his kisses as wet as her *yoni*.

Her hand grew a will of its own as it eased down his chest to his groin. His *lingam* was small, but fiercely stiff. She first pulled her hand away from it, but Dipaka encouraged her hand back down over it. Preeti wanted to stop, but his forbidden hardness felt good in her touch, and her *yoni* yearned to be filled. As Dipaka unravelled her sari, Preeti surrendered any resistance.

She had recently taken to denying her husband, willing him to become a poet and a master of words with her own silence. But Anil's only poetry was the occasional plea that she open her body to him. She denied him, making any convenient excuse. Despite the fact that Anil's need had now been growing like bamboo in spring, she continued to deny him.

Now, Dipaka's hardness was to Preeti as a cup of finest rice to a starving peasant. She stretched nude across Dipaka's large, soft bed. She opened her legs just enough as he removed his garment and kneeled between them. As he entered her, his *lingam* felt like one of Anil's fingers, but not as strong. Then it became as strange as a poison root would feel in her mouth. Though she was hungry for the filling and needed to be sated, she hated the terrible bitterness. She began to feel she must cast the small man away from her body, and yet the magic nub at the entrance to her *yoni* caved under the insistence of Dipaka's deliberate fingers.

Her soul willed him away though her body could not, and it was as if the Goddess heard her plea. Dipaka lasted for less than ten beats of her fluttering heart before his *lingam* suddenly sprang from her *yoni* and exploded across her tight stomach.

Guilt shadowed over her like a great black veil. Dipaka tried to console her as she smeared his hot white juice from her body and hastily dressed. "Preeti, please, stay at my side. I am sorry that it did not last. I must love you yet again! I will caress you with my hands!"

But for all his poetry, Dipaka had shown that he did not know her heart. He certainly did not know she was grateful that he had released so easily.

Chanda had once come to her to help Preeti find that hole in her heart, and it seemed that this elegant small woman had indeed done so mightily. She had brought her Dipaka, a man who Preeti thought would certainly fill that hole with joy. No, she did not want to love him in the body, but she wanted to fill that hole. But the hole was now filled with the heavy weight of an obelisk stone. Dipaka's *lingam* singed her *yoni* as poison burns a throat, as fire burns flesh.

Anil's words were few and only of the practical sort. He did not seem to appreciate the joys of music. Sounds to him were just sounds, where to Preeti they were all music, and all sacred.

She recalled this as she walked back to the house of her husband, shrouded in her shame and her soul choking on the sudden infidelity, how Anil and she had made love sometimes twice a day until Chanda came. Preeti recalled how she could hear the song of the bird, the sound of the river, the cackling of monkeys, the plodding of footsteps and be in joy.

She had known joy before Chanda, but somehow she had become convinced that she had not known a single joy since her marriage. It was true that his silence disturbed her, but this had suddenly grown like the roots of a banyan tree in her chest. Dipaka had grown this feeling like tending a garden of the most insidious weeds.

Preeti sought out Chanda to help pull the black veil from her heart. She thought that Chanda would help her understand how she might cleanse herself after this most ignoble assignation. Chanda had been so understanding.

But Chanda was as cold as the bitterest winter in the north mountains. "Preeti, you wanted music and poetry, Dipaka gave you that."

"But he took things I did not want to give."

"Did you think he would give you his poetry for free? I have no more time for you, silly woman."

This rattled Preeti's ear as if her head had been inside a bell as it rang. Preeti was not wise in the world, but her wisdom grew manifold now. Dipaka's only objective was seduction. Chanda was no more than a vehicle to carry him across the threshold of Preeti's propriety. She was the earth to anchor Dipaka's deadly root.

Chanda waved Preeti off as if she were the lowliest servant. She ran from Chanda's house until she came into sight of the large, elegant home of her practical husband. A torrent broke in her eyes. She was as a great storm, fearful and dark, until she composed herself.

Her husband came to her that night and tried again to convince her that, as his wife, she must fill his need. Now she refused, not because she wanted to change him, but because she was unclean.

As Preeti approached the home of her husband after cleansing in the river goddess' offering, she considered what she might say to explain her absence. Perhaps she should just tell the truth, or at least part of it, that she needed to bathe in the Ganges.

But she was surprised when she entered the sleep chamber to see her husband, his enormously warm body big and stretched naked over the bed. His dark buttocks curved like two powerful mountains, then cut to a fine dark valley, only to swell up to the mighty ridges of his shoulder blades. He looked so handsome. He was indeed a beautiful man, with long lean muscles powerful enough to challenge a tiger. He rolled onto his back, and his *lingam*, huge and swollen, glistened purple in the slits of soft morning sun that incised the chamber.

Preeti felt so badly that she had denied him, and she now wondered why he did not take his need into his own hand and find some relief. He was certainly entitled. Indeed, he would be entitled in taking a servant girl at any moment he wished, and yet he had not.

The feeling of guilt, like poison expelling from her stomach, made Preeti feel dizzy, but her need made her feel strangely powerful. She stripped the plain sari from her body and approached the bed.

"Preeti, my wife," Anil said, his eyes open. A smile curled over his lips, seeing that she was looking upon his stiff *lingam*. It became obvious he worried that she might yet again deny him. Preeti thought to be playful, but knew it would be far too cruel, especially with what she had done the previous day. She smiled broadly, displaying her white teeth, then she lay to his side and began to caress his *lingam*.

It was as hot as fire and felt magical in her cool hands. Anil's hips moved into the soft strokes of her palms, which massaged his foreskin, then polished the shiny head beneath this hood, which circled it like the sari had circled her body. She twisted his *lingam* from side to side as she stroked, and his voice emanated from a deep place in his chest. The harder she twisted it, the more he moaned. He grabbed her body and held her tight while she stroked him in her strong hands.

Her *yoni* flowed like the sacred river and she eased beneath Anil and spread her legs wide. Her starving need had only grown since the awful dalliance with Dipaka. She closed her eyes as she always did when she made love, listening to the sounds of their connection. She prayed to the gods that the image of her small lover be forced from the backs of her eyelids like an uninvited guest removed by the hand of a burly servant. But it seemed Dipaka wanted to stay.

Preeti opened her eyes and held the gaze of Anil. His dark eyes, bathed in golden sun flexed, and Dipaka was as if he had never been.

Preeti's whole body writhed. Carried on a deep breath, her voice began the song of the broken flute just as she had heard it, right or wrong. The tip of Anil's thick *lingam* entered her and she continued to hum, knowing that while it might not be the right song for the old man, it was right for her.

Anil smiled. "The song is beautiful, my wife." He penetrated her to full depth.

Her heart leapt. She had never thought to give a song for Anil because he was so quiet.

Her body was perfectly matched to his. His size could be confidently folded inside her long waist. She savoured his contours as his swollen balls slapped the bottom of her *yoni*. Anil propped himself up with his arms spread wide, his thick muscles bulging to hold his chest so near that his hairs tickled her smooth flesh. Despite the desperation that Anil certainly felt, he was slow in his loving. A starving man savouring every bite of finer food than would be found on a prince's table, and this was something Anil knew a little about.

The great *lingam* slid in and out of Preeti, but she resisted the urge to close her eyes and just listen to the sounds while savouring the sensation. She forced her eyes to stay locked deep within his, tightly connected. There was a massive power in his gaze. It stole her breath as he slowly pumped. It was the gaze of a hungry tiger prowling near a river. Anil's deep, black eyes penetrated into her soul, and she felt as if the cleansing from her soul that started in the Ganges was being expedited. She dare not take her eyes from him as his *lingam* stretched her *yoni* in stroke after magnificent stroke.

Suddenly, she drew her left leg up along his thigh, across his hip and to the great muscles beside his ribs, then she curled her knee to his chest. His mouth gaped open and his eyes widened in surprise. Preeti could feel a smile she would never be able to restrain open on her face. After several strokes, she drew her left leg back down, then hooked her toes under his thigh while her left leg travelled up until her knee rested atop his heart, and she counted ten great throbs. She began alternating this motion again and again, feeling his hardness curl at different magical angles like the stars suddenly loosed and curving from side to side in the sky.

Anil's usual silent loving gave way as his deep voice announced his pleasure. It was a pleasure so broad that it consumed Preeti beyond the significant pulse in her *yoni*. She made her moves stronger and faster until her hips began to hurt, but she pressed on. Even the pain was joyful, as the pain of curling Anil's *lingam* in her writhing grip seemed to bring him the greatest joy. His voice became louder and louder, as if he were a great bell announcing a festival. It became a yell, and she watched every mighty turn of his face, even as the glow of deep release exploded from her depths.

Her legs collapsed to his sides and the sweat on her body continued to drain. She fought for breath, as did he. His body was a magnificent, weighty heap above her, a fallen statue carved by the greatest master, crushing her breasts and her waist and her groin. She gripped his chest so tightly that he lost his breath. His *lingam* finally softened, but remained for a time cradled softly in her deep *yoni*. Finally, it was pushed gently from her, and he rose up on his arms and looked down her body admiringly.

"Were my *lingam* a flute, you would certainly have broken it, my wife."

"That was never a concern for a good flute that plays the sacred songs right, my husband," Preeti said, and she flashed a bold smile.

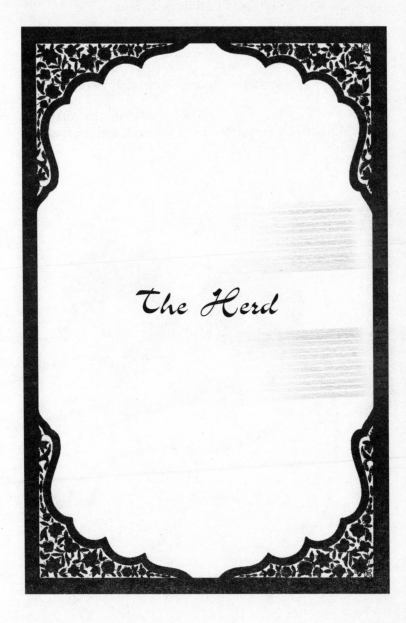

The Herd

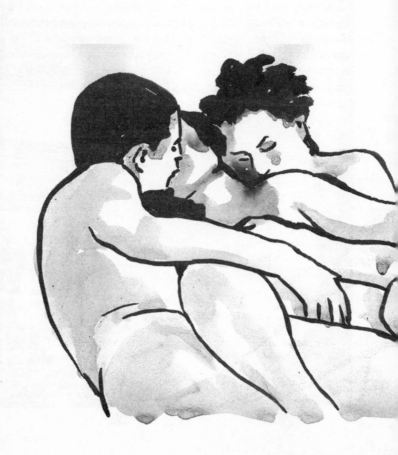

The Herd

Goyuthika
Kama Sutra

During the Gupta dynasty, when Vatsyayana compiled his *Kama Sutra*, it was not unheard of for a prince or a king, not only to have many wives, but to have relations with many of them at once. The civilizing of sex which is advocated in the *Kama Sutra* means that a man had already gained control over his senses, and would therefore be able to participate in a sex marathon without being completely overcome and exhausted. He could control himself, indulge in foreplay, eroticism and sensuality. Sexual intercourse was not the only weapon in his arsenal. Touching, kissing, embracing, nibbling, playfully slapping and marking, could go on for hours if the king so desired.

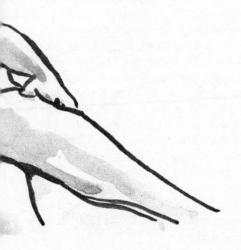

The Tale of the Playing Elephant

as told by Teresa Noelle Roberts

All customs start somewhere. What follows is the tale of why, when one man and several women play together, they imitate the antics of animals, making each other laugh even as they make each other cry out in pleasure.

Once, long ago in India, there were three friends who were unfortunate in their marriages.

Meena's parents had chosen for her a man in the prime of his life, but tragically, he had been felled by a stroke after they had been married for only a few weeks and now she was more nursemaid than wife. Jaimala's husband longed for a houseful of children, but it seemed unlikely to ever happen; his preference for the charms of other men was so strong that after three years of marriage, he had succeeded in lying with her only a handful of times. And Adarna might be most unfortunate of all, for she had been happily married to a man she loved and who loved her. But her beloved had been gone more than a year on a journey that should have lasted no more than a few months – enough time that Adarna knew he had likely met with a fatal accident, but not enough for her to accept this sorrow and move on.

The three women were wise enough to realize that, being young, healthy and frustrated, they were all too likely to fall for the first rogue who plied them with clever words and soft caresses. And so they made a pact: they would keep each other from making the mistake of taking an unworthy lover, one who did not know tact and honesty and the myriad ways of pleasuring a woman. (If one is risking not only reputation but karma, it's best to think it through carefully and be sure the joy gained is worth the risk.) If one of them started to falter, the others would do everything in their power to strengthen her resolve and judgment.

Sometimes that meant holding the one who was having the worst day as she wept, or weaving flower garlands and giggling like girls, or talking far into the night.

And sometimes the three women would find some place that was private and quiet. And they would loosen their sashes and their bright wrapped garments would fall to the ground like mounds of flowers and the three women would entwine their limbs and lie down together, the heavy silk of their long dark hair enveloping them, but not disguising how they made love to one another. Soft lips kissed, and round, ripe breasts pressed together, and hennaed hands petted and caressed, and plump golden thighs scissored. Soon it would be hard to tell where one woman began and the next started. Soon the air filled with the mating cries of some curious creature – cooing like a dove, then rising to a sharp pitch like a monkey or howling like a panther.

And if it was not quite what any of the women craved, for all of them preferred men's bodies to women's, still it was the blessing of another human's touch.

One day when the scent of flowers mingled pleasantly with the spicy fragrance of saag paneer and korma, and smoke from cooking fires, and the warm, earthy smell of the neighbourhood cows, the three women made their way to the river. They balanced dirty laundry on their heads, but their path took them far from the place where the other women gathered to wash clothes and gossip. All of them had been feeling the itch, had been cataloguing men whose eyes made promises while their mouths made small talk, had been fantasizing about what had been, or what might have been, and they knew they were reaching a point where one of them might do something regrettable if she didn't have some release for her tension.

And that was their plan for the afternoon.

Like many good plans, it worked, but not at all as anticipated.

As they rounded a bend in the path, Jaimala put her hands out, stopping her two friends. "Listen," she mouthed.

Something was splashing about in the river.

"Young elephant," Meena whispered, but shook her head almost as quickly as she'd spoken. Elephants travelled in herds, and while that was enough noise for a solitary elephant calf, it wasn't nearly enough for the calf and all his friends and relations.

Then they heard a noise that no elephant could make: laughter.

The hearty, raucous laughter of a young man.

"If boys are sporting here," Adarna said, "we should go."

"Definitely. We should go have a look," Jaimala proclaimed.

Adarna grinned. "Tempting. I swear I've forgotten what a well-built, well-hung lad looks like, let alone what one feels like."

"At least you knew," Meena said with a sigh. Even in good health, her husband had been on the scrawny side, with a *lingam* that, while functional, did not impress with its size and beauty.

"I'd love to take a peek," Jaimala said. "As long as it's not my husband and his latest lover." Then she shrugged. "And if it is, what matter? They're both handsome men, and I might as well take what pleasure I can find from them."

So quietly, they followed the sounds down the path. Setting their laundry bundles down, they parted the undergrowth on the riverbank.

Only one young man was sporting in the water – but that one was well worth a stolen look.

"Holy gods," Meena exclaimed in a fierce whisper. "That's Vikram! I'd heard he's in town because his grandmother is looking for a bride for him." Vikram, orphaned as a lad, had been sent to live with his father's brother in a neighbouring village.

"Vikram?" Adarna said. "Can't be. He's just a boy and that's a man. A beautiful man."

"Not any more," Meena said. "I can't remember how long it's been since we've seen him, but he's all grown up."

"And he looks like Krishna," Jaimala breathed.

He was just on the verge of manhood, not a boy any more, but barely old enough to be seeking a wife. Still, he had a man's stature, paired with a boy's coltish grace and soft-edged beauty. His golden body glistened with water, his damp curls glinted in the sun as if they were woven with jewels, and whatever trade his uncle was training him in had given him lean, strong muscles.

While seeing a man's bare chest was commonplace – only in the coolest weather would a man cover himself with more than a jaunty drape to accent the width of his shoulders or hide any paunch – seeing a fine one unexpectedly was a pleasure, one heightened by the naughty sense that they were spying.

He wasn't exactly bathing, and he wasn't exactly swimming, just splashing about. He looked good doing it, though, and the women were happy to watch his antics in hopes that he'd step into shallower water and give them a still better view. Such a fine young man must have an equally fine *lingam*, but the water hid it.

He ducked under the water, then popped up and squirted water from between his teeth, with his arm cocked at a funny angle in front of his face.

"What in the world?"

"Elephant," Adarna said, giggling softly. "He's playing elephant like a child. Guess he's still a boy at heart."

Jaimala tried not to laugh out loud.

She failed.

First Adarna joined in, then Meena.

Vikram froze, his arm still in "elephant trunk" pose, and stared at the riverbank. He probably couldn't see the three women, but he'd obviously heard them. A flush ruddied his cheeks and he grinned sheepishly, like a child caught in a prank.

Then he pulled himself together, apparently trying to cover his embarrassment with good manners. "Good afternoon, ladies," he said and took a step forward in greeting.

Which brought him into shallower water.

His *lingam* was as well formed as the rest of him, and if most of Vikram looked like he wanted to crawl under a log and hide when he realized the show he was providing, his *lingam* was completely unembarrassed. If anything, it swelled with pride at the idea of having an audience.

And then Jaimala was moved to do something that surprised even her.

She stepped out from the underbrush and dropped the light cotton *uttariya* that shielded her head and upper body from the sun, baring her glossy black braid and the soft but strong lines of her shoulders, making it impossible to ignore her lush breasts. "Mind if I join you?" she asked. "That looks like fun, and it's so hot and sticky."

"Jaimala, what would your husband say?" Adarna whispered urgently.

"He'd be in the water already – and in Vikram too, if the boy would have him. And your husband's lost on the Silk Road and Meena's, poor man, doesn't remember his own name half the time." She took two more steps towards the river, started unwrapping her skirt. "But we're here and hot and sweaty and we might as well go for a swim like we'd planned." She tactfully didn't mention they'd planned for rather more than swimming.

She swayed her way to the water's edge, walking like a goddess moving among mere mortals, and, once there, she unwrapped her draperies and posed naked but for her necklaces and earrings, and the bracelets on her wrists and ankles.

She could have been one of the statues in the temple come to life, naked and sacred and giving her beauty as a gift.

Even to Meena and Adarna, who had seen their friend naked many times, Jaimala seemed to glow with erotic radiance. Vikram stared, stammered something inaudible. He was grinning from ear to ear, but it was a slightly terrified grin.

Adarna thought, and she thought fast.

If Jaimala were left to her own devices, she might do something she'd regret later. Vikram was delicious, but taking a very young lover who hadn't been properly tutored in the discreet way to carry on an affair could lead to gossip and heartbreak. Jaimala would be as much of a scandal as her boy-loving husband. More so, because fair or not, the world was always harder on women who had ill-advised love affairs.

So they had to stay and keep an eye on Jaimala.

Of course that meant keeping an eye on Vikram as well, but if she and Meena were there to remind Jaimala of their pact, that was all anyone would be keeping on him.

Just eyes. No hands, no lips and certainly no *yonis*. Just a little flirting and banter that would be good for their spirits and the young man's ego.

"A swim sounds delightful," Adarna said. As she started to undress, she turned to Meena, trying to convey what she was thinking.

Luckily, Meena seemed to understand. "We walked out here so we could relax and cool down while we washed our clothes. We might as well."

And soon all three women were naked and in the water.

Vikram's eyes grew wider, his face flushed darker – and his *lingam* got bigger and harder. For a moment, he was frozen on the spot, his straining, twitching *lingam* the only part of him moving.

Then he chuckled and started splashing the three women. Under this playful cover, he and his swollen *lingam* retreated into deeper water.

The fire of Jaimala's lust cooled a bit in the face of the more immediate need for playful revenge. Older than Vikram or not, she was not so old that she'd forgotten the cardinal rule of water fights: keep them going until everyone involved is wet, laughing, and gasping for breath. "Ladies," she said, "get him!"

And they did.

At first they were just splashing.

Then Vikram dunked Jaimala.

Adarna had resolved there would be no touching, but some things were not to be borne, so the three women ganged up and dunked him.

And it was all innocent and playful, and yet it wasn't, because every time Vikram looked at the women, his eyes were full of desire as well as mischief, and every time the women looked at him – or at each other, for that matter – it was the same. And when they touched, even in jest, they all felt the heat.

Then, somehow, they fell into doing elephant imitations – spraying each other and trumpeting and laughing like children. "If we're all elephants," Vikram said between bouts of laughter, "that makes me the bull elephant and you the cows. And you know what that means."

"You protect us fiercely from hunters and tigers?" Adarna suggested, trying desperately to lead them back to safer territory.

Vikram snorted.

"In any case," Jaimala said, drawing closer, "you're not a calf any more, but I'm not sure you're the lead bull yet. One of the young ones around the fringes of the herd, perhaps, waiting his turn with the females."

"That's not very kind."

"Answer me honestly," Jaimala said. "Do you know what to do with one woman, let alone three?"

He sputtered. Looked away and then looked back again, meeting each woman's eyes before he answered. "One woman, yes, although I'm sure I still have much to learn from the right teacher – or teachers. Three women would be a challenge, but it would be a challenge I'm willing to die trying to meet."

And something about his earnestness and charm won them. Or perhaps it was the playful antics they'd shared, a welcome respite from the difficulties of their lives.

Jaimala looked at Meena and Adarna. "What do you think, my friends? They say that when you're ready to learn, a teacher will appear – so perhaps this was meant to be." Not that she knew so much of what transpired between men and women herself, but she knew how to satisfy a woman's lust in various delicate ways that might not occur to a young man with an insistent *lingam*, so she was sure she could teach him something.

Meena thought of the few times she and her husband had made love before he'd fallen ill. She'd learned just enough of the pleasures of the flesh to know what she was missing. But her husband was not nearly as handsome and virile and full of energy as Vikram. And she thought of her long restless nights spent tending to a man turned prematurely old and impotent and crippled. "You're right," she said. "It's a sign."

Adarna took the longest to ponder her decision. For her, taking a lover would mean admitting she didn't believe her husband was coming back. On the other hand, theirs had been a passionate marriage; when they weren't making love, they were walking around in a daze of sated lust, with love bites on their throats and foolish grins on their faces. Her heart wasn't ready to let go, but her body insisted that it was time – not time to give up praying for her husband's return, but time to let herself live.

She took a deep breath, tried to say yes, found she couldn't speak and simply nodded instead.

Tears filled her eyes but desire filled her body. And before she lost her nerve, she wrapped her arms around Vikram and kissed him on the mouth, biting at his lower lip until he moaned and ground against her.

A heat she thought she'd never feel again surged through her, and if it made her want to weep, it also made her want to sing.

Meena's arms circled her waist. Meena's hands slipped between Adarna and Vikram, one cupping Adarna's breast, the other toying with Vikram's flat nipple.

Jaimala was behind Vikram, reaching between his legs to cup his testicles.

Vikram bucked forward, pushing his hard *lingam* against Adarna, rubbing it between her legs until she was trembling so hard she could scarcely stand. It would be so easy to wrap one leg around him, open herself to him, let him push inside her *yoni* so she could once again revel in the feel of a man inside her, the pleasure of male and female joined.

But that wouldn't be fair to her friends. They'd shared joys and sorrows and orgasms. They'd share Vikram properly.

"I think," she whispered, "this will work better on dry land."

On the riverbank Adarna instructed Vikram to lie on his back. Vikram, being a clever young man, grinned and said, "And then I can have my hands free for the others."

Jaimala smiled. "I have a better idea. I can kneel across your face. You'll be able to lick between my legs as if you were licking mango juice off your fingers, which is one of the most wonderful pleasures a woman can experience." The three women shot heated glances at each other, for they had licked each other to climax many times and just hearing Jaimala's words made them remember that delight.

"Don't be too greedy, Jaimala," Meena said. "I'll want a turn at that."

"I'll make sure you all have a turn at everything," Vikram promised. "This is a taste of paradise for me and I want to make sure it's the same for all of you."

And for all her doubts before they'd actually got started, Adarna didn't hesitate to straddle Vikram's narrow hips and sink down, with a lascivious twisting of her hips, onto his *lingam.*

And it was not her beloved husband's, but it filled her almost as deliciously – to be honest, it was an even nicer size, even though it didn't feel as perfect because it wasn't part of the man she loved – and for a few seconds she was troubled by guilt.

Then her long-starved body took over and she began to move on him, swaying her hips and riding him hard, grinding her tenderest flesh against him, stroking at her own nipples because his hands were busy with the other women. She closed her eyes and let the sensations fill her. With her eyes closed, she could pretend. Pretend it was her husband inside her. Pretend it was the best of all possible worlds, that he had come home safely to her but sympathized with her beloved, lonely, sexually deprived friends and was making love to all of them.

A cry of pleasure made her open her eyes.

Meena had taken one of Vikram's hands and had put it where she needed it, riding three of his fingers as if the fingers were a *lingam.* With her own delicate fingers, she was stroking herself, making sure to squeeze maximum pleasure from the moment. She was obviously close to her release already, writhing and panting and making small noises that Adarna knew well from times when her hand had been the one bringing her friend to climax.

Jaimala was sitting on Vikram's face, crying out encouragement and occasional instructions. Her nipples were hard and dark and her face was contorted with need and desire; to Adarna she'd never looked more beautiful.

Adarna leaned forward to kiss her friend and, as she did, her body found exactly the perfect angle against Vikram's, the angle at which his *lingam* stroked all the most sensitive points inside her and her clitoris and the lips of her sex ground against his pubic bones. Kissing Jaimala and pinching at Jaimala's nipples, Adarna rode Vikram faster, unable to stop herself, pushing herself towards the satisfaction she craved.

And as she reached it, she clamped down around Vikram, the muscles of her *yoni* milking at him. His hips bucked up, and he cried out his pleasure against Jaimala's soft flesh, and something about that brought her off. Meena, who'd already been close, tumbled after them.

"So much . . . for everyone trying everything . . ." Meena panted. She sounded petulant, and understandably so, for the pleasure Vikram had given her was the closest in kind to what she could give herself alone in the dark.

"Don't worry, beautiful ladies," Vikram said. "With such loveliness around me, I'll be ready to play again in no time."

Adarna slipped off him, glanced at his still-hard *lingam*. "I'd say you already are."

Jaimala laughed kindly. "My husband, who sadly for me is an expert in such matters, always says that younger men's great advantages are beauty and inexhaustible energy. It seems he's correct."

For many hours, the three woman and Vikram continued to sport in every possible combination. Sometimes he took one from behind, like an elephant with a female or a bull with a cow, while she licked at one of her friends and he caressed the other. Sometimes he and one of the women fucked while the other two assisted, licking and nibbling and caressing in various ways until they were frenzied with desire. Once the women lay one on top of the other and he entered their *yonis* in turn – teasing, but delightful. Once Jaimala, who'd learned of such things from her husband, thrust first one slim finger and then two into Vikram's bottom while he was plunging into Meena, making him growl and buck and scream like a wounded panther and explode with fierce joy.

And when they needed a respite, they would go and swim and splash and play, pretending to be elephants and water buffalo and cattle and other creatures, just because they were feeling young and giddy and happy to be alive.

Finally, though, it grew late and even a young man's energy wearied and the lust of three long-denied women grew sated.

The four of them dressed again and wandered back towards town, smiling and laughing together as lovers do.

As luck would have it, they ran into one of the town's biggest gossips, a widow who chose to spread rumours about other people's lovers rather than take one herself and find a more pleasant way to pass her time. "Well, don't you all look happy?" she said, a venomous edge to her voice. "What have you all been up to down at the river?" It was clear her sharp eyes had taken in the still-dry laundry, the love bites and scratches, and the dreamy smiles of those who have just made love. "Playing a bull among the cows with young Vikram?"

And Adarna, thinking fast, answered, "After a fashion, yes. We'd gone down to bathe and ran into Vikram, who was fooling around like boys do – even boys who are nearly grown. The next thing we knew we were all splashing each other and imitating elephants and mooing like cows and . . . just playing."

"Childish, I know," Meena said, "but good for the spirits. You know what hard work it is looking after my poor husband, and playing like a little girl did me a world of good. You should try it sometime, my dear."

"Indeed you should," Jaimala added. "You need more fun in your life."

The gossip sputtered and tried to think of something catty to say.

Then she looked at Vikram. The handsome lad grinned and winked at her and suddenly she was smiling back and looking much prettier and less irritable than she had a few seconds before.

"You have a point," the gossip said. "Perhaps my friends and I will go down tomorrow morning and see if playing elephants is as much fun now as it was when we were children."

And somehow the three friends never lost their good name, and when, several months later, Adarna's husband finally made his way home (his adventures are another story) not even the worst gossips breathed a word to suggest that she'd been anything but a model of propriety.

But Vikram settled in that town, although it was a long time before he married.

And among the widowed and unhappily married women, "playing elephants" and "bull and cows" became remarkably popular pastimes.

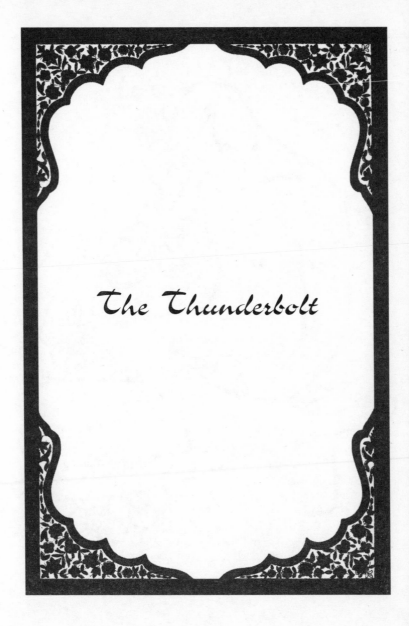

The Thunderbolt

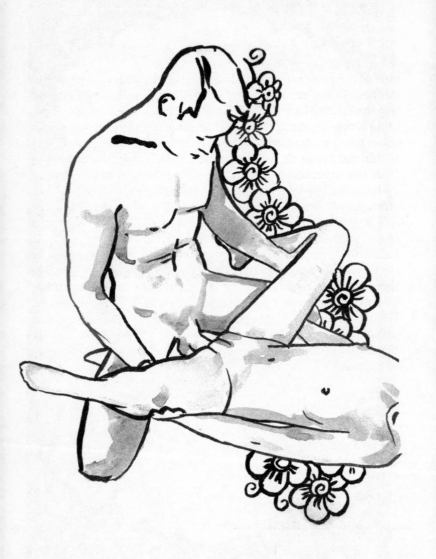

The Thunderbolt

Nirgbata
Kama Sutra

One of the responsibilities of a man is his arsenal of thrusts and strokes. These are to be studied and employed to seduce and win the hearts of women. This particular stroke has a hint of the same cruelty that may be found in some of the slaps (especially those using instruments). There is definitely a sadomasochism within the *Kama Sutra*, but it seems to be something stemming from the true nature of men and women's desires, rather than violence for the sake of violence (throughout the *Kama Sutra*, attitudes of nonviolence are encouraged).

The "thunderbolt" is also named the "buffet", "giving a blow" and a "blast of wind". It occurs when, during sex, the man withdraws his *lingam* completely, and even moves away slightly so that he is a small distance from his lover's sex. He then, however, moves with speed and, in one smooth, somewhat violent thrust, sinks his erect *lingam* back into his lover's *yoni*. He is to plunge back down into her vagina fast and hard. Some translators even go so far as to say he should "fall brutally downward", and they compare the strike from his *lingam* to that of a dart.

The Tale of the Thunderbolt

as told by Nikki Magennis

The day was cold, the air as sharp as a blade. Bhanu strode across the courtyard to the stables, and felt the frozen-hard ground through the soles of his fur-trimmed boots. When he swung himself onto his horse, he was grateful for the animal's warm body between his thighs. Hunting was hard in the cold season, the mountains around his home still wrapped in snow and the animals asleep or hiding deep in the forests. But Bhanu tired of the palace and soft cushions, grew irritable at the servants who scuttled under his feet. He thirsted for the dark tangle of the wood, the black earth and the thrill of the chase. More than anything, he relished escaping from the bustle and gossip of the court.

He knew he was the subject of many of the jokes whispered in the marble halls of the palace; Bhanu was twenty-seven and still unmarried, and people said that he spent too much time chasing deer and not enough chasing girls. The truth was that none of the perfumed women that visited the court stirred him. They came bedecked in jewelled saris, dripping with gold and pearls, their reddened lips stained with betel. Pushed forward by their eager parents, the girls smiled sweetly and lowered their eyes. At feasts and festivals, Bhanu watched the crowd of hopeful princesses indifferently. Their kohl-rimmed eyes and painted feet amused him. Like peacocks, he thought, beautiful to look at but with fickle temperaments and sharp claws.

He preferred to hunt, alone in the mountains. On that winter day as he rode towards the indigo-blue forest, Bhanu breathed in the sharp, sweet air of freedom and shivered with relief. With his bow over his shoulder and a full quiver at his hip he felt as though Shiva himself were riding alongside him. Bhanu took a shaded path through the dhok trees and headed uphill to the deep pool where the deer came to drink. Already he could hear the roar of the water, so much more pleasing to his ear than the jangle of the courtiers' stringed instruments. As he drew closer to the river, though, Bhanu pricked up his ears. There was an unfamiliar sound dancing through the trees, more playful than birdsong and brighter than the sound of the river – he heard laughter. The voices of girls. Bhanu slipped from the saddle and led his horse closer, stepping delicately to avoid cracking twigs. He moved like a panther, slipping silently through the trees.

Beyond the fringe of the tree trunks, Bhanu saw a sight that took his breath away. A group of eight girls moved like sparrows bathing – splashing and leaping and calling out from the shock of the cold water. They were a blur of brown-skinned bodies, writhing waist-deep in the river, with the glint of gold at their wrists and ankles. Bhanu was dazzled at the sight of so much ripe, naked flesh. Among the riot of girls, though, he noticed one that roared the loudest and splashed the hardest. She wore no jewellery – his eyes slid over her sleek, unadorned flesh as if it were carved out of amber. Her breasts were full and high, her hips and thighs shaped with the strong curves of a cat. Bhanu noticed her small nipples tight from the cold and the gooseflesh that stood out on her arms. She thrashed and flailed at the water, her mouth wide and her eyes screwed shut. Her face was heart shaped and her long loose hair hung to her waist; wet, it clung to her body in black inky streaks. And her voice – Bhanu thought he was hearing music for the first time as he listened to her laughter.

At that moment, Kamadeva, the god of love, loaded his bow. The string was made from bees and the arrow tipped with a lotus flower. He took aim at Bhanu and fired a shot straight into his heart.

Did Bhanu feel it? He felt afire – as though he'd swallowed hot coals and his whole body were burning.

Forgetting his huntsman's garb, he walked forward from the shelter of the forest. As he broke cover, screams rang out and there was a flurry of splashing as the women ran to where their clothes lay on the bank. Only one stayed where she was. She turned her heart-shaped face to look at Bhanu, curious

and defiant, a half-smile playing on her lips. Though the
water must have been icy, she didn't move but stood in the
whirling current of the river and met his stare with bright
brown eyes.

"What are you doing here?" The words fell from his mouth
before he could think, his voice unintentionally harsh. He
sounded like the arrogant prince he never wanted to be, Bhanu
thought with anguish, yet his eyes couldn't stop roving over the
girl's small, firm body: the high pointed breasts and the neat
arrow shape of her pubic hair.

"Praying to Krishna," the girl said, bold as a monkey. She
had her hands on her hips now, and although her teeth were
chattering she showed no trace of fear. Behind her, the other
girls yelped and giggled, whispered behind their hands and
stared at Bhanu as though he were the incarnation of the god
himself.

"For marriage!" called one, provoking another rush of
screaming laughter among the gaggle.

Bhanu ignored them. The girl in the river, who was now
shivering so much that her breasts shook, transfixed him. He
unfastened his fur-trimmed cloak and waded into the water. As
he approached, the others shouted and ran for the safety of the
forest, where they disappeared into the dark shadows between
the trees. Bhanu hardly noticed, for since he had first seen the
girl it was as though nobody else in the world existed. He
wrapped his cloak around her narrow shoulders and pulled it
tight over her nakedness.

"What is your name?" he asked, and this time his voice was
gentle.

"Mira," she replied.

"You're shaking," Bhanu said. "It's too cold for swimming!"

She looked up at him and her eyes glowed like embers. "So
warm me," she said, pushing past him and climbing onto the
shore. Bhanu watched as she lay on the bank, propping her head
with one hand and grinning at him.

"What's the matter, huntsman, scared of a naked cowherd?"

Bhanu blushed under his fur hat.

"What are you waiting for?"

Bhanu scrambled over to where she lay, and knelt in the snow.

"It's so cold I'm burning," Mira said. She reached out to touch Bhanu's face. After a moment's hesitation he caught her hand and kissed it. Closing his eyes, he took her fingertips to suck one at a time.

"Rubbing will work quicker," she said, moving his hands to her breasts.

Bhanu felt himself grow hard. He bent to kiss her mouth and it was as though the spring blossom burst into life around them, so sweet were her lips. Rolling on the grass, they drank each other in, their hips already undulating like snakes.

When Bhanu's *lingam* slid between Mira's legs and inside her, the frost on the grass under them melted. When she bit his shoulder and scratched at his back, the sun broke through the clouds. And as they cried out, reckless in their urgent joy, the birds stirred in the winter trees. Life sang out around them, rising from the earth like sparks, catching the trees alight, and spreading until the whole forest burned with sap and buds and spring.

They returned to the palace on horseback, Bhanu holding Mira on the saddle in front of him. She was still wrapped in his cloak. Her clothes, the cotton rags, were left on the banks of the river. That day, instead of taking home a deer, the prince brought the girl he'd chosen to be his wife.

The wedding was planned immediately, to the shock and agitation of the local gossips. The court ladies took charge of Mira's preparations, tutting at her rough hands and unbrushed hair. She had no dowry, they said, and no manners either. They shook their heads.

"A bride with no jewellery!" said the court poet, as she combed the tangles out of Mira's black tresses. "But we must make sure you are adorned just as the wife of a prince should be." She tied Mira's hair back and pinned a brooch at the knot.

Mira laughed out loud at the thought of herself as a rich lady. Bhanu had ordered a lavish trousseau that filled her chamber – saris and sandals and the sixteen kinds of make-up, as well as anklets and necklaces and vermilion. The vivid silks and the glittering gold were dazzling, and she felt itchy in her new clothes. The bracelets on her ankles made her feel like a falcon chained to its perch and she longed for spring grass and damp earth under her feet rather than cold marble. As the servants swarmed around her, Mira sighed.

"I'd rather be playing in the river," she said.

The lady helping her dress gave a bark of laughter. She tugged at Mira's sari and sucked her teeth. "Not easy, making a diamond from such a rough piece of rock. Give it time, though, and you will learn how to behave."

"Bhanu loves me," Mira said, "more than any diamond."

"Love and marriage are not the same thing," said the lady. "You are not a cowherd any more, girl. Hold still or you'll smudge your make-up."

A servant approached and knelt before them to apply the henna to Mira's hands. As they traced the patterns over her knuckles, Mira tried not to shake. She held her hands out in front of her, fingers spread wide.

Four hundred guests attended the party, keen to catch a glimpse of the prince with his cowherd. They were delightfully scandalized by Bhanu's bride – her evident poverty and peasant's manners. Even though she was dressed in silk, they said, you could see she walked like a barefoot country girl. And even though her hands were painted with henna, the ladies whispered that you could see the dirt under her fingernails.

Bhanu was in rapture the whole day. He loved the way Mira held herself, tensed like a cobra before it strikes. He loved her full lips, her brown eyes and the thought of making love to her on his soft, silk-covered bed.

After the ceremony Bhanu took Mira by the hand and led her to their bedchamber. The floor was strewn with flower petals and the heavy perfume of sandalwood filled the air. He pulled her towards him, but she twisted out of his embrace.

"What's the matter?" Bhanu asked.

Mira tugged irritably at the black beads on her wedding necklace. She moved to the window and pulled aside the silk curtain. "I can't see the moon," she said.

"Mira, my sweet, come to bed."

"I'm not tired."

"I'm not suggesting we sleep."

"I don't want to make love with you!" Mira cried, grabbing a handful of the curtain and ripping it from the window. "Leave me alone."

Bhanu, bewildered and confused, withdrew to his old quarters. He slept on his own that night. Mira sat up till dawn, wrapped in her rich silk clothes and adorned in her gold and pearls.

Over the summer, Mira became pale and sullen. She barely spoke to Bhanu, and refused to sleep in the same bed as him. Most of the time, she sat in her room, watching the sky. Though he brought her sweetmeats, flowers, jewellery and paintings, nothing seemed to interest her. Not pomegranates or lotus flowers, not a parrot or sherbet or musical instruments. Most of the time she sat as still as though she were carved out of wood, muttering under her breath, but sometimes Bhanu would enter her room to find her rocking back and forth, her eyes empty like those of an ascetic. If her husband tried to caress her, she would lash out and scratch him, and soon he learned to keep his distance.

As the days became hot and the gardens blossomed, Bhanu's worry deepened. He became frantic with longing for Mira. More than anything he wanted to feel her skin against his again, warm and yielding. He found himself staring at the servant girls as they did the laundry, the transparent cloth of their wet saris as the water splashed over their laps. Instead of riding into the mountains to go hunting, he paced the hallways of the palace, waiting for his wife to call for him.

The summer stretched out and sweltered, the landscape grew limp and scorched. Bhanu forgot the kites of the sun festival that year, and he ignored the Holi celebrations, shutting his doors to keep out the sounds of revelry. In the courtyard the ladies of the court ran riot, squirting men with coloured water and throwing flower garlands around the necks of the ones they wanted to take to bed. In the evening the whole palace seemed to overflow with the sounds of love – women's sighs and men's grunting. Bhanu's thoughts dwelled only on the silent room where Mira sat, watching the peepal tree in the garden and counting the clouds.

When the skies became heavy and Shravana approached with its hot storms and the promise of the monsoon, Bhanu could bear it no longer. He ordered his horse to be saddled and made preparations for a hunting trip. The rivers had shrunk to thin trickles in the summer heat, and he would have to travel high up the slopes to find the cool springs where the deer drank.

As he climbed onto his horse, there was a commotion from the palace courtyard. Bhanu turned to see Mira, in a whirl of yellow silk, running towards him. Servants followed her, shrieking with anxiety, and Bhanu saw she had left a glittering trail, dropping her sequinned shoes and her jewellery piece by piece on the grass. When she reached him, she was wearing only a top and her *dhoti* – a slight wrap of silk around her waist that she had tucked up between her legs.

"Take me with you," she said, and her eyes flashed darkly. Bhanu hesitated. Servants clucked round Mira, fussing over her and tugging at her arms. She stood as straight as a bullrush, watching her husband. If he took her into the forest, would she slip away? Bhanu felt his skin turn clammy at the thought.

Finally he reached down to help her climb onto the stallion. Sitting behind him, she wound her arms through his and held on tight. Bhanu felt a rush of love at her touch, and kicked the horse's flank to send them into a fast gallop.

Ahead of them the hills were pale and ragged, their peaks brittle under the heavy skies. Bhanu could smell the storm in the air.

"It may be dangerous," he shouted over his shoulder to Mira. "If you want me to, I'll turn back now." She only squeezed him harder, and Bhanu rode onwards. As they climbed, he felt the air thin against his face and heard a low, melodic sound that seemed to come from the hillside. Mira was singing. Quiet at first, but as they neared the forested slopes of the mountain, her voice grew stronger. Bhanu slowed to hear her better, for the sound was making his heart thump in his chest.

"Faster!" she cried, pushing herself against his back as though to urge them onwards. "Higher! Climb higher!"

"The storm is coming," Bhanu shouted back at her, pointing to the angry clouds massing around the peak.

"Chase it," Mira replied, and her voice was sweet and husky in his ear.

And so they chased the storm, weaving through the trees as they grew sparser, urging on the horse as it tired and picked its way gingerly over the rocky ground. The sky overhead grew darker. Sweat glistened on the stallion's flanks and he snorted air through his nostrils, labouring hard to carry his passengers up the steep incline. A cloud of black flies surrounded them, emitting a low buzzing note that irritated Bhanu's ears. There was a crackle in the air, and the birds were quiet and still in the trees.

"We must stop and find shelter," Bhanu said finally, when the horse had slowed to a weak, stumbling pace and the daylight had turned to an eerie purple glow. As soon as he pulled on the reins, though, Mira slipped down and scrambled upwards. Though her feet were bare and she winced as she climbed, she kept going, running over heather and shale towards the mountaintop.

Bhanu didn't even stop to tie his horse – he sprinted after Mira and reached out to catch hold of the trailing yellow silk of her *dhoti*.

"Wait," he called, desperation in his voice.

Mira only laughed, and ran higher. Soon the two of them broke free of the last straggling trees and were exposed on the craggy slopes of the mountain, like two beetles against the dusty rock.

The first lightning was an electric sheet of blinding white light. The thunder came close on its heels, shaking the earth underfoot and roaring in Bhanu's ears. Among the crackle and the groan, he heard Mira's high laughter and saw her standing spine-straight, spellbound by the storm dancing around them. The wind caught her hair and whipped it around her, transforming her into a dervish in the unearthly light.

Bhanu saw his chance and leapt forward to catch her. He brought her tumbling to her knees, crying out as she fell against the sharp rocks, and held her tightly round her waist. Overhead the lightning smashed into jagged forks, flitting over the mountain's peak and striking the highest rocks.

Bhanu crouched over his wife and tried to keep her low to the ground while avoiding her scrabbling, scratching fingernails. It was like trying to hold onto the lightning itself, he thought. Her skin was electric, and she seared his heart with her wild energy. Mira lit up his life, but she threatened to leave Bhanu's heart charred and smouldering. While he held her and felt the quick writhing of her limbs against his, his *lingam* swelled. It pressed against her buttocks and slid over the silk of the *dhoti* tucked between her legs, giving Bhanu a rush of pleasure that was the first he'd felt since the day on the river bank. He clasped her closer and reached to feel her breasts, hanging loose in her robe like ripe fruit, and moaned as his hands closed over them.

A low rumble of thunder stirred around them then and Bhanu felt that the storm had entered him. He could not stop himself. He gripped Mira roughly, dug the points of his nails into the soft skin around her nipples. The lightning grew fiercer as he mauled her, the thunder came louder and faster. His stiff shaft butted against her buttocks as though knocking on a door.

Bhanu untied the knot that held Mira's *dhoti* and the silk unwound to reveal her bare flesh, the colour of pale river mud.

Between her thighs he could see the glint of her wetness, and knew she was as inflamed as he. He took hold of his wife's thighs and tugged her towards him, sinking to the ground and yet not feeling the rocks under his knees.

It took a moment to free his *lingam* from his garments and let it stand proud in the storm-stirred air, the flesh of it dark and crossed with veins. Bhanu moved forcefully, barely aware of their turbulent surroundings. All of him was concentrated on the deep secret of his wife's body, the firm feel of the muscles in her kicking legs and the promise of the sweet little mouth between her thighs.

The sky was midnight blue as he pulled Mira backwards to impale her on his sticking-out *lingam*. The air turned black as the tip of him nudged at her slit and drove deeper, stretching her lips around his shaft. Around them the sky fought with itself, but Bhanu felt only the raging heat, the beautiful silkiness and the fiery tightness of her *yoni*. She twisted and bucked and Bhanu thought that he himself might shatter like a dry tree when lightning crashes through it. Mira lay on her elbows, pinned onto his shaft as he pulled her back towards him. She wailed as he entered her and her hands raked at the ground. Bhanu gripped her thighs and moved her as he pleased, sawing back and forth into the delicious deep embrace of her.

The storm howled around them. Hot wind whipped their flesh and grit stung their faces. The thunder seemed to come from inside the earth, an angry roar that shook the mountain, while the lightning leapt and cracked wildly, trying to jump back into the sky. Mira's hair was filled with static and strands of it waved around her, like the goddess Kali when she dances her dance of destruction and rebirth.

A bolt of lightning struck a rock no further than a hare's leap away and Bhanu felt it sear his flank. Mira shouted – whether in terror or ecstasy, he couldn't tell. She moved like a river surging against a rock, her inner flesh flowing and pressing against Bhanu's *lingam* as it swung deep into her belly. They had a rhythm like drums, moving away from each other only to charge back harder and slam their bodies together, letting the electric pleasures fill them until they felt on the brink of spilling over.

Bhanu tensed as Mira ground against him, all the power and desire of his body concentrating in one white-hot surge that started at the soles of his feet and rose steadily, inexorably upwards. As the clouds struck together a boom resounded and echoed through the mountains, while hisses and sizzles from the tortured lightning flashed on either side of them. Bhanu and Mira pounded at each other, lost in the furious blood of their lovemaking, climbing towards orgasm.

It came from all around them, finally, splitting the sky and turning everything black and white in a moment. Bhanu's mouth opened to let out a scream, and Mira's cries were swallowed like a sparrow's in the howl of the storm. He surged into her, flooded her with his seed and drenched her with fierce and ecstatic love. Had Kali crushed the world underfoot at that moment, neither Bhanu nor Mira would have noticed anything other than their booming heartbeats, their vast expanding bliss.

Afterwards, as they sagged to the ground and lay over each other limp and soft, they heard the rain singing far overhead. Fat raindrops splashed on the couple's naked skin, soothing their flesh. It hushed them as it fell, warm and heavy and drumming the ground lightly like an army of happy women dancing. The monsoon had arrived.

"We can go back to the palace." Mira had to raise her voice over the sound of the rain. "But bring me here, again, Bhanu, to the mountain. I need the sky above me and the earth beneath me."

Rain soaked their hair and clothes, ran down their backs and dripped from their eyelashes. Bhanu kissed the top of his wife's head.

"We'll hunt together, my love. We'll hunt the birds and the fish and all the creatures of the forest, and at night we will hunt for stars. The earth will be our bed and the sky will be our blanket. If you wish you can run naked over the mountains forever and I will follow, for all along I have been chasing your heart and I will never stop."

The rain continued as they climbed down the path from the mountain, drenching them in its warm embrace. When it stopped, suddenly, drops hung from their earlobes and fingertips like bright diamonds.

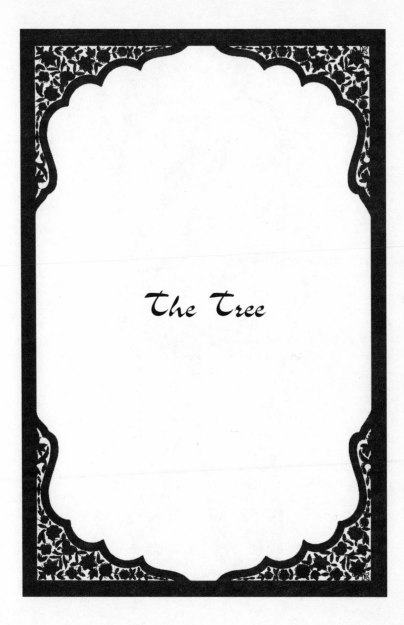

The Tree

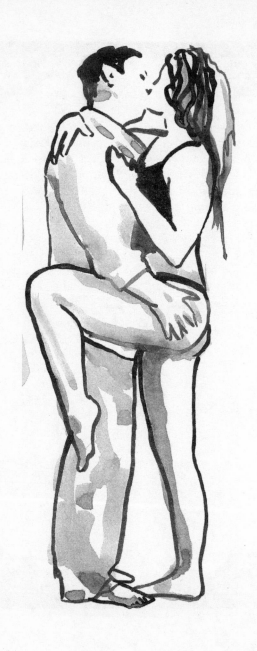

The Tree

Vrisrkshadhirudhaka
Kama Sutra

With her foot on her lover's foot and the other on one of his thighs, the woman passes one arm around his back, kissing and cooing to him all the while. She places her other hand on his shoulder. It becomes affectionately apparent to the man during this gentle attack on him by this woman, that she wishes to climb up him as if he were a tree. She wants a kiss and she will stop at nothing to have it. But she takes her time and bends around him, caressing his back. Nuzzling her foot against his, she strains up every once in a while for the kiss and pouts when she can't reach him. He smiles at her, and the game starts all over again. She clings, she climbs, she sighs. This is one of the embraces done during foreplay.

The Tale of Kakali and the Climbing Tree

as told by EllaRegina

Kakali thought she was a monkey. The townspeople summarily ignored but tolerated her; she was let alone in honour of her dead parents. They had been well-respected and left no other children; she lived in the house of an uncle and aunt. Kakali was not the kind of young woman for whom a husband could be easily found. Her mind was her own and the strange habits she cultivated bewildered the neighbours' sensibilities.

She cared not to wear the traditional female clothing or adornment – except for a pair of *kinkini*: anklets with tinkling hanging bells – and was not bare-breasted or diaphanously garbed like other women, preferring to cloak her body in garments of her own invention. Interpretations of men's dress, they combined the military furnishings of elephant drivers with regal costumings: a short-sleeved *cholaka* [jacket], decorative bands at the neck, hem and sleeve edges, and short billowing muslin drawers (of which Kakali was exceptionally fond) – laughing monkeys delicately embroidered between blue stripes – that gathered tautly above the knees, bound in glittery ribbons woven with threads of real gold, fastened at the waist by a knotted silk cord worthy of a rajah. She assembled this attire herself, stitching together odd pieces of material given her in pity by a handful of local merchants.

The loose raiments allowed Kakali to enjoy the activity that occupied most of her days, and sometimes parts of her nights – climbing trees. She could, in fact, outscale the small, clever, flat-furred she-monkeys who were her sole companions during these ascents. She favoured one tall tree in particular, which rose defiantly like an upright arrow in what had been a forest bordering the kingdom, until it recently saw fire – no other tree survived and tigers roamed the carbon ruins, deer having run away from the charred remains. All bark was burned off this solitary phoenix, giving a sheen to the hard, dry surface of the wood beneath, and making for a challenging climb. Its limbs were stripped of flora since the blaze, leaving stalks the length of a child's forearm, providing rungs for Kakali's nimble, slippered feet to grip, toes arched like a turtle's back.

She would face the tree, plant her right foot on the lowest welcoming limb and her left foot on a rung of greater altitude for leverage, and then, grasping the grey-brown tree trunk as if hugging her lost parents, she would hoist her lithe frame aloft, her boyish hands using the higher rungs to pull herself farther from the ashen forest floor, repeating this sequence of manoeuvres until the tree's peak was reached. Ambling skywards, she emitted a warbling singsong, fulfilling the promise of her name [the voice of a bird in Sanskrit]. She would often pass avian creatures in spiralling mealtime flight, engaging them as if she were part of their flock.

Kakali had never been with a man and despite her fierce independence and single-mindedness she was filled with loneliness and a longing she could not identify. As she climbed the tree she would stop at certain rungs and, in a dreamlike state, rub their tips into her *yoni*. The drawers adorned with monkeys parted in front, and Kakali would grip a rung with her yawning pink flesh, hiding all motions within the ballooning fabric. She knew that women of the royal harem gratified each other similarly, perfecting their lovemaking skills in lieu of an absent monarch, by means of bulbs, root vegetables and fruits bearing a certain shape.

When especially moved she could spend much of an hour with one rung, rhythmically swaying, cooing in a soft uneven tone as if conversing with starlings. In Kakali's initial climbs, although she was quiet, the sound carried due to a lack of surrounding foliage and the height at which she stood, and her whimperings shortly attracted the attention of young boys playing nearby. Before long she had an audience comprising half the adjacent village, but Kakali was thoroughly unaware – climbing, piercing herself in blind abandon with the amputated limbs. However, had she noticed the crowd gathering below, mocking her, she would not have given heed; so, without a reaction to which they could respond in further jest, the villagers ultimately lost interest and minded their own affairs.

Within several weeks of her congress with the tree, soft green buds sprouted from its limbs, adding to Kakali's nameless pleasure. She took more of the stems inside herself with each climb, the plump and succulent young growth massaging her *yoni*'s virgin walls and tickling the swollen red bulb atop its opening. Sometimes she held onto rungs left and right with both hands and feet while resting almost her entire weight on one protuberance between shuddering thighs, thereby granting her quivering nub all the pressure gravity provided. In these hours she had no sense of time, just an oblivion of pure physical bliss and movement, the sun warming her smooth copper-coloured skin.

Akshan was a young man who tended goats. He would sit on the nearby hillside, a betel leaf between his teeth, and dream. He used to survey the forest while in thought but now it bore a lone towering skeleton, regularly holding a female figure wearing men's apparel, swiftly heading towards the clouds, tree limb by tree limb, in effortless pursuit. The goatherd noted Kakali's private moments with the stumps and at first averted his gaze so as not to intrude, though he was many deer leaps apart and wholly unobserved by the tree-climbing girl. However, after some weeks, he yielded to the pull and fascination Kakali had over him and watched her as one absorbs a blanket of stars on a clear night. He was moved by the need he sensed, which in turn encouraged something within his own body, keyed to her motions, in sympathy. Akshan would not attain final paradise, as she seemed to, but kept that part of himself steadily and evenly awake. He was enchanted by her, charmed, and could not break the stare, perhaps realizing the promise of his name [eye in Sanskrit].

Kakali would eventually return to the ground and walk back to the town for nourishment and rest. One evening, when the subject of his vigil was safely out of sight, Akshan approached the tree and examined the rungs within his grasp, smelling their fragrance mixed with Kakali's scent, licking the treewood of the ripe sap she had left, freshly redolent of cumin and baking bread and something else – unidentifiable – which stirred him again, immensely. He looked upwards at the trunk with its several dozen rungs pointed outwards like spindles against the darkening sky. He put his hand around one, gripping it as if an oar, and jumped back in surprise, having received a splinter. He thought not of himself and this small pain, but of the alluring orphaned monkey girl, and what she must be enduring with her amorous arboreal thrusts.

Akshan felt for Kakali, deeply, and wanted to make her daily launchings less hazardous. He, too, was an able climber, with an agile sinewy body, the colour of sandalwood. He removed a small blade from his waistband and began working, commencing with the rung of lowest station, then moving to the next highest until he arrived at the treetop, capped by a nest of birds in slumber. He toiled all night and into the dawn. The goats bayed below but he feigned deafness. At long last they slept and he focused solely on what he was doing, a rung in one hand and sharp metal in the other, his even motions lit by a full golden moon. Akshan felt a pressure in his *lingam*, and stretched out for himself that stone which projects, liberating it from sweltering muslin confines, letting cool breezes graze his warmth. He regarded himself – rigid with desire – while he continued to work but would not touch his stiffness; instead of abating it kept presence as sentry until his task was done. And, when descending to the sleeping goats – a blue jay passing on his left side; a good omen – his *lingam* was also dormant behind striped orange gauze.

The following day brought showers and Kakali did not come to the forest. She remained in her room practising a variety of the 64 arts, many of which – despite her peculiarity and resistance to conform to what was expected of her – she had mastered under her aunt's tutelage. She had an abundance of gifts.

Of course she could sing with her birdlike voice in a haunting cadence. She played the lute. She danced. She could do all three at once. She invented songs playing musical glasses filled with water. She wrote and drew. She was especially adept at arranging flowers on the ground. She strung garlands. She could bind a turban but since her beloved father's death had no opportunity. She enjoyed acting and gave performances to nobody within the walls of her small room. She knew magic and sorcery. She was quick and dexterous in manual skills. Although fed by others she was a master of the culinary art and also made lemonade and sherbets.

As was apparent by her singular creations, she was adept in tailoring and sewing. She fashioned parrots, flowers, tassels and knobs out of yarn and thread. She solved riddles and enigmas, mostly in her own head for lack of playmates or willing companions. She was an excellent mimic, with a specialty for animal languages. She read aloud, chanted and intoned. She handled a sword and quarterstaff. When given the rare occasion she excelled with a bow and arrow. She understood architecture, the art of building.

She knew about gold and silver coins, jewels and gemstones. She was well versed in chemistry and mineralogy. She could garden, knew how to treat the diseases of trees and plants, how to nourish them and determine their ages. She estimated the tree on which she climbed almost daily to be 186 years, 7 months and 25 days old. She taught parrots and starlings to speak and genuinely enjoyed their conversations.

She used various body ointments and dressed her long black hair with unguents and perfumes before gathering the locks and weaving them into a perfect braid.

She understood the art of writing in cipher. She could speak by changing the forms of words – by altering their beginnings and ends and by adding unnecessary letters between syllables. She knew languages and the vernacular dialects. She framed mystical diagrams, addressed spells and charms and could bind armlets. She excelled at an assortment of mental exercises, especially putting into verse or prose sentences that were portrayed by signs or symbols. She composed poems from a vast knowledge of dictionaries and vocabularies.

She could modify and disguise a person's appearance, especially her own; she could also transpose the appearance of things – making cotton to seem as silk; coarse and common things to seem as fine and good.

Her skill in youthful sports and gymnastics was innate; she had always been a monkey. She was able to deduce the character of a man by his features. She partook of arithmetical recreations. She created artificial flowers and delighted in making figures and images out of clay.

Akshan walked his goats by the burned forest – herds of wild elephants running through the rain – and admired his night work, hoping the weeping sky would soon stop its lamentations, and so deliver to him the beloved object of his desire.

The next day the skies were as clear and blue as a cat's iris. Akshan claimed his greensward perch and waited for Kakali to materialise. When the shadows cast by the tree onto the ground crawled several man-lengths to indicate mid-morning, the monkey girl appeared, walking at a rapid pace, her long wavy hair undulating with her gait, ankle bells jangling, drinking the juice from a coconut. When she had drained the hairy orb of its liquid she flung the empty vessel in a grand arc like a rock into water, and it alighted some yards beyond her favourite tree, now in silhouette owing to the strong sun, flooding her eyes with a temporary blindness.

As she approached the tree Kakali noticed it to be somehow different, though she could not determine the exact change. The new buddings were gone – that she perceived. The lower rungs without flora were unmolested and she took foothold, beginning her climb. As she progressed, the higher rungs gradually came into view, one at a time. They had all been carved – whittled – likely with a sharp metal utensil, obviously by a master of the craft. Rung stems closest to the tree torso were left untouched but outward areas of measurement – three or four finger lengths to the broken tips – had been sculpted, each one resembling the others but no two identical.

The shape was distinctive: a long cylindrical shoot finishing in a sleeve, retracted to some degree, over a rounded bulb with a slightly opened eye – a cap resembling mushrooms she had picked among fallen leaves when the forest and her parents were still alive. The configurations mostly adhered to the natural bend of the limbs' growth, perpendicular to the tree trunk, but some had been manipulated to angle vertically in a slight curve, or towards the side like a waving flag. These were finely detailed representations of *lingams*.

Kakali knew they were *lingams* because she had beheld a cluster of them once – on a summer morning before the loss of her parents – when she accompanied her father on his daily walk to bathe in the sacred river waters. After spreading a thin cotton square over the grassy bank, for his daughter to sit upon while she outlined nature verses, he disappeared behind a leafy tree to disrobe and wade into the muddy water.

The hours grew.

As Kakali wrote she heard murmurs coming from the river. She glanced up and saw, through a web of thin branches, a huddle of unclad men standing in shallow water, talking and laughing, playfully splashing one another. Her round brown eyes followed the sweep of long fleshy pendulums – like elephants' trunks – swinging between the men's legs, and the wrinkled bags, a set behind each dangling pendant, all varied in size, shape and colouring and unlike anything she had observed on a human body, not realizing she had only viewed the female form – her late-bloomed and ever-boyish example and the more topographically advanced versions of her mother, her mother's maid and those of varied friends and relations. Kakali was enthralled.

The men were not aware of her gaze upon them and when she finally detected her father's voice – singing in the distance, getting closer with each syllable – she lay down on the sun-kissed cloth and gave pretence of a nap, lodging fevered hands discreetly between her shut legs in response to the new fire and excitement she felt there after having just witnessed such a spellbinding picture.

Kakali climbed steadily, noticing that the *lingams* grew in size – girth and length – the higher their location. She felt the familiar itching in her flushed nub and opened the slit of her drawers, sliding one of the *lingams* into her damp *yoni*. The carving was perfectly smooth and she could feel the round mushroom cap as it stroked her inner walls. She held the tree tighter and forced herself onto its wooden appendage, a rhythm establishing and taking over, as usual throwing her into a condition somewhere between delirium and oblivion.

She withdrew her wetness from the shiny peg and edged higher, reaching a *lingam* that was larger, if only by a slight increment. She repeated her dance, one arm around the tree, her opposite hand clasping a *lingam* above. She turned her head sideways, resting it on the trunk while her torso ploughed itself in delight, eyelids fluttering down like curtains. During this abandon Kakali knocked into a nearby *lingam*, startling herself for an instant, but reacted as naturally as a fish swimming with a river's current: she leaned in, opened her lips and sealed them around the entity, pulling it inside her mouth, licking its length, sucking it, retreating and attending to the mushroom cap, her tongue a darting wick into its carved eye – juices leaving her openings, each in *lingam* congress; one above and one below.

Akshan watched from afar, with pleasure, pride and astonishment, his own *lingam* as hard as those he had spent countless hours moulding. He took out a reed pipe and began to play. The instrument was dressed with extracts of seven different plants – a green potion ensuring, as with Krishna's bewitching flute, that once its lilting notes penetrated her ears the monkey girl would become, irrevocably, his.

Kakali clambered higher, almost dizzy and feeling faint. She paused to compose herself, firmly grabbing a pair of *lingams* so she would not plummet to the base of the tree. With her breath caught, she ventured to a group of sculptures several notches in size greater than those her virgin *yoni* had already sampled, which would dilate her still. She was insatiable, and realized that somehow and by someone she was being given a lesson – remotely – on the art of lovemaking, an art she took to as a soaring hawk owns the skies. She travelled from rung to rung, *lingam* to *lingam* – her *yoni* stretched slightly wider with each in accommodation – adjusting her position to the individual shape presented her, adapting her movements, her speed, her passion, to match each one.

Hours elapsed; it was nearing sundown. Kakali had experienced almost every *lingam* the tree offered yet there remained one, at the very top – by the nest of birds, now vacant while the feathered ones crossed the sky gathering their evening repast – which beckoned her, in an almost audible bellow. She reached it in her final climb and soon found herself standing eye to eye with what was clearly the Brahma of *lingams*, pointing boldly, decisively to the east. He had been given special attention. Veins were carved along the side, raised – bloodless but undeniably alive – in bas-relief. A meticulously chiselled triangle of abundant coiled hair tufts hung above the *lingam*; the mushroom cap and its winking slit were more refined than on the other specimens. The root of this limb – on all other rungs left in a raw state – had been crafted into duets of hanging pouches, like those Kakali had seen on the men in the wading river one past summer day. Lastly, to the right of the *lingam* – incised exactly and deliberately into the tree's surface – was a name, presumably that of the woodcarver, etched in a clear and florid script: A-K-S-H-A-N.

Kakali caressed the remarkable object aimed like an arrow at her brow. She stroked its robust span in admiration and cradled the bags with her hands. As if under a spell, she bent to meet the *lingam*, opened her mouth as wide as she was able and took the formidable expanse between her cheeks, wrapping it with her playful tongue. She moved her head from the base of the *lingam* to its tip, leaving a trail of moisture – sucking it, at first gently and then with more hunger, as she would a mango had her stomach not been filled in many days. Kakali imagined this *lingam* belonging to a real man and gazed upwards, conjuring a beautiful face the hue of sandalwood – having even features and dark brown lotus eyes, almost indistinguishable from black; surrounded by curly hair the colour of night falling to shoulder level; and a full mouth, the shade of a pale pink apple – an image which then vanished, replaced by the indigo sky with its small clouds afloat, shaped like cotton batting.

She climbed half her body's height farther, and guided the wet *lingam* into her *yoni*, her vesture disclosing stains of excitement. An odour of cumin and baking bread and something unidentifiable reached her flared nostrils. As she planted herself upon the carving a cry escaped her, a weeping sound over which she had no control. It was not an utterance of pain but rather of profound contentment, her *yoni* dilated and gorged, holding the length of wood snugly.

This *lingam* filled Kakali's interior like no other – her *yoni* a fitted gauntlet; it poured into her private crevices as liquid clay into a mould, leaving no point untouched – the mushroom head striking her innermost boundary. She took care to move upon it slowly, to savour each minute contour transition along its solid form. Kakali enveloped the tree with both arms and one leg in a hug, enjoying the delicacy of her carefully timed propulsions, put her forehead to where the bark had been, kissing and licking the spot. She lodged her tongue in a knot, turning it into a pair of full moving lips, the shade of a pale pink apple, mottled by one freckle on the upper, near the corner of the mouth, beneath which stood two uniform rows comprising straight glistening ivory-coloured teeth.

As Kakali gambolled with the *lingam* scores of tree knots transformed into dark brown lotus eyes, almost indistinguishable from black, that followed her every movement with a resolute intensity. In a half-trance, distantly, she heard a simple yet captivating melody which instantly filled her with a desire for whoever was its creator. The sylvan floor became ever far removed – the tree was growing, shooting upwards with each of her thrusts. The empty bird's nest drifted off, untethered. Vines erupted like snapping serpents from the burned wood and wrapped themselves around Kakali, lacing her into a protective cage as the tree barrelled towards the orange sun. She danced with force upon the *lingam*, lost in a dream, moaning, cooing – trumpeting howls she didn't know herself capable of making. She travelled beyond the birds, writhing and bucking at a faster pace. At once a wave of pleasure moved through her, round buttocks shaking like tree fruit, and a word passed her lips in a scream loud enough to wake the doves: "AKSHAN!"

In that moment the tree vaporized – becoming a column of sky – and Kakali ceased to maintain her usual form, breaking from the arborical metamorphosis as the arrow of Kama, the God of Love – a garland of jasmine, hibiscus flowers and mango blossoms – spearing the ether with great velocity; buoyed by the spring wind, Kama's powerful ally, heading in the direction of the nearby hillside and landing – a fragrant bolt of lightning accompanied by jingling bells – in the body of Akshan himself as he sat amidst a circle of goats, the shaft piercing his heart.

The earth was quite agitated. A blue mist filled the air, veiling the scene, gradually dispersing and revealing in its departure the semi-clothed figure of Kakali – round cinnamon eyes fringed by lashes covered in lampblack, her face radiant as the moon, bee-stung lips, teeth lustred as pearls. Jasmine and hibiscus flowers wove through her long hair, a chaplet of lotus blossoms reining in twirled ringlets, and splendid kadamba petal necklaces of celestial bouquet draped as garlands across her small, black-nippled breasts. She sat with legs crossed, facing Akshan, his pose a mirror image of hers, ripe mangoes strewn about them like luscious stones, making a beautiful patterned blanket spread upon the ground – a parrot, a peacock and a flamingo mute witnesses to their encounter.

Kakali examined Akshan closely. He was not unfamiliar. She reached out to touch his beautiful sandalwood-tinted countenance with its even features, dark brown lotus eyes, almost indistinguishable from black; her hand lightly brushed curly hair the colour of night, cascading to his shoulders. She slowly moved a finger across his full mouth, a shade of pale pink apple, tracing a freckle on the upper lip, near the corner, beneath which stood two uniform rows comprising straight glistening ivory-coloured teeth.

She addressed the goatherd, uttering his name in a manner combining both question and declaration. He nodded in assertion, confirming his identity, avowing that they had made each other's acquaintance in the tree.

They glimpsed the now-barren forest, hearing confused shrieks of scampering monkeys. Looking moonwards, Akshan noted the positions of different planets and the twenty-seven stars, reciting their influence and how they can direct people through forests. He showed her a pair of human beings – a man and a woman – cut from the leaf of a tree. Kakali blushed, as did the goatherd, and they rose together, as if already having knowledge of one another's rhythm. Akshan was tall and sturdy, his body stiff as a pole, much like her forest diversion, and Kakali knew of only one thing to do: she placed her right foot on the left foot of Akshan and her left foot on his right thigh, passed one arm around his back and the other encircling his shoulders. She made slight singing and cooing noises, wishing to climb him like a tree for a kiss, mounting herself onto his muscular frame. Akshan bent his head down to meet her lips and they exchanged breaths. There was no time. The moon was stopped in the heavens. The couple strengthened their embrace as the goats watched them in silence.

Kakali felt a hardness behind Akshan's clothing. He released his *lingam* for her. It was the king atop the tree, only the colour of skin – throbbing in gentle but unwavering forceful tremors – with raised blue-green veins, a tuft of curls above and the pendulous bags ripe figs underneath. Kakali seized him gleefully and caressed the familiar shape. A bit of dew emerged from the narrow aperture at its tip. Akshan put one hand over that of Kakali as she held him. His other fingers loosened the knot of the corded belt tied around her slender waist – unwinding in several revolutions. The drawers it had secured unfastened and fell away, bringing the sight of her *yoni* to his craving eyes, and the smell of cumin and baking bread and something unidentifiable to his flared nostrils. He stroked her secret places, as the elephant rubs with its trunk.

Kakali felt weak with the pleasing sensations she knew from her tree frolics. Akshan took his *lingam* and slowly herded himself into Kakali's *yoni* – opening like a flower – warm and wet with her ardour. A cry emerged from within as she melded herself to him without hesitation. Akshan found a home in her body, driving forwards and piercing the lotus. Once his *lingam* was inside her she could feel its pulse and hold it for a hundred heartbeats. She contained him completely, the fit as perfect as it had been on the tree. He was poured into her like water in a jug. But this time she was filled with burning solid flesh – not unyielding treewood – the swollen mortal limb of a real man yearning with carnal desire and love for her.

Kakali enthroned herself upon Akshan's *lingam* in an intimate cling, and he responded to the encouraging moves of her hips, the entreaties of her glinting *yoni*, gripping him as a vice, with a churning, as of cream, haunches aflame, both of them lost in the same reverie – moaning, cooing, gasping, wailing, exhaling sounds that animals made; and of thunder, of sighing, of weeping, of something falling into water. Kama's fire, transformed by nature into black bees and the very amorous cuckoo, buzzed and sang as the lovers' mouths met again in an entwining of tongues like cobras, mimicking the joining sparks of *lingam* and *yoni* below.

They writhed and they bucked, blind with passion in the heat of congress, mixing into one as salt into water. Akshan's *lingam* a relentless flute, a brisk sparrow going back and forth continuously inside Kakali's *yoni*; his powerful arms holding her up as he whispered suggestive words. They enjoyed themselves in vigourous fits – kissing, biting, scratching – limbs enlaced, uniting the two organs as closely as possible, until they both naturally derived pleasure from the act they performed; their desire quenched, shaking like tree fruit, Kakali's ankle bracelets ringing out joyously as she once more, tremblingly, called Akshan's name.

And, as Kakali felt, for the first time in her life, the sacred fire, the bursting life force of a man's jewel, his seed – kindling, fluid and abundant – coating the walls of her *yoni*, its semen also falling, heating her belly in a way far more satisfying than any meal, she realised with certitude: never again would she enter a forest path, but instead would climb Akshan, her living, loving tree, ardently, ecstatically, intensely – in all the ways that she knew how – infinitely and forever.

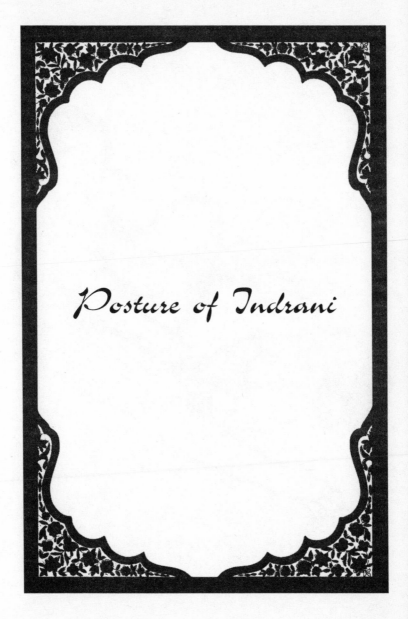

Posture of Indrani

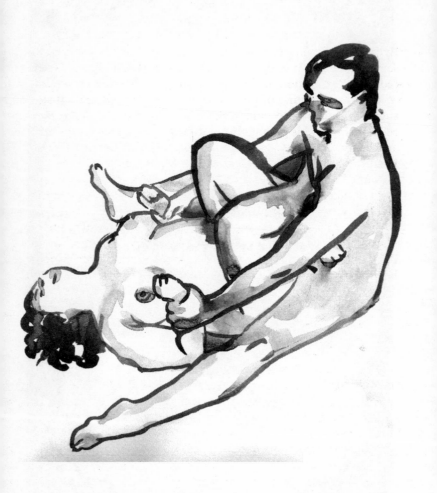

Posture of Indrani

Indranika
Kama Sutra

Every size of man, from the hare to the elephant, is able to find sexual satisfaction with every size of woman. The Kama Sutra reduces the question of size to a passing, easily solved problem. With a simple tilting of the pelvis or a pressing of the thighs, it suggests that orgasm can always be achieved. It is the love relationship that is paramount, not the purely sexual one. There are many positions designed to solve size differences. The Posture of Indrani is a particularly effective one.

Named after the spouse of Indra, the King of Heaven, this position allows even the smallest *yoni* to be penetrated by her lover's *lingam*. In this position, the woman engages in congress with her thighs bent on themselves and held on either side of her body. It is a useful position but takes practice. The lover, in turn, encircles her thighs with his thighs and forcibly widens her further. He might even open her with his hands.

The Tale of the Wife of Indra

as told by Miranda True

It was the type of night that inspired men to draw their swords in the name of love while women studied their shields for the cause of virtue. A soothing scent of lavender carried through the breeze, perfuming everything it embraced. From all around the nightingales began their chorus, the same songs that had set the scene for generations of lovers. On the edge of the water, a mating duel played out.

First, he conquered her lips with his own. Next, his hand invaded her flesh, exploring every hill and valley of her body. Overwhelmed by the fragile perfection of their surroundings her defences collapsed. She mounted her own attack, wrapping her legs around him until she could feel his desire press against her. They united as one, taking their time through every position their heart could imagine. She cried out in devotion under the touch of her beloved and as she reached her apex a crack of thunder sounded and they both fell dead. The death spread out like a ripple in the water. Pillows of green grass withdrew, turning brown and brittle. Swollen blossoms that played in the breeze snapped shut and fell to the ground. The lakes dried up leaving muddy graves for the animals that had called them home.

This is how the world ended.

Nobody knew exactly why the plague had happened, but there was no question as to who was behind it. For whenever some type of disaster befell Earth, it was known that Indra was the cause. When the Creator was moulding the planet, he took the remaining clay and sculpted its ruler, a god with the power to control the very elements of existence. Indra and the planet were twins, and like most twins they shared a unique connection; what Indra felt, the Earth put into action. Indra was angry. The bleak state of the land made that clear. The real mystery was what had caused this anger.

Indra was respected as the King of the Gods; worshipped by all creatures, from the lowest spider to the Great Lord Shiva. They gave offerings in his name; built statues in his visage. There was no word that was more respected or honoured than that of Indra, yet, he had still decided to turn his back on his devoted followers. Some people responded by desecrating the shrines in his honour, but anger is easier on a full stomach. As people began to see themselves wasting away from starvation, they became obsessed with finding a way to please Indra once again.

Some sacrificed animals in his name. Others opted for human offerings. The loveliest women in the village would call out to him, promising to exchange the jewel of their virginity for an end to the plague. Dressed in the wedding gowns they had been saving since girlhood they'd make the trek to Indra's temple, never to be seen again.

"It's not much of a loss," the old women of the village would tut. "Only a whore would treat love as a commodity."

Most of the parents believed that it was sex that had got them in this mess in the first place; that the plague was punishment from the gods because of the permissive children, who dared to kiss before the bonds of marriage. The grandparents thought it went back further, to the way their own children had held hands prior to the wedding ceremony. Whatever the cause, everyone was hurting now. Hope was dwindling as quickly as their bodies. As the desperation grew, the offering to Indra became more ostentatious: golden bowls, decadent jewels and, most precious of all, the last remnants of food.

Sachi's mother prepared a plate of overly ripe fruit, the only thing left from the prosperity of the past. Their soft skins split open with the slight caress of the knife, oozing sweet juice onto the plate below. The older woman worked precisely, starting with the freckled red strawberries, then the fuzzy kiwis and, finally, the soft, yielding mangoes.

"Can I have a taste?" Sachi pleaded.

Although she was a woman, with gently sloping hips and pert breasts to prove it, she still had the attitude of a child, looking for momentary pleasures without thinking of the long-term consequences. It was the nature of woman to be sacrificing for others, but Sachi never learned how to deny her desires. More than one person had described her as a force of nature, unstoppable and unpredictable. It was not a compliment. Maybe it was better if the plague did take her life, her mother thought, since she was not the type of girl that men would choose to marry. Yes, they'd fantasize about her when they were in the marriage bed, but never take her to the altar.

She handed the offering to Sachi. "Take the plate to the temple of Indra. It is the most precious thing we have to offer, and we will give it to him. Then pray that he forgives us for whatever our offence was."

"What makes you think Indra even wants our rotten fruit? How will you feel when we give up our only food supply for nothing?"

"How will you feel if we do nothing and get the same result?"

Weak from hunger, Sachi refused to argue with her mother, and balanced the tray on her head as she began the walk to the temple.

Her steps took their own rhythm as she rolled her hips back and forth. Sachi knew she was beautiful, her face was a perfect heart topped off with thick black hair that fell to her waist. There was always the faintest trace of a smile on the pink lips of her mouth, and her brown eyes seemed bottomless with no hope for escape to the one who fell into them. There was a time when the simple act of watching her walk would have drawn a crowd. She liked it when men watched her, the way their eyes narrowed and their breathing grew rapid. The men were gone now; they'd gone into the jungles looking for a meal, but ended up becoming one.

As she approached the temple she couldn't help but stare at it. It was carved from a single block of marble stone, a task that had taken three generations to complete. Inside there was an altar, covered with dried rose petals and illuminated by a soft orange candle glow. A life-sized statue of Indra presided over the room, with ruby eyes looking down on the gifts presented to him.

Sachi slowly removed the plate from atop her head and placed it before the ten foot tall statue.

"I offer you these gifts," she whispered, feeling silly as she talked to herself. "Please take them as a sign of our forgiveness and . . ." The futility of the act, an offering of fruit to the God who could make trees bloom with a touch, washed over her. Speech became pointless. Faced with a hopeless situation, she reached for the guarantee of momentary pleasure. The strawberry was soft in her fingers as it tried to slip away. Its texture was rubbery and the flavour non-existent. But the memories it invoked, the days spent playing in fertile fields without a care in the world, made her mouth water

"You have stolen from me," a deep voice boomed.

Sachi looked up and saw the statue of Indra had come to life, and now stood before her with blazing red eyes. The food fell from her hands, hitting the floor just as Sachi did, bowing on her knees before the King of the Gods.

"Have mercy, Lord Indra," she stuttered, "I did not mean to offend you."

Indra's anger erupted; the Earth responded by shaking violently. "I don't care about your intention. Your actions tell more than your words. Once again, you have proven that your race specializes in deception and blasphemy."

"I am truly sorry," she pleaded. The ground continued to quake, and Sachi thought only of her frail mother and the ramshackle shack that they shared. Her eyes filled with tears at the thought of anyone else being harmed because of her actions. She stood up to try to make eye contact with the great God, but he towered over her. "Please," she begged, "let me atone for this sin. I will give you my very life to make things right."

The ground settled. Indra seemed to smile, or was it a trick of shadows and flickering candlelight? "Do you realize what you are doing?" Indra bellowed. "Are you aware of what you have agreed to?"

Sachi's voice was thin as she tried to speak. "I am prepared for whatever you wish. My life belongs totally to you." Her eyes closed as she waited for a death blow, but it never came. Instead

Indra chuckled slightly. When Sachi opened her eyes he was nude and standing without shame before her. Sachi had never seen a naked man before, and she couldn't help but stare at this perfect specimen.

His skin was the colour of the earth, deep tan, with muscles that were carved from stone. Sachi's eyes came level with his chest, and she allowed them to trace the muscular canals down his stomach and along the deep V at his thighs until her focus came to his manhood. Her inexperience marvelled at how it stood so straight in defiance of gravity. There was a stir in Sachi's loins, a quivering of the flesh that she had never experienced before. A small butterfly had emerged from the cocoon of her womanhood and was starting to flutter for the first time. Sachi's face flushed pink as the ticklish feeling subsided, overtaken by confusion. "What is it you want from me?" she asked.

"To worship me." It was such a simple request, but one that many before her had been unable to meet. However, Sachi was obedient, and pleased Indra by sinking to the ground and pressing her head against the cool stone of the temple floor. There was no pretence to this one; no coy games or flowery praise. In the eyes of the God, submission was the most beautiful attribute, but the deity couldn't help but be stirred by her beauty. From above he could see her shapely frame spread on the floor, her round backside pressed towards the sky. She had a crown of thick black hair that acted as another appendage, flowing softly down her back and swaying back and forth with her body. He wrapped his hand in the thick tangle of hair and pulled her upright until her face was directly in front of his staff.

"Worship me," he repeated, pulling her towards him.

Sachi's lips pressed to the head of his massive erection. Slowly, she slid her lips around the tip, surprised by the contrast of soft velvety skin and rock-hard muscle. Like a calf feeding from the udders of a mother, she began sucking gently until a thin milky fluid began seeping into her mouth. This small sustenance made her take Indra deeper into her mouth and suck more vigorously. The fluttering of her groin was spreading across her body. The buds of her breasts had grown hard and were aching as the thin cloth of her gown rubbed against them. Her body was taking over, pulling the God's great phallus deeper into her mouth. The lust overcame her natural gag reflexes as his quivering manhood pushed at the back of her throat. Sachi let her eyes flutter open for a moment, her gaze fixing on the hairless valley of his pelvis. Curiosity begged her to look up, to see the great God's reaction to the explorations of her mouth, but she didn't want to appear unladylike. The warnings she had always heard about the evils of lust, and the duty of women to always be pure, swirled around her mind. Sachi pulled away and let her hair shield her body.

"Just as I expected," he frowned, "another ungrateful mortal."

As Indra walked past Sachi, she allowed her hand to run down her body and pause as she felt a fiery heat coming from her female flower.

"What are you doing?" he snapped. She quickly put her hands to her sides, but realized he hadn't seen her shameful touching. He was motioning her to join him outside the temple, where he was preparing his elephant for travel. Indra was so large that he wrangled the mighty beast with the ease that a mortal man would prepare a stallion. With one quick motion he mounted the elephant, gently calming it with a pat to the head. He looked at her and shook his head. "Come along. It is almost sunset."

Sachi stepped towards her new master. Indra saw her tremble as she walked and he felt a quick stab of pity. She is just a simple village girl, he told himself, and she must be overwhelmed. Just as quickly he felt anger as he realized that she was trying so hard to appear brave, another mortal deception.

But Indra was only half right; Sachi was trying to hide her feelings from the God. However, it wasn't fear that caused her to shake as he lifted her up and held her against his chest. It was desire. The elephant began to walk, slowly rising and falling with each step and rocking Sachi deeper into Indra's arms. He was holding her close to prevent her from falling, but if she closed her eyes, she could pretend it was more. A lover's embrace.

But he wasn't her lover, he was her God. The feelings bubbling up through her were completely wrong, and yet so natural. It was unexpected. Men were always the ones who were described as lustful and needing. When her mother would talk about the duties of a wife, she always mentioned lovemaking in the same dutiful tone she used when describing the best way to sweep the living room. Women were to be efficient lovers, who would satisfy their husbands' desires quickly and then get back to their more important duties. Men were the ones who burned with desire, and women the ones who quenched the flames. At least that was what everyone said, and while Sachi could feel wetness between her legs, it seemed more likely to spark a flame than eliminate it.

The rocking of the elephant stopped, and Sachi opened one eye, to glance up at Indra's expressionless face. They were standing in a muddy swamp with sticks and branches lying on the ground. Acid rose in the back of her throat as she noticed dozens of bodies spread out before them. Some were in such a state of decomposition that only their bones remained, but other, looked as if they were just sleeping in their lace bridal gowns.

"Where are we?"

"This is the place where man first betrayed me."

Indra waved his hand and the earth came back into bloom. Water filled the lake, bringing pink lotus blossoms to life on the bank. The most weathered pair of bones came together and grew muscle and flesh, until they took the form of lovers, joined as one in the beauty of nature. The woman was on her knees, rocking back and forth as her lover took her from behind. They were both nude, although her smooth rounded figure shielded him from view, except for his face which was buried in her thick black hair, the soft strands muffling his grunts. She was bucking back and forth like a wild animal, being pushed up as his manhood impaled her, and then pulled back down by his hands

on her shoulders. The soft orbs of her breasts bounced up and
down with the movements, and she reached up to steady them,
massaging the pink buds with her fingers.

"I saw her through the overgrowth," Indra explained, "And
at first I thought she was praying. Instead, I see this blasphemy
going on before my eyes."

As if on cue, the woman began screaming the words she had
whispered before as her lover thrust deeper inside her. "I want
you. I need you. I belong totally to you. There is nothing else I
need." She kept repeating these mantras until her lover took
one final thrust and then ceased movement, holding her still
against his body. Indra waved his hand again, dismissively, and
the scene returned to death, except for the lake. It had been so
long since she had seen water that she had to touch it, just to
prove it was real.

"You may bathe, if you wish. Some of the others have chosen
to."

"What happened to the others?" she asked, although she
feared the answer.

"They were unable to worship me properly. And so I had to
kill them." There was no malice in his voice, which scared Sachi
even more.

"I will take you up on your offer," she said, trying to buy
time. As she disrobed the aching of her body became almost
unbearable. Everything felt more intense. The breeze that
moved past was like a hurricane, sweeping her away. The soft
current of the liquid became a second skin. She had never felt
more alive, or closer to death.

Her body ached for sexual conquest. Under the cover of the
water she could finally reach down, and explore her private
temple. Sachi had never touched herself in that way, but the
need for contact was an itch that demanded to be scratched. The
water hadn't doused its heat, warm as she placed her finger
against the slit. With eyes focused on Indra, who was still
looking away, she broke the seal and felt the honey-coated lips
of her womanhood. It was slick, like oil, and her hand glided
smoothly along the outer circle. When she reached the top there

was a small nub that made her quiver as she touched it. Involuntarily she gasped, and Indra looked up at her. Sachi never looked away from him while she continued her exploration, going deeper into that silken cavern until she could no longer reach.

Realizing that she would be unable to fulfil her hunger, the fog of lust lifted and terror took over. "Come now," Indra commanded. "It is time."

Sachi moved slowly, her death procession. Her thick black hair covered her breasts and fell to her waist, reserving some modesty. The air was cool against her naked skin, but as Indra removed his clothes, it was warm again.

"Lie down," he demanded, and Sachi was obedient.

The dead grass stabbed into her back which made it easier to ignore her growing desire. Indra placed his body on top of hers, and slowly slid his sword into her waiting sheath. It was a tight fit, and he didn't go much deeper than where she had been able to reach on her own. Once inside he didn't move, instead lying still as his weight comfortably merged with her. He was so much larger than her and covered her completely, like a warm blanket. He was in a push-up pose, his hands on either side of her head, with rippling muscles coming up to his chest. She wanted to lick them, to feel those hard muscles in her mouth, like another part of him had been earlier in the day. Inside, she could feel him sitting right outside the deepest core of her being, and it threatened to explode if she didn't open it herself. But she couldn't. Sex was evil and wrong. It was the message of her parents, society; even this greatest God Indra seemed to agree. Sachi told herself to behave like a proper lady, and not to let herself go, or it would be the end of her life.

Mind and body warred for a moment, until she decided that a satisfied death was preferable to these tortures in her lower heart. Slowly, Sachi pulled her legs up, one on each side of him until they were in a V. Sachi yelped in joy as he sank deeper, but she wanted more. She reached up, grabbing each leg at the knee, to pull them tight to her chest. With her legs doubled up against each other she was fully open, and Indra fell gently into her deepest part. Like a dam breaking, her female essence covered him and he began to slide out of her. But she was still not satisfied, and so Sachi reached up and wrapped her arms around the great God's neck to pull him close again. "I need you," she cried out to him. "I am yours now, and belong to you fully."

And he answered her prayer. With his full intensity he moved in and out of her, his expanse gently grazing the outer bud of her lotus flower, taking her to higher levels of pleasure with each pass. Each touch built on the one before until she could no longer stand it, and could feel herself falling and a great tumult of ecstasy. Her body quaked uncontrollably at the release, and a moment later he joined her.

As the two were intertwined in satisfaction, something re-remarkable happened. The Earth sprang back to life. It started beneath them, the grass becoming soft and green, but then it spread out until all the world was full of life again. A soft rain began to fall, signalling the end of Indra's punishment.

"You have succeeded," he said, hoarsely.

"I thought you were going to kill me. I gave into my lust and . . ."

"You worshipped me completely," he explained. "I have had towers built in my honour, and lives sacrificed in my name. I've been prayed to and held in esteem. I thought I was loved. But the day I found that couple, I realized that it had been nothing compared to the passion they held for another. Over the years, some have tried to show me worship. But it was never close to what I saw that day. Until you. You have shown me greater love than I could have ever hoped for. And so, I release my curse on your people, and my hold on you."

Sachi's heart caught in her throat. "I don't want to be let go. I want to remain yours forever. Please, let me worship you for eternity."

His answer came in a kiss, as his mouth met with hers just as he grew hard inside her again.

This is how the world began again.

Indra made her a goddess and kept her forever in the heavens as his bride. Never again did he curse the Earth, for her prowess kept him forever satisfied. Her openness to the gift of sexuality was what had saved all of mankind, and so the gods decreed a book be written to let everyone know the innate good that came from the art of pleasure. Featured in this book of love was the position Sachi had demonstrated when she pulled her knees back and opened fully to him. They even named it for her, calling it Indrani, or the Wife of Indra. When performed correctly, it is said to make a man feel like a god. The most important key to its success isn't the physicality, but for the woman to allow her sexual need to be evident. Anyone can contort their bodies into an image, but only those truly skilled lovemakers can allow themselves to be overtaken by their desire. To be fearless in the face of passion is the most important lesson of the *Kama Sutra*.

Ratiratnapradipika

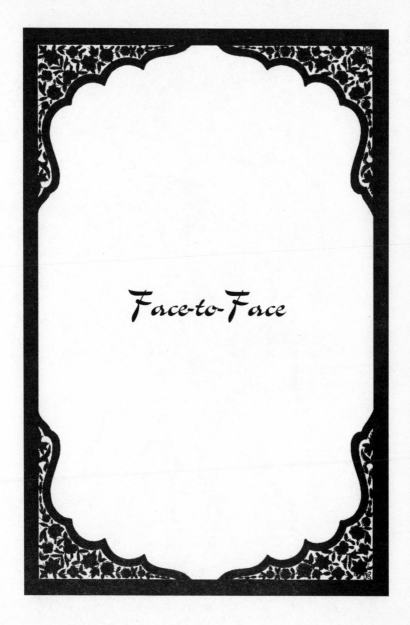

Face-to-Face

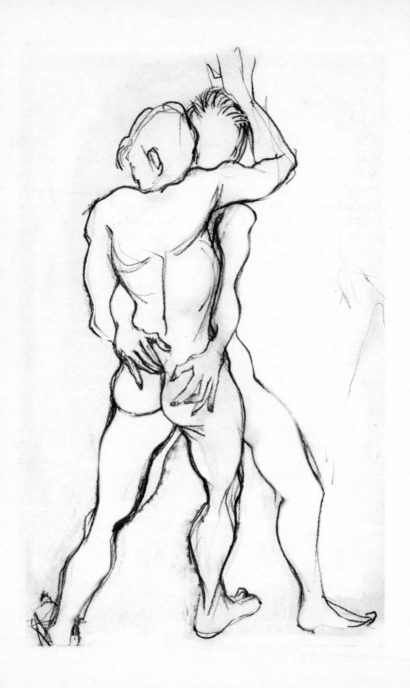

Face-to-Face

Sammukha
Ratiratnapradipika

When the woman is feeling bold, she might lean, fully clothed, against a wall, in casual conversation with her lover, perhaps outside, but away from prying eyes. Perhaps he wouldn't be aware of anything amiss. He would notice, however, her glorious smell, the jasmine perfume she always wore and the gold bangles on her wrist, the way they jangled and clashed together as she lifted her hand to slip an unruly wisp of hair behind her succulent ear. He would notice their closeness, he might even be imagining their coupling.

Then, without a thought for consequence, and staring deeply into his eyes, she shifts quietly, so as to plant her feet as wide, then wider, just like Maharaja Praudha Devaraya's *Ratiratna-pradipika* love text has taught her. She wants him face-to-face, crushing his mouth to hers, pushing inside her thighs, roughly, to press his hard shaft against her. She wets her lips and watches him, still speaking, oblivious. She plants her feet further apart, tilts her pelvis (just like her sister had explained to do the position correctly). She is inviting him inside. She stares at him and begins pulling up her skirt with one hand while with the other she undoes the first two buttons of her blouse. She wets her lips again and lets her hair down. He is looking at her strangely. Hm, isn't he going to be surprised?

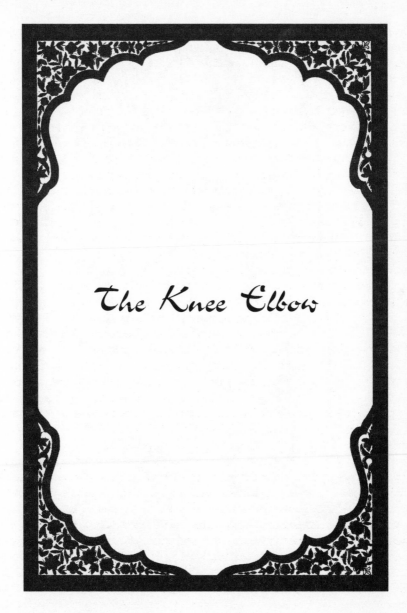

The Knee Elbow

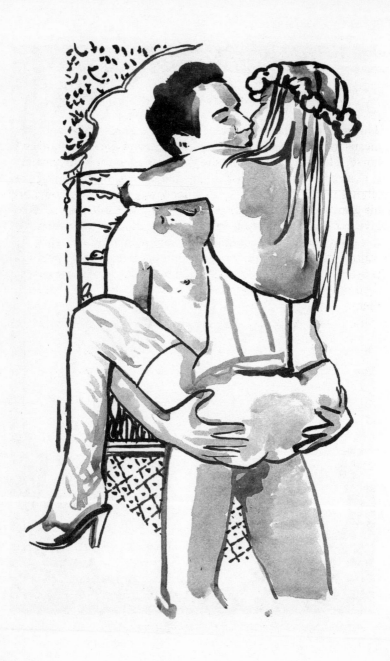

The Knee Elbow

Janukurpara
Ratiratnapradipika

This position calls for a strong man and a smaller woman. This means the woman will probably be a deer and the man a bull or a horse. This is a high union, and so satisfaction for both partners is assured. The man must lift his partner up by threading his elbows under her knees (so that her lower legs swing down off his arms like a doll's legs) and then grasp her buttocks so as to give her some support. This position might be a little scary for the woman as she is completely at the man's mercy, while he controls the thrusts and the depth of penetration. This position is probably best suited to a love union, where the partners know each other very well and there is a great deal of trust between them.

The Tale of Janukurpara

as told by Colleen Anderson

It is said that it all began just before the great *nāga* worship in the month of Shravana. The sun glares down and flattens the earth with heat. Little moves but the warmed bodies of the *nāgas* that slither and hiss, gliding over rocks and terraces to lie coiled in the sun. It is unwise to disturb those sinuous bodies for the *nāgas* do not like surprises.

Amrita did not particularly like the *nāgas* but she was not overtly afraid of them. Rather, she envied them their freedom and wished she too could shed her skin when needed. She was not a princess but still of noble birth and had all the duties and luxuries dependent on being in such a position. Jewels and the richest silks were hers, as well as the finest honeyed meads, and any richly flavoured food the cooks could devise. But she could not walk freely beyond the garden walls, nor shed her sari and breast band as the women of the villages did when it was very hot. In the privacy of the walls she was allowed to wear a breast band and a simple cotton sari over an underskirt.

Still, the fabric stuck to her and made her uncomfortable. Amrita clung to the shaded seats though the air was only a touch less stifling.

It was there that Sheshdhar found her once again, the most beautiful flower surrounded by musk rose and lily, clematis and blue poppy. He was naught but a gardener and performed his duties exceptionally well, though he had been reprimanded twice for trying to talk to the noble family. Still, as only any creature loving of nectar could, he was drawn to Amrita.

Her kohl-rimmed eyes of rich golden amber matched her skin. Her full and deeply crimson lips begged to be kissed. But it was the roundness of her breasts, and just like those ancient Vedic sculptures they crested down to a slim waist and voluptuous hips, that just made his hands itch to travel over her contours. So smitten was Sheshdhar that even Amrita's voice sent shivers along his skin.

Surreptitiously, he glanced about, looking for those who always guarded Amrita. She was not the only daughter of this cousin to the Prince, but she was the rarest blossom, both beautiful and intelligent, a prize sought by many above a gardener's status. Sometimes love shoots the sweet flower-tipped arrow at gods and mortals alike and it can cause chaos to ordered plans. Sheshdhar moved closer to Amrita whose eyes were closed against the heat. He had cut a long slender stalk of papyrus and now lowered the bushy ended frond towards the languishing woman.

It brushed over her bosom and Sheshdhar's heart quickened as if his fingers had touched her. The frond slid along her cheek, and her brow crinkled ever so slightly as she reached up to brush the annoyance aside. When it repeated she opened her eyes. Sheshdhar grinned at her and bowed.

His smile caught the light and it was if the shadows lightened when Amrita looked at him. He saw her chest flutter like a butterfly's wings alighting on a bloom, and wished to place his lips upon that pulse. "Come walk with me, Amrita. I will show you all manner of birds and animals."

She glanced quickly across the gardens and whispered, "Go away, Sheshdhar, or you will get in trouble."

He placed his long, strong fingers over his heart. "I am already troubled that you will not spend a moment with me."

Standing in one fluid motion, Amrita straightened the end of her cream-coloured sari and walked slowly away. "I cannot, for you know I am promised to others."

And yet she was reluctant to leave the sight of him. His hair was such a lustrous black it seemed to hold the night sky, sparkling as if stars kept their secrets there. And his eyes – they were so deep a brown with green flecks that she was sure the very plants were given birth in such realms. Each time before when he had come close she had stared into his eyes, had fallen in and wanted to float in those pools for an eternity. His brows were like those of a crested serpent eagle, swooping, strong, noble as the fine lines of his nose. She wanted to touch the curve of his brow, the turn of his lips and the sculpted planes of his cheeks. But a lady of her station did not do such things.

Amrita could not touch, so she left, visions of Sheshdhar's lips haunting her.

Sheshdhar knew the meaning of perseverance. He had watched many a spider rebuild its web when he and the other gardeners had cleared brush and weeds. Just so, he remembered the day when he had come upon the pit dug to catch a wild boar that had been ravaging the field. At first he thought it empty till he heard the hissing of a cobra. Squatting down, with hands on his knees, Sheshdhar peered into the pit at a magnificent six-foot long *nāga* with the largest hood he had ever seen. "Ho, fellow, you have wandered into the wrong place. But do not worry, handsome, it's not your time. I'll help you out."

Rash in some things, Sheshdhar moved carefully, aware that vibrations and movement would warn the cobra. He slid into the hole, not that deep for a man, a few feet from the cobra. Then before the *nāga* could pinpoint his location, Sheshdhar struck out with his hand, grabbing the cobra behind its hood. It hissed furiously, opening wide its mouth to reveal wicked-looking fangs. But Sheshdhar laughed. "Oh yes, you would be a killer but I am no threat to you and I respect you for your strength."

Using his other hand he pushed himself up to sit on the pit's ledge, the *nāga* all the time writhing like a ribbon burning in flame. Then Sheshdhar leapt to his feet and walked over to the stand of oleanders. Bending over, he lowered the cobra amongst the creepers, then let go, moving quickly out of reach.

The cobra should have slithered quickly out of sight, finally safe; instead it turned its black eyes upon Sheshdhar and moved out of the bushes. Puzzled, Sheshdhar backed up. He could easily stay out of reach from a *nāga* but why was it coming towards him? He stopped and so did the cobra. Then its hood swelled, the brown, black and white hues shining brightly in the sun. It moved into defensive stance, two feet of sinuous serpent rearing into the air, but it kept growing, reaching higher towards the treetops until it hovered a good three feet above Sheshdhar's gaping mouth.

The *nāga* spoke. "You have proven yourself brave and an ally. You may ask a boon of me."

Sheshdhar stared at the cobra towering over him, which could have easily exited the pit. "I . . . I don't understand."

"There is nothing to understand. It is the way of gods and you have proven yourself an ally of the *nāgas*. What boon would you have of Shesha Nāga?"

Swallowing, afraid to raise any more questions of the lord of serpents and try its patience, still he asked, "May I ask it at a later time? I can think of nothing I need now."

If the *nāga* had eyebrows, they would have risen. Shesha regarded the human a while longer in silence, swaying languidly back and forth, its forked tongue darting in and out. "Very well. When you wish to use it, swish the grass back and forth with a stick and call the name of Shesha, and I will grant your boon."

This was how Sheshdhar came to be swishing the grass, far into the fields of the estate of Amrita's father. The hunger to taste so exquisite a flower filled Sheshdhar. As he worked each day he thought only of Amrita: the elegance of her hands and feet, the sway in her step, the brightness of her laugh, her sweet dewy breath. Each night was worse, raising in him a fever of visions that were not assuaged even with his hands stroking the desire from him. Even as the pearly fountain erupted from this shaft, still his mind burned with his love of Amrita.

And so he called upon the King of Nāgas and asked his favour. It would be a subtle thing in two parts. "I need only for you . . . er, one of your people to pursue her, but not harm her." Sheshdhar outlined the details and Shesha agreed, giving him further instruction on how to call the *nāgas* when the time came.

Again, Shesha regarded the man before he slithered away. "You are an interesting ally. Many would ask for riches or power but you ask only for the help of procuring a woman's love."

Sheshdhar sighed, a small smile playing over his lips. "She is worth life itself."

The airless days continued and Amrita found it hard to concentrate. Her irritation sent the servants scattering, sometimes to bring her cooling drinks of pomegranate or a fan or just to leave her be. Only the gardens and the one great fountain offered any reprieve, but everywhere she saw Sheshdhar. Sheshdhar raking clipped foliage, his muscles moving like music beneath his bronze skin. Sheshdhar cleaning the fountain, his laughter like a rich trumpet call. Sheshdhar glancing at her and wriggling his eyebrows, the ivory shine of his teeth snaring her gaze.

Amrita frowned. These sights did little to cool her down and her head began to ache. Feeling stifled, she walked the perimeters of the domain, her fingers trailing over the rough marble walls, as if trying to pull any lingering coolness from the stones. Distracted by sensations and heat, Amrita didn't notice the hissing until she was almost upon the *nāga*.

She froze, a squeak escaping her. It was never good to surprise a *nāga*, especially in the hot season. Slowly, she backed up, one hand at her throat. But even as she inched away, the cobra followed. Amrita's heart thudded in her chest, making it hard to hear. It should be going its own way but it wasn't. Foolishly she moved towards the wall and realized too late that the cobra had her cornered. She didn't dare move to the right or left for it could strike faster than deception. The *nāga* advanced and all she could do was scramble up the wall, no wider than a hand span. Long ago the wall may have been used to protect the estates from marauders. These days it mostly kept out wandering cattle. Although it was little more than five feet high, Amrita was not sure that she was safely out of the *nāga*'s reach.

Glancing over the wall's edge, she saw the other side made the barrier more effective with formidable thorn bushes covering a span of five feet. It would not be possible for her to leap over them without being severely gouged on the brambles and sharp-edged rocks beneath. Amrita's saffron sari had unwound in her evasion of the *nāga*. If she could reach it, she could throw it over the cobra's head but it too lay beneath the *nāga* and Amrita was stuck.

Amrita and the *nāga* stared at each other. She was too far for anyone to hear her calls and the day was long and hot. If she fainted from the heat, she would probably fall to the *nāga*'s bite. Sweat collected and trickled between her breasts as the underskirt for her sari clung to her damp legs. Sighing she tried to balance on the hard stone ledge, keeping her feet pressed against the wall, teetering precariously when she heard a distant shout.

Amrita yelled and the *nāga* hissed. She waved frantically with one hand and quickly grabbed the ledge again. Over the rise a man ran. As he neared, Amrita saw who it was. "Sheshdhar! Be careful; there's a *nāga* at the wall and it is very angry."

Sheshdhar stopped and looked around. He wore only the wrapped *longhi*, tucked between his legs like baggy pants. He bent down, then arose with a long stick and warily approached. "Don't worry, Amrita. I'll take care of this but don't move, in case there are others."

Swishing the stick through the grass from the side, he cautiously drew nearer the cobra. Noticing the shadowy stick, the serpent swayed in time to it but slowly backed away. It eventually moved towards some bushes, then deflated its hood and slithered on its way.

Dropping the stick, Sheshdhar ran up to Amrita. He grabbed her about the waist and looked into her eyes. "Are you all right? It didn't bite you, did it?"

She shook her head, hands on his bare shoulders, her fingers zinging with the feel of his hot flesh. "No, no. I was scared but I'm fine." A breathless moment filled her when all the land surrounding them seemed to wait in anticipation. Amrita keenly felt every texture, from the rough stone beneath her legs to the smooth suppleness of Sheshdhar's muscles.

Sheshdhar stared up into her face, the line of worry being replaced with relief. "Ah, Amrita." Then he did the unthinkable and buried his head in her lap, his hands ruching up her underskirt.

She meant to shout, "Sheshdhar, how dare you!" and push him away, but her fingers dug into his shoulders and her cry of indignation became a call of supplication. "Oh, Sheshdhar . . ."

Amrita yearned, yet could not give in. Not now, maybe not ever, not under the bright stare of day.

Sheshdhar's tongue darted like that of the serpent he had banished, seeking blindly yet knowingly up Amrita's firm thighs, ever closer to the valley of hidden nectar. His tongue touched the first dark fronds and Amrita gasped.

Sheshdhar's eagerness was his undoing. He moaned as he licked over the little fleshy bud, mingled with the salty yet sweet elixir of Amrita's sweat and her arousal. "Ahhh, Amrita, you are a delicious flower and I must have you."

Had he stayed silent Amrita's mind would have swirled down into sensation, unable to shape the harsh words. But Sheshdhar opened that door and as a lady of virtue and station her instincts flared into being. "No, Sheshdhar, you cannot. Stop this before the guards come and skewer you."

She grabbed a handful of his wavy hair and forcefully pulled his head up, his lips shiny with her juices. Biting her lip, trying to still her breath, she said, "This isn't right. Let me down from the wall before I fall."

The moment was gone as the sounds of the world encroached once again on their interlude. Silently, Sheshdhar lifted Amrita from the wall, his hands lingering on her slim waist. Then he retrieved the river of her saffron sari and Amrita pleated and tucked it back into place.

Walking back to the manor, Sheshdhar trailed a few steps behind. "We are destined, you and I. Can you not feel it?"

Without looking back, Amrita shook her head. "I am destined for an allied marriage. You are destined to take care of the land. We have no future. Every gardener and goatherd wants to get under a girl's skirts."

"It is far far more than that," Sheshdhar said tersely. "I think you know it. No matter where we end up, we will not be parted. We are of the same soul."

Amrita walked away, head bowed, acknowledging nothing.

Two nights later Sheshdhar once again called Shesha Nāga and requested the last part of his boon.

Shesha, swaying slowly above the head of the man, looked down upon him and said, "It will be as you ask and then your boon is fulfilled."

Sheshdhar bowed. "Thank you, oh King. You found favour with me and I will always honour you and your people for what you have granted me."

And so it came to pass that on the hottest and longest day of the year Amrita was like the ocean, in a constant state of motion. Her pacing only partially abated the emotions that roiled within, pulled by the currents of her fate. Dressed in her lightest sari of sheer crimson (for she felt as if her blood boiled out of her), draped over the smallest breast band and thinnest underskirt, she walked the perimeter of the manor house's inner garden. Back and forth she went until her father irritably said, "Go, Amrita. You drive us all to distraction. Go for a long walk."

Amrita closed her eyes, her nails biting into one palm. She had placed herself in this inner cage for she feared what would happen. But now she must meet her fate.

And walk she did, filled with dread and anticipation, but nothing happened. Eventually lost in deep thought, trying to avoid how fate tore her in two, Amrita grew careless of her surroundings and the time. Her hunger was not for food and so she never felt any pangs as the sun rose higher and higher and then began its descent.

It was still bright and hot, and only the most discerning eyes would have noticed the thinnest pinking of the sky. Amrita, staring at her feet as they moved assuredly along, first heard the odd sound. A rustling, a swishing that grew in tempo. Puzzled, she stopped and looked up. The golden grasses behind her rippled like the ocean, but there was not even a baby's breath of breeze. Squinting, she looked about and after a few moments saw a cobra slithering towards her. And another. And another.

There was a whole sea of serpents coming towards her. What was this? *Nāgas* didn't migrate. But Amrita had little time to ponder the anomaly. She had to get out of the way. Frantically looking around, she spotted a sturdy and thick-limbed bodhi tree but it was some distance. The *nāgas* were nearly upon her, approaching from two directions, so she ran.

Unlike the cobra of the other day, these were determined and coming upon her fast. She ran around the tree, seeking a purchase up into its branches. Finally, leaping up to grab one limb, she found a hold with her feet and began to climb, but her sari had unravelled, tangling itself. Quickly Amrita pulled it off and dropped it, grabbing for the next branch. Several *nāgas* reached the base of the tree and began, slowly, to inch their way up the trunk. Amrita reached higher, her breath coming in gasps, not caring that her breast band had unravelled and dropped. The *nāgas* were after her and she didn't know why.

When she was high enough for a moment, she began to scream for help but she was afraid nothing would save her. There might have been a shout but she only had eyes for the branches beneath her and the serpents wending their way forward. Afraid to crawl onto the thinner limbs, Amrita tried to break off a branch, but nearly unseated herself. A cobra neared the branch she perched upon when she heard a piercing whistle.

Then there was thrashing and bellowing beneath the tree and when she looked down she saw the bronzed body of Sheshdhar moving as if in a war dance. He whipped off his pale *longhi*, which had wrapped his hips, and snapped it at the *nāgas*, causing them to drop from the tree and for some reason slither off hissing.

When Sheshdhar snapped the long end of his *longhi* at the last cobra furthest along the tree, it harmlessly dropped to the ground and moved into the tall grass.

"Amrita," he called softly. "They're gone, come down."

She held tightly to the branches, her hair dishevelled, the fine fullness of her breasts as tempting as any succulent fruit. Her thin underskirt outlined her hips and legs. Sheshdhar could only stare, feeling the heat of his shaft rising like the cobras he had chased off.

"Come down," was all he said and held his arms up to Amrita.

Gradually, silently, Amrita made her way down the tree, hanging on to the branches above her head for the bark was slippery. She stood nearly upright, her arms grasping a limb above her head, giving an enticing allure to her breasts peaked by deep russet nipples. Her feet sought purchase on the sloping trunk. It was then she seemed to realize Sheshdhar's splendid nakedness.

"I . . . I can't."

"You can," he replied as he gazed upon her wild splendour.

It was then that her feet slipped and Sheshdhar grabbed her legs beneath the skirt, lacing his elbows under her knees. "Let go, Amrita."

The touch of Sheshdhar's strong arms along the length of her thighs, the heat of his body against her, and then his lips kissing her legs was too much for Amrita. Her hands, slippery with sweat, lost their hold and to avoid falling backwards she grasped the muscular gardener about his neck.

Sheshdhar reverently kissed and sucked Amrita's breasts.

"Ah, Sheshdhar, no."

"Yes, my flower, yes. I have loved you since I first saw you." He grabbed her buttocks, opening her to the heat of his staff, a *nāga* that would not be gainsaid.

Amrita felt the velvet heat press into the hot petals of her labia. It was as if she was a lotus in bloom and, giving up her last shred of resistance, she slid slowly down his shaft, till they were meshed, flesh hotter than the day, lips to lips, elbows to knees, interlocked in magnificent rhythm. Their gazes locked and Amrita bowed her head to taste Sheshdhar's lips.

Sheshdhar raised her up and her muscles flowed like liquid pulling her down. They moved like the silent glide of *nāgas*, up and down, in and out, ecstasy and love rippling out from their core until they cried in great spasms of pleasure, rocked from head to toe.

And still, Sheshdhar, holder of *nāgas*, drank of Amrita's elixir. Perfectly joined, they stood silhouetted against the sunset as the full moon rose on the longest day. Fused as one, they made love again and again.

It is said that Shesha, King of Nāgas, looked upon the union and if a serpent god could smile, he did so, naming their position *Janukurpara*, for are not the *nāgas* known for blessings of fertility? They also say that if you stare towards the trees at sunset on the longest day you may still see Amrita and Sheshdhar joined as one in their love for they represent the union of opposing forces leading ultimately to harmony in the universe.

Smaradipika

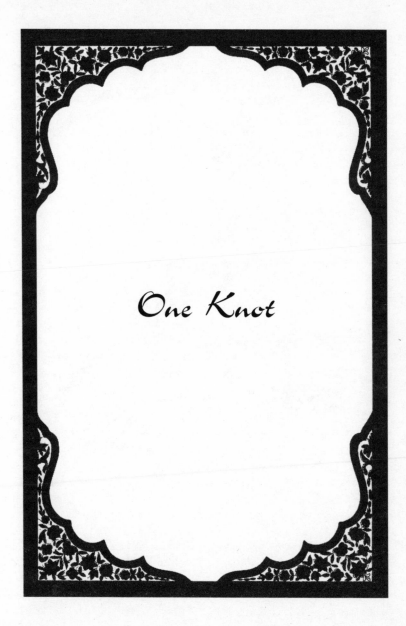

One Knot

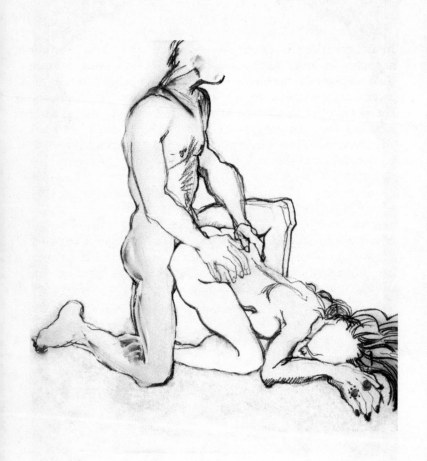

One Knot

Ekabandha
Smaradipika

In archery, there is a position where you kneel down on your haunches in order to shoot your bow. In this position from *Smaradipika*, the man gets down on his haunches and tells his lover that he is like an archer, shooting an arrow into her heart. He asks her to come and sit in his lap so she might be an archer too, and shoot an arrow back into his heart, the heart she's already won. When she ventures near, not as timid now, but bolder and sure of his love for her, with a trace of a haughty look on her lovely face, he pulls her down onto his lap, laughing and gentle, but firm. When she stops squirming, he loosens the knot of her sari. Bending his lover forward until her small breasts press against her thighs, he caresses her all the while. Then he tells her again that he is an archer and that he is going to pierce her with his love arrow. Kissing her neck, he tells her he loves her. Then, in this position, from behind, he takes and enjoys the woman, pressing her close while he enters her and she gasps.

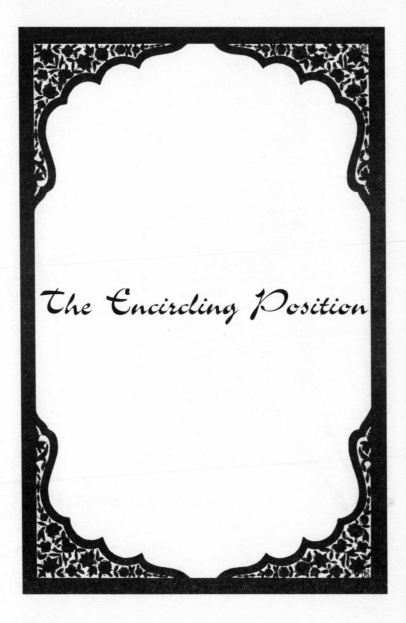

The Encircling Position

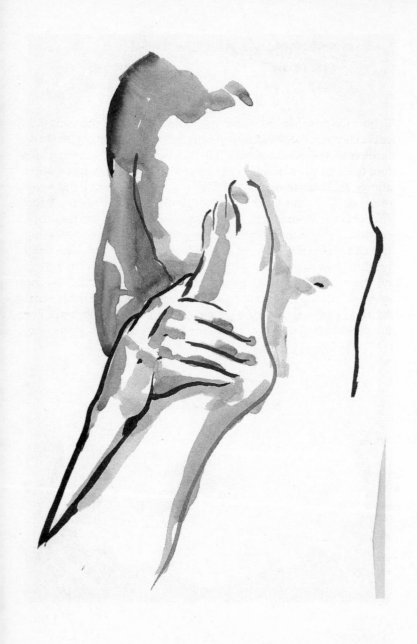

The Encircling Position

Veshta
Smaradipika

A novelty position from the *Smaradipika*, one of the medieval sex texts composed sometime in the fourteenth century after the fashion of the *Kama Sutra*. The act of a woman pressing her foot to her lover's heart is very sensual and loving. The position allows the couple to hold a steady gaze throughout the love-making. The man leans slightly against a wall at his back and supports the woman's raised hips during congress. As the name suggests, the man encircles the woman, almost encompassing her and enveloping her, as she presses her foot to his heart and he thrusts into her *yoni*. She is able to feel the skin of his chest on the sole of her foot (something that is not afforded by too many of the sex positions) and can perhaps even feel his heart beating with the passion and the exertion of the act. The affection between the couple is apparent in this loving position.

The Tale of the Legend of Veshta

as told by Joe Filippone

The pale lavender blue light from the full moon was the only source of light for Aseem as he made his way home. He tried to walk in a straight line but every step he took felt as if he was walking on rolling waves during a storm at sea. He stumbled several times: over rocks, dirt, his feet, the air. Even when he tried to walk as slowly as possible, he still couldn't stay upright for more than three steps.

Aseem had never drunk as much as he had that night. He felt ashamed, a man who came from a family as wealthy as his, drinking like a peasant. Even though he didn't like the way the alcohol made him feel, he still wouldn't have changed anything about that night. It had been special. A rejoicing with all of Aseem's male friends celebrating his marriage to Veshta, the most beautiful girl in the village.

All of the men had been in love with Veshta, doing everything they could to get her attention but Veshta hadn't given any of them one iota of attention. Until her eyes fell on Aseem. And his hair, black as ebony, which fell just above his shoulders and only barely covered his eyes. He was tall, almost six feet, with muscles well proportioned over every inch of his body.

Like every other man in the village, Aseem had had his eye on Veshta for as long as he could remember. The thing that had attracted him, and every other man, was the air of mystery that exuded from Veshta. Her eyes, dark pools, were all she allowed the world to view, choosing to keep the rest of her body, even her hair, hidden from the world by means of a dark blue dress, which even covered her feet, and a pale blue veil.

Aseem hiccupped as he tried to increase his speed to get home and begin his wedding night. Tonight was the night that he would be able to unwrap the greatest gift in the world. He had been anxious to get home to Veshta for many hours. His mind had been painting a picture of what he thought she would look like naked. Both him and his man-root couldn't wait to get home and find out how accurate that picture had been. Nothing could distract him from his journey. That is, until he heard the chanting.

He stopped and turned to the source of the chanting. It was soft. Delicate. Feminine. It reminded Aseem of a bird manufactured in heaven. He slowly made his way towards the chanting. He didn't know why but his heart started to pump faster and little droplets of sweat seeped out of his pores as he made his way closer and closer. He took a step and fell in the dirt. Not bothering to get up, he crawled along the ground like a serpent. Slowly. Silently. He didn't want to disturb whoever it was that was chanting.

Aseem had to shield his eyes from the glow of the candles that were coming from the temple of Shiva. He could see her illuminated by the reddish-orange shadows of the many candles she had placed around the temple. Her eyes were closed. Her head thrown back. She was completely nude. Aseem's breath caught in his throat at the sight of her. Curly black hair guarded the entrance to her most sacred temple; breasts, round like the sun; nipples standing erect from the cool breeze that blew in from the outside. Her hair, black as the night sky, swept back and forth as she moved her body in time with her chanting.

Aseem didn't know what came over him. He got up and moved towards the temple. His feet were silent. The girl didn't even know that an invader had intruded on her nightly ritual. Aseem felt as if he were being manipulated by a higher power controlling him with strings. He moved towards the girl. Closer. Closer. Closer. Timidly he reached out a hand and clasped her round, full buttocks. The girl jumped, startled by the foreign touch and turned around so fast she almost knocked herself to the ground.

"Hello." Aseem's throat felt tight and constrained; he could barely get the word out.

The girl didn't speak. She opened her mouth to yell for help but no sound came out.

"You're very beautiful." Aseem smiled brushing her cheek with his finger before clasping her breast in his hand.

"Please." The girl found her voice. "Don't."

But Aseem did not listen. He grabbed the girl and kissed her. She protested, not only with her voice but also with her fists, but it was no use. Aseem was too strong and seemed to have a thousand arms.

Aseem felt ashamed. He didn't know what had come over him. After he had spilled his seed, he had run from the temple, realization sobering him up. His feet were a blur and didn't stop until he had got safely inside Veshta's huge home. He leaned against the door, panting. He didn't want his new bride to know that anything had happened.

"Aseem, is that you?" Veshta's voice called from her bedroom.

"Yes."

"Come to bed. I've been waiting hours for you."

He made his way down the hall to the bedroom. Slowly. Scared that Veshta would be able to tell what he had done. Timidly he opened the door and walked into the room.

All of his fear and shame disappeared when he saw Veshta lying naked, seductive, on the bed. Aseem's eyes traced her body, drinking in every detail. She was more beautiful than he had pictured. Her skin was a rich chestnut colour. Her breasts, as round as melons, were the largest he had ever seen. Her nipples, a dark cinnamon colour, had sharpened into hard little knobs. His eyes travelled lower and he couldn't believe what he saw. The entrance to her woman's temple had no hair guarding it. Her legs were spread wide, giving Aseem a perfect view of everything.

"Does my body meet with your approval?" she asked smiling like a temptress.

Aseem could only nod his head affirmatively for a large lump had caught in his throat.

Veshta smiled at the power she had over her new husband; it was a power she had always possessed. She slowly crawled towards the foot of the bed.

"Don't just stand there, Husband. Undress. Let me look upon you as you have looked upon me."

Aseem did as he was told. Lust filled Veshta's heart when he pulled off his shirt. His skin was darker then hers, the colour of mocha. His chest and arms were well muscled and sparsely populated with hair. Her lust boiled over, she could feel the moistness of desire seeping out of her woman's temple when he stripped off his pants. She licked her lips at the sight of his man-root standing proudly at attention.

"Very nice." Her voice was low and husky. "Now get in bed, Husband, and show me if you know how to use that tool."

Aseem tripped over his feet as he rushed to the bed. Veshta ran her hands over Aseem's body. She could feel the heat of desire exuding from his pores. Running her fingers through his hair, she took the lead, drew him close to her and kissed him fully. Aseem didn't think it was possible but he felt his man-root grow even harder and thicker with the throbbing blood of desire.

Pushing him onto his back, Veshta got on top of him and slowly, painfully, rubbed her body back and forth across him as she continued to kiss him. Aseem could feel her breasts and hard nipples pressed against him. Her body was just as hot with passion as his. His hands were caressing her back. As they continued to kiss, his hands grew bolder and travelled lower and lower until they reached her round buttocks. She moaned approvingly into his mouth as he kneaded her doughy cheeks.

"Let me show you something a servant boy taught me," she whispered in his ear before gently biting his ear lobe.

She turned around until her mouth was inches from his man-root. Aseem smiled, he now had a perfect view and easy access to her woman's temple.

"Now we will be able to give each other pleasure," she said as she lightly stroked Aseem's length with her finger.

Aseem's back arched and he felt a tingling in his toes when Veshta opened her mouth and swallowed him whole. Aseem smiled as he stuck a finger inside her most intimate temple and rhythmically thrust it in and out; the way Veshta made love to his man-root with her mouth told him that she had had much practice and would not disappoint him in bed.

Aseem clutched Veshta's thigh and gently licked every inch of flesh around her *yoni* before growing braver and sticking his tongue inside her. Veshta's body tingled with a small tremor. She let out a low sigh. Aseem grinned mischievously at her private entrance and increased the thrusting of his tongue, even swirling it around inside her. Veshta closed her eyes, enjoying his oral pleasure. She continued to move up and down his *lingam*, giving his whole length ample attention. She liked the feel of him in her mouth.

"Husband," Veshta moaned breathlessly, "your tongue is wonderful within me, but I need to feel your man-root inside me. Now."

Veshta rolled off of Aseem, got on her back and spread her legs wide. Aseem climbed on top of her and was all set to enter her when the room rumbled with a voice filled with anger.

"Stop!"

Aseem and Veshta looked around in fear. Their eyes popped out of their heads and almost fell to the floor when they saw who had appeared in the bedroom: Shiva, the very angry god.

Shiva had witnessed what Aseem had done to the girl in his temple and it had angered him. After Aseem had left, the girl had prayed that Shiva take revenge. Shiva had loved the girl. She was his most faithful follower. She had vowed to always remain a virgin to show her devotion to Shiva. Hearing her prayer for revenge, Shiva knew what he had to do.

"Aseem." Shiva's voice reverberated off the walls. "You have committed the darkest crime of all. You have soiled my most loyal follower. You have soiled my temple. You have soiled yourself. For that, you and your wife will forever pay. I will make you both untouchable. When you lie on top of your wife and stick your man-root inside her it will feel like the cobra's fang is penetrating her. But that is just the beginning of my wrath. If you two should ever find a way to reach simultaneous pleasure, you will both die instantaneously."

That was all he said. For as quickly as he had appeared, he was gone. Aseem and Veshta looked at each other with fear.

They didn't know if what they had seen was real or a hallucination.

"Was that true?" Veshta asked.

"I don't know."

"Lie on top of me. There's only one way to find out if what he said was true. Or if he was even truly here."

Aseem got back on top of her. He took hold of his *lingam* and started to guide it into her *yoni*. He had just got the tip inside her when she screamed.

"What's wrong?" Aseem asked pulling out quickly.

"It felt like the cobra's fang was inside me," she explained with tears in her eyes. "It was just like he said." She pushed him off her, got off the bed and began to pace around the room. "Now we will never lie together. What is the point of even being married? All because you couldn't control your lustful desires."

"Please don't be angry," Aseem tried to reason with her. "We will find a way to lie together."

"How?" Her voice was tear-stained. "You cannot lie on top of me. We can never achieve mutual pleasure. You can't outsmart an angry god."

"I'm sorry. Really I am." He got up and embraced her. "This is all my fault."

He held her close to him. She clutched him. They kissed. She didn't know what came over her but she put her legs around his waist. His hands were under her, gently caressing her buttocks. It was several minutes before they realized that his man-root had somehow become embedded deep inside her.

"There's no pain," she said surprised. "Only pleasure."

Aseem thrust in and out of her a few times to make sure. Veshta moaned but it was quiet cries of pleasure. The two lovers smiled at each other. They had found a way to outsmart a god.

"I am not on top of you." He grinned.

Veshta screamed in pleasure as Aseem thrust in and out of her, hitting every pleasurable spot her woman's temple possessed.

"Aseem—" her voice was breathless "no man has ever given me this much pleasure before."

Her legs encircled his waist tighter. She kissed his shoulders, sucked on his neck. Her hands became entangled in his hair. She tugged his head back giving her greater access to his neck.

Aseem's hands squeezed the flesh of her buttocks. He pushed her against the wall and thrust harder into her. He pressed his body hard against hers. They were so close, it was as if he wanted to meld them into one being. Her breasts were flattened against his chest like rose petals that have been pressed into a scrapbook.

Veshta's ankles caressed Aseem's buttocks, increasing his pleasure. He continued to thrust in and out of her. The sounds of their lovemaking echoed throughout the bedroom. Veshta let out a low animal-like growl and clutched Aseem's hair tightly in her fist. She could feel her pleasure boiling over, beginning at the tips of her toes, causing them to curl, before spreading throughout her whole being.

"Husband!" she cried out as she felt pleasure overtake her.

Her desire poured out of her woman's temple, staining Aseem's skin. At the same time, Aseem spilled his own seed deep inside her and kissed her deeply.

The servant girl knocked softly on the door the next morning. She opened the door and peeked in. She had heard the sounds of passion coming from the room the night before. They sounded so vigorous, she deduced that Veshta and Aseem were probably dead from exhaustion.

She looked around. The room was empty. She felt disappointment rush over her. She had been hoping to see Aseem naked. He was very good-looking. The servant girl had made up her mind that if she didn't get a look at his naked form that morning, she would hide in the closet that night to see him.

She turned around and that's when she saw the rug. It hadn't been there last night. Maybe it was a wedding present from Aseem. The servant girl blushed, feeling lustful tingles enter her woman's temple as she looked at it. There was a man and a woman embroidered on the rug; they looked strangely like Aseem and Veshta. Her legs were wrapped around his waist, her hands clutching his hair. His hands were clutching the flesh of her buttocks, supporting her. His man-root was deep inside her woman's temple, deeper than the servant girl had ever thought possible.

The lustful girl left the room, forgetting all about finding the newlyweds. She rushed down the hall, looking for the very handsome servant boy, eager to try out the position she had seen on the rug.

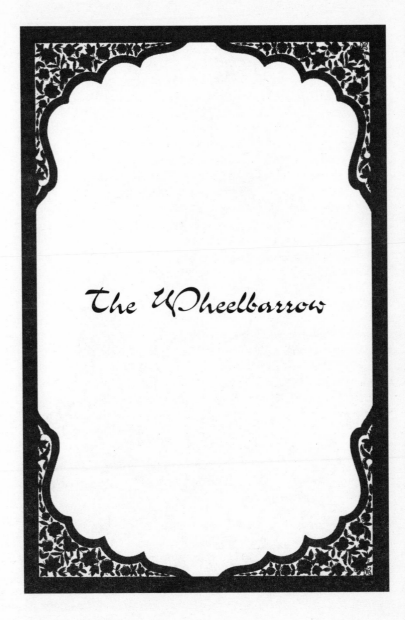

The Wheelbarrow

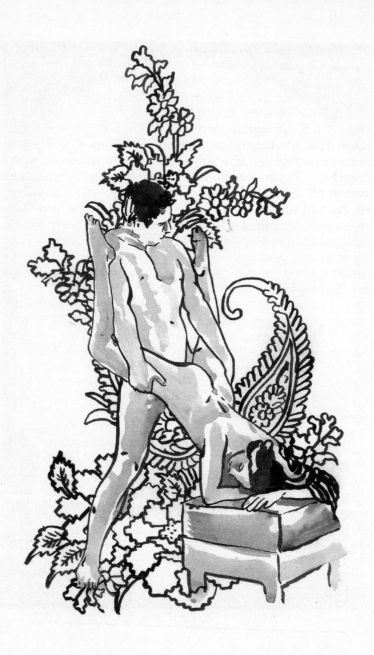

The Wheelbarrow

Kulisha
Smaradipika

Use of the appropriate vigorous strokes by the man is a necessity here. Once the woman is in the position, backwards, and with her feet in your hands as if she were a wheelbarrow, the penetration depth that you can achieve is highlighted. The woman must simply hold on as the man is totally in control. He can add further variations to this position if he wishes by opening up her legs or holding them in a more closed position, tight to his hips. Orgasm should not be a problem for either party in this position. The woman can look back over her shoulder if she wishes to, gazing at her lover as he enjoys her. Sensual additions add much to these positions.

The Tale of Unleashing the Thunderball

as told by Carmel Lockyer

Aditya stared at the furrows he had dug with the village plough. The soil was drier than flour, more powdery than talcum. Neha was bound to blame him for the failed crop; she always did. It had been a mistake to marry her, despite the old matchmaker's claim that "their marriage would be like sun and rain". There was too much sun and too little rain – the marriage was a misery. He wanted to throw himself on the ground and cry, hammering his anger into the earth with his feet and hands, to push his hips into the dry dust and force it to submit, but a man had his pride. He turned his back to the village.

Neha stared at the seedling pepper plants, their leaves pointing earthwards in despair. She watered them three times daily, carrying the precious liquid in a jug and building walls of dry soil around each plant to hold the water in, but it wasn't working. The rice crop was already dead; she would have to let something go to buy dried rice. She had only one gold bangle left of her wedding dowry and she would have to sell it before the week was out. Aditya would grumble – after nearly two years of marriage, her husband always grumbled. She straightened her back, feeling her sari binding itself to her skin with sweat – her hips, thighs, belly, buttocks, all swathed and rubbed by the hot, wet fabric. She plucked at her waist, wanting to unwind the yards of cotton and walk naked, to soak her feet in the water around the peppers, to lie on her back and point her nipples at the baking sun. Such things were not possible, so she lifted the end of the sari, wiped her forehead and stooped to collect more water.

When all the plants had slaked their thirst, she walked back to the little house she shared with Aditya. Things could have been worse, she could have been living with her parents-in-law, like so many girls did, but Aditya's mother was dead and his father had become *moksha* – travelling the country with a pilgrim's begging bowl as soon as they were married. As she waited for Aditya to return from the fields she cooked fish curry and *palappam*. She had dreamed of marrying a farmer, raising crops and a family in Kerala's rich and sometimes fierce landscape, but her dreams had died, like the rice plants.

Aditya left the plough outside the headman's house and walked to his own bungalow, pausing to pat the village elephant, which had been tethered outside his own house when his father had been headman. He knew his father had expected him to take on the job, but with the failed harvests and his dry marriage, Aditya had felt he was not fit to lead his neighbours. The elephant flapped its ears and listened intently to his words, which was more than Neha ever did.

Back in his own garden, the peppers were trying to lift their leaves in the evening cool but the effort was too much for them. He understood their feelings. Outside the house he poured water into a brass bowl, kicked off his sandals, lifted his shirt and unwound his *mundu*, finally standing naked as he lifted the dipper. He poured water in thin streams, watching its silvery passage over his body, washing dust away and cooling the hidden, dark parts of his body that had chafed during his work with the plough. The cool teasing of the water made him wince and harden at the same time, and he looked down at the purple bulb of his glans, rising like a night flower.

Neha watched from the window. Her husband's body – stocky and powerful – had once aroused strange feelings in her: curiosity and a hot itching to understand the way his masculine parts worked and what they might do inside her. But something was wrong between them – never once had he roused her during sex. This was not the way things should be, but it was Aditya's job to put it right, not hers. Even so, as she saw his *lingam* rising, curving into the air as the streams of bright water parted around it, she felt her own body heating, sweat prickling between her legs where she removed the hair, heaviness in her breasts, as though something needed to be squeezed from them. She sighed and leaned against the uneven mud-brick wall, pressing her body to it. Every night, as she watched her husband wash, she found the same brick, a little more protruding than its neighbours, and rubbed herself against it.

Aditya thought about his wife as he washed. How many nights had he stared down at Neha, as she lay beneath him, her *tilak* of red dye like a third eye in the middle of her forehead, her eyes closed as though he didn't exist? Her body was a fine thing, that was undeniable. Her breasts were round and soft, her hips lissom and her buttocks as tender as the best *paneer*. Her skin was the colour of *masala chai*, and her hair smelt of coconut. And yet she lay as passive as the seeds in the fields – inert and sterile. He pushed past her into the house and ate the fish curry she'd cooked for dinner, then fell asleep almost immediately, crowding her into a corner of the *charpoy*.

It was hot and dry again the next morning. Neha made *appam*, the sticky rice pancakes eaten for breakfast, and laid them in front of Aditya with small bowls of pickle. He ate slowly, refusing to look at her. A parakeet screamed in the tree outside, splitting the heavy air with its cry. Aditya was so startled he knocked an *appam* from the banana-leaf plate to the floor.

Neha frowned. What to do? If she threw it away he would accuse her of wasting food in a drought year, but if she put it back on the table he would say she was showing no respect to him. She bent, picked up the pancake and broke it in two. One half she laid on the leaf, the other she threw out of the window in the direction of the bird. Aditya stared out of the window, then at the broken *appam*, then at her.

"Are you a mad woman? Has the heat cooked your brain?"

Neha lifted her chin and stared him down. "Are you a man? Has the heat cooked your *lingam*?"

Aditya pushed the table towards her, its weight seeming nothing to him. When his arms were fully stretched and she was almost pinned in the corner, he rose, suddenly very dark and strong. "Are you a wife or a mattress? You need not answer,

I know you are a mattress, lying beneath me like a dead thing, stealing my strength and soaking up my passion but giving nothing of yourself."

"A mattress?" Neha laid her own hands on the table and braced herself to speak as loudly as possible. "If I am a mattress, what are you? Are you a plough? Yes, exactly. A clumsy, heavy thing that turns the earth but cannot plant a seed!" Her fingers found the metal pickle dish and she knocked it to the floor with a dramatic gesture.

Aditya roared like a water buffalo and swept the table clear with his arm, sending *appam* and banana leaves flying. He grabbed Neha by her sari and pulled her round the table, dragging her to the tin mirror over the washbasin.

"Look!" he bellowed. "See how bad a wife you are!"

Neha glanced in the mirror and saw their angry faces, open mouths yelling, eyes hot. Aditya looked just like Pushkara, the villain in the Kathakali play they had seen in Trivandrum the week they got married. Pushkara had shown just such a face when he caught his brother's new bride alone and prepared to ravish her. What had the heroine done? Ah yes . . .

Neha lifted her hand and slapped Aditya's cheek.

He blinked, seemingly unaffected by her blow, and transferred his grip from her sari to the back of her neck, marching her across the room to the bed. She found she couldn't break free – it was like being held by giant pincers. Aditya pushed her down on the *charpoy*, wrapping her long hair around his left hand like a leash. "Now we shall see what happens to a wife who strikes her husband."

Neha glared up at him as he loomed over her, one hand pinning her down by her hair, the other gathering up folds and swathes of sari cloth and shoving them towards her waist so her legs and belly were bared. The world outside the bungalow fell silent as birds and beasts responded to the oppressive atmosphere by rushing for shelter, but the couple failed to notice.

Aditya gestured and Neha parted her legs sullenly. He lowered himself onto her with such force that she gasped, and he grimaced like Pushkara. "So, my wife can make a noise in bed after all!"

Neha scowled and closed her mouth tight. Aditya's *lingam* was pushing between her thighs and she tilted her hips grudgingly to let him in, as a wife must, just as he found the way for himself, thrusting into her with an ill-tempered cry. The sky lit blue as brilliant lightning flashed over the fields. Aditya thrust again and Neha gasped at the force of it. He closed his eyes and shoved into her, releasing her hair so he could gain purchase for his thrusts. Lightning flashed again, making his face dark but his teeth gleamed in the momentary glare. Neha stared up at him – it felt as if he was stretching her body to its utmost, as though the head of his shaft was pressing against her ribs. Her hand crept down her body, touching her sternum, her belly, her navel, trying to find the point inside her where his deepest touch arrived.

Aditya opened his eyes and looked down. Neha's face was dark and relaxed, as though she was simply resting. He admired the lushness of her mouth, her lips soft and lax, before remembering his anger and intensifying his thrusts. As he penetrated her more deeply even than before, he saw her eyelids flicker in the electric light that split the sky. The line of her mouth changed, becoming an upward curve. He ignored the lightning, repeating the thrust and saw a smile emerging on her face. Aditya paused, his bad mood wiped away by Neha's response. All the gentle ways and sweet caresses he'd tried since their wedding day had not produced this result. He braced his arms, lifting his hips high above her, watching as the gleaming length of his shaft slid into view until only the very tip remained in contact with the dark folds of her *yoni*.

The sky flashed again as he forced himself down, slamming his body into hers, onto hers, with a force that he regretted immediately. Not so his wife – as he watched, her smile became wide and greedy and her hands, formerly quiescent, moved – one to settle on his hip, the other to form a first just above her pubic bone.

Neha had found the place, and in her discovery had found something else. If she pushed down hard, a strange hot sensation rose from under her fist and spread through her body. If Aditya pressed down with all his power, that feeling became a heavy ecstatic pleasure. She put a hand on her husband's hip and pushed up, encouraging him to lift away from her so she could experience his descent again.

Aditya hovered, staring down the length of his torso to his *lingam* in the turquoise flash of the silent lightning. His shoulders knotted with the strain of holding his body in the air but the effort was pleasant and the reward great. Beneath him Neha opened up her body, pointing her breasts to the ceiling with her back arched. He lowered his head to tug one nipple with his mouth. Neha groaned, a faint musical sound. "So my wife can make a noise in bed after all," he said softly and Neha opened her eyes and gave him a look of such joy that he nearly lost control of his body. Reciting the 108 names of Krishna under his breath, he held still, quelling the desire to empty himself into her. As usual, thinking of the God disciplined his unruly *lingam*. Krishna had pleasured an unknown number of milkmaids – surely Aditya could satisfy one wife! He plunged down, forcing the air from Neha's lungs with his weight and power.

Neha dug her nails into Aditya's flesh as though to force him even deeper into her. This was better than her vague dreams, or pressing herself to the rough wall. The new, strong Aditya made her body tense with pleasure. As he rose, she opened her eyes, watching his stern face as he hovered above her, then looked down to his *lingam*, glistening as it slid into view, dark purple and more swollen than she had ever seen it. Her body was sure of what it wanted – as Aditya moved away, her thighs opened wider until her feet barely touched each side of the narrow *charpoy*. Her hips pressed down as his rose, widening the distance between them, but her back arched, lifting her breasts like temple offerings. She sighed gently and smiled again.

Aditya had got to name 56, Mayur – the lord who has a peacock-feathered crest – when he thought of something. He rose to his knees and gripped Neha's ankles firmly with his hands. "Hold on," he said, grinning, and twisted her body so that one foot rose over his head as the other descended. Neha rotated on his *lingam* and came to rest face down.

"Ugh! What are you . . .?" she said, trying to untangle her arms and lift her upper body from the *charpoy*.

Aditya descended, splitting her like an arrow hitting the target. She yelled, and what she yelled aloud was "Yes!"

But nobody heard, not even Aditya, because as his body met hers, the skies split once more with blue light, but this time with the light came the sound of a thunderbolt and immediately after the crashing meeting of flesh and flesh, earth and sky, came the monsoon rain. It poured so fast and hard that it was like a waterfall. No individual drops could be distinguished, only sheets and walls of water.

Aditya felt the temperature drop – the skin on his back prickled with the sudden chill – but it was a minor consideration beside the intensity of his pleasure as he knelt above Neha, holding her ankles in his hands as he prepared to descend. Now he moved faster and Neha began to cry out, short low sounds that drove him crazy, punctuating his own desire, reminding him that she was capable of more than he had guessed and that his release must wait, and wait.

Neha gripped the edge of the *charpoy* with both hands, bracing her body with her grasping fingers and her forearms, as her lower body was raised by Aditya's strong arms high into the air, her spine bending, her feet higher than her heart and her legs spread wider than the *charpoy*. She lowered her face to the bed, bracing herself to receive him.

Aditya stole a glimpse and then closed his eyes against the lovely view, the delicious curve of Neha's spine, her buttocks proud and taut in mid-air, her legs straight and muscular, her ankles imprisoned by his hands. The head of his shaft was twitching to enter her again, the darkness of her *yoni* invited him to plunge forward, but he kept his eyes sealed against her, counting under his breath until she spoke.

"Aditya, husband . . ." She could feel him poised behind her, what was he waiting for? "Please . . ."

It was all he had waited for, the sign that Neha was ready. He fell on her like a warrior, sinking to the hilt in her body, thrusting forward, hammering on her like a devotee ringing a temple gong.

Neha heard strange sounds through the sensations that were vibrating into the marrow of her bones. There was one like thunder, and another like a bell or a gong, and there was a drumming too, as if a thousand barefoot men were running silently through the village. For a second she lifted her head to try and identify the noises, but then Aditya pushed deeper and she lost any sense of where she was, only knowing that she must make him do that again, and again.

Aditya heard the *charpoy*'s metal frame banging against the wall like a muted bell, but the heavy pattering of the rain didn't attract his attention because he was too busy trying not to hear his wife, his lover, his darling Neha begging him to move faster, push harder. If he allowed himself to be distracted then he would lose control and it would all be over. He began reciting the names of Krishna again, "Achala, Achutya, Adbhutah . . ." He didn't hear the thunderbolts that split the sky above the village, nor the rising monsoon water that swirled along the gutters and rushed into the fields from the raised road. He did hear Neha begin to gasp and moan, and took her cries as his rhythm to thrust, and thrust.

Neha felt the pleasure turning into something much stronger, a hot liquid swirling that she'd never imagined possible and as she gripped the bed, gritting her teeth to try and make the moment last longer, she came.

Aditya felt Neha's body vibrate and heard her low cries become higher and more vociferous as her orgasm broke. He followed it with his own, bellowing aloud into the storm as he came.

Neha thought her heart was still drumming when she woke up several hours later, until she separated her own breathing from the rain pounding the roof. Aditya was a warm solid presence beside her and she pressed herself against him. He stirred and woke and reached out for her . . .

The rain stopped just before dusk. They dressed hurriedly, keen to see how their neighbours and crops had coped with the downpour. Neha slid her gold bangle over her wrist, wanting to mark the occasion in a way Aditya would understand.

Outside, the pepper plants sat in a lake, each leaf lifted to the evening air. Aditya examined them. "All it took was rain to make them stand up properly," he said.

"All it took was your *lingam* standing up properly to make rain!" Neha replied and then ran shrieking down the path as he chased her with mock growls. There was something serious behind her joke though, she thought, and as they approached the village she slipped to one side, wanting to watch his reactions. The villagers were tending vegetable patches or even planting rice in their fields despite the lateness of the hour, while the new headman weighed out *annas* of seed and yelled at people in his debt, "There is no excuse now the rains have come. I want the money you owe me – bring it tomorrow. If you cannot pay, I will take a share of your harvest."

Aditya stopped in the path. "My father would never have soured a day of happiness with such carping," he muttered. "Nor would he have broadcast who was so poor they couldn't pay their debts." He looked for the old matchmaker, but her hut was empty.

Neha moved in front of him, speaking loudly. "Mr Headman, perhaps the rains won't come again – perhaps your rudeness will scare them away."

There was laughter from the villagers and the headman blinked. "Oh, the wife of Aditya speaks and what rubbish falls from her mouth – no wonder she is usually silent."

Neha touched her bangle. "It is not rubbish, it is truth. Since you became headman, the rains have avoided us."

"Oh, but they are back now, so you are once again talking nonsense."

Neha looked at the mud path, sensing Aditya behind her, his rising anger making lightning crackle across the sky. She held out her arm. "I am talking sense, and I am willing to wager my gold bangle that you cannot say when it will rain again and Aditya can."

The headman laughed, eyeing the gold. "It will rain tomorrow night, as it does every night in the monsoon. You are a fool – and you will owe me your bangle."

"But you must bet something too." Neha spoke loudly enough for the whole village to hear. "You must gamble an election date – two months from today."

The headman frowned, glancing at Aditya, who stared back, as impassive as the village elephant. "Very well."

"Now listen." Neha turned to the villagers. "Our headman says it will rain tomorrow. Aditya says it will not." Aditya looked surprised, not having said anything, but nodded. "Aditya, who truly knows when the rain will come, says it will rain the day after tomorrow, starting at . . ."

"Noon," Aditya supplied.

"Noon? The rain starts in the evening, always," the headman couldn't resist saying.

"Noon," Aditya repeated.

Neha turned aside. "Where is the matchmaker, we came to . . . thank her."

There were wide grins in the dusk as villagers guessed what thanks the young couple had come to offer, but a voice spoke up from the gloom. "She's gone, she left the village as the rains arrived, said something about it being time to move on."

Neha frowned and looked at Aditya, but he was talking to the elephant, whispering that in a few weeks it could come home where it belonged, once he had been elected headman, like his father before him.

Aditya and Neha walked home, hand in hand. "I will spend tomorrow night at the temple, giving thanks," said Neha. "That way we cannot be tempted."

"Be home by midday," said Aditya, smiling to himself.

"Or you will strike me with thunderbolts?" Neha teased.

"Something like that," her husband replied.

Srngararasaprabandhadipika

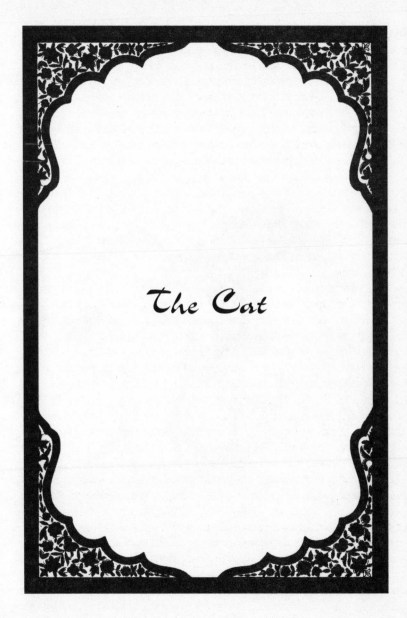

The Cat

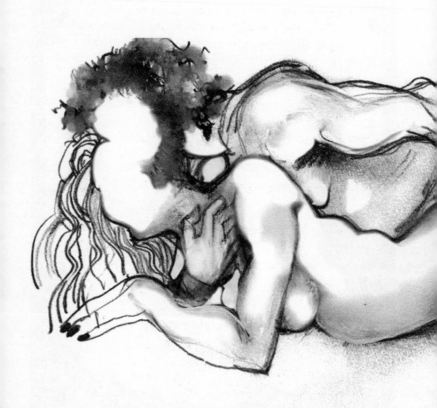

The Cat

Marjara
Srngararasaprabandhadipika

The cat position from the obscure love text *The Light of Love* by Harihara is one of the favourites of all the 64 listed there. Lying on her stomach, naked but for the flowers in her hair, the man seizes her ankles in one hand, lifts them as he penetrates her from behind, tilting her chin up so he can gaze into her eyes as his lingam enters her yoni. The woman acts like a cat in heat, making the appropriate mewling noises.

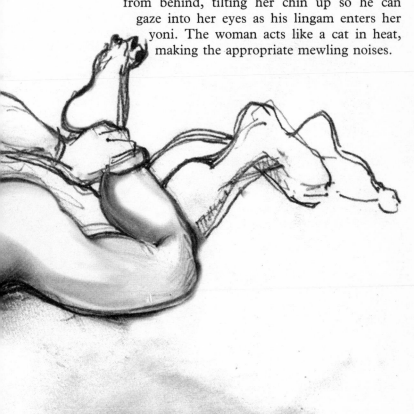

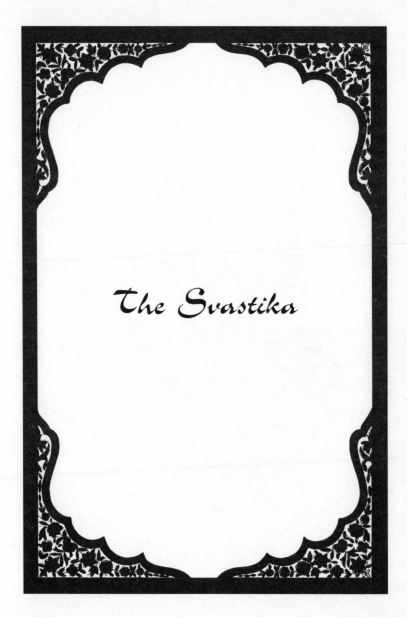

The Svastika

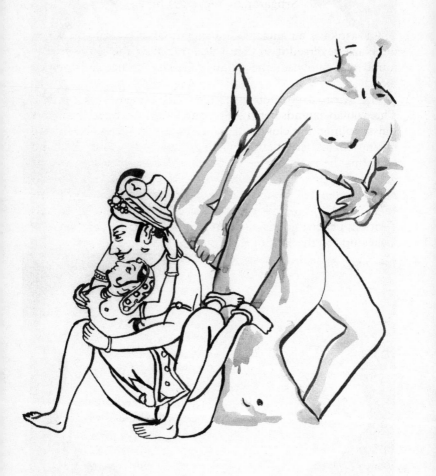

The Svastika

Svastika
Srngararasaprabandhadipika

The svastika is an ancient Indian symbol of good luck. When the Nazis reversed it so that it was travelling the opposite way round (anti-sunwise), the pandits called it sacrilege and doomed them.

The svastika position resembles this ancient luck symbol. The woman extends her right leg and wraps it around the man's waist, pulling him close. She makes sure that her ankle ends up resting on his left thigh. The man then follows her lead and performs the exact moves so they both end up in a basic shape like a svastika with groins touching. Penetration is then possible, as well as all the forms of scratching and marking, particularly suitable to this position because of the angle. In this position, penetration is moderate but the closeness and novelty makes up for the lack of depth.

The Tale of Absolute Being

as told by K. L. Gillespie

The stars are bright tonight and appear as a canopy, winking in the sky before the sun has fully set. They vie for my attention, glittering, full of life and promises in the face of the dying sun. But the sun smiles knowingly. After his rest he will be refreshed and the moon and the stars will be no match for him. They will soon disappear in his glory as he cartwheels across the sky. He will sleep soundly tonight.

The Purandar Valley stretches into the darkness and from my hut on the side of the hill I can see for miles as I idle away the hours on my flute, content to know that my sheep are grazing safely around me.

Rumours of a hungry tiger have reached my ears but there has been no sighting of her in these parts. Tonight I pray she will be someone else's problem and I stoke the fire again, just in case.

In the mouth of the valley I can see the lights of Narayanpur flickering as the village prepares to sleep. One by one the lamps are extinguished and the windows disappear. Except one and in that window I know my Suvali, my love, is waking from the slumber I left her in.

I have loved Suvali since we were infants playing in the dust outside the houses of our parents. When we were six we married behind the temple, our witnesses were the stray cats and dogs of the village, her veil was a sack and our rings made from grass stalks. Eleven years later we were married by our families and this time her veil was made from silk.

Many moons have passed since that day and with each sunrise my love has grown stronger. She is my life and I live for just one thing, to be possessed by her, to kiss her neck, to look into her eyes. This is my reason for living. She was the reason I was born and in a few more hours I'll be heading back down into the valley and into her arms.

The sweet music of my fellow shepherds winds through the valley like a daisy chain, connecting us in the darkness, keeping us awake and alert. I wander down to my flock, picking some mountain dates on my way, and count their fleeces by torch-light. All present and correct and a calm envelops the hillside as I head back to my hut.

The hill is matted with flowers. Chickweed, datura, sweet snow and wind flowers dance on their stalks in the gentle breeze. Columbines embroider the earth's carpet and their beauty reminds me of Suvali. I pick some for her, a gift to celebrate our reunion. Just as I reach for one last bloom some-thing catches my eye in the night sky.

Just a glint in the distance to begin with, a shooting star I thought at first, but within moments I knew this was something else.

Seconds later, the sky cracks open and I am blinded by a burning light, like a manic sun in the night sky.

It spins at speed through the air like a celestial chariot, lighting up the pastures. So close to me that the jets of steam streaming from it, bent by the force of its journey, appear like the four arms of the svastikas that mark the ancient temples, the image of Brahma's own footprint.

Chaos falls upon the hillside as the other shepherds run in fear. Some run to their huts for shelter, shaking in their skin, sure that the mighty light in the sky is a harbinger of doom. Others ring bells to wake the village but their warnings go unheeded, blown into the next valley by a crosswind and my townsfolk sleep on, unaware of everything that is happening in the sky above them.

At first I too am rigid with fear as it hurtles towards me and I pin myself, flat on my back, into the hillock beneath me, desperately trying to shelter in the Earth's warm soil.

But as the mystical cross whirs across the sky I am transfixed, beguiled with wonder as it tears by, so close, yet so faraway. I reach out and it is as if I am holding it in the palm of my hand and I feel like a god.

I am no longer afraid. I feel alive, honoured and blessed and I know that I have to share this with Suvali.

I run down the hill as fast as my feet can carry me, bursting with the weight of my news until I arrive at our home and while I struggle to control my breath I catch sight of Suvali through the window. I cannot drag my eyes away. She is naked and beautiful beneath her chiffon veil and I can see the gentle curves of her body disappearing into a shadow that nurses a half-made basket between her crossed legs.

A twig cracks beneath my foot and she looks up and sees me watching her. A smile dances across her face and she beckons me inside.

The room is decorated with flowers, fragrant with scents and dotted with candles, our very own universe. She kisses me and that one kiss surpasses the magic of the miracle I have just seen.

I take the basket from her and kneel on the floor in front of her. She snakes one leg around my waist and pulls me closer. I mirror her.

Sweet jasmine floats in a bowl nearby, and I dip my finger in the scented water and anoint her breasts with its cloying essence.

I kiss her forehead, her eyes, her cheeks, her throat, her breasts, her lips. Her mouth tastes of sweet, ripe pomegranate.

It's a kiss that kindles love, a kiss that awakens the deepest possibilities in me.

Her eyes are as deep as oceans and there is such naked promise in them, such electricity in her touch, and the heat in her kiss warms my blood, chasing out the cold night air from my lungs.

I whisper in her ear and breathe in her sanctified love.

I can feel her nails gently digging into my skin and her teeth drag down my neck and I repay her by making my mark on her breasts.

She tightens her leg round my body like a creeper, cooing under her breath, an embrace like a mixture of milk and water.

I grasp her hair and pull her head back, tenderly dragging my nails down her throat, her breasts pressed tight against my chest. She whispers in my ear and her voice is as sweet as a thousand angels.

Her silken thighs await my firm yet gentle touch. Her cloven inlet is moist with hunger and her velvet tunnel is throbbing with need. Her scarlet chalice rears and she slowly lowers her *yoni* onto my erection.

We rock gently into each other, moving closer and closer until I am fully inside her.

Our bodies became one, our legs flailed out like the tails of the comet, the limbs of the holy svastika, we became the life force, the four winds, the sun moving round the Earth. We have become the inward and the outward, we have become one sky.

My head swirls like a whirlwind of leaves, the rhythm of love beats in my mind and the melody of our being swamps all else.

The room revolves, enveloping us in a kaleidoscopic miasma, and like a whirling dervish I'm taken to a different plane.

I cannot tell where I end and she begins. Our souls fuse together and in that moment I know her. Every pore, every pulse, every thought, every fear. I am within her and she is within me. We have reached the root of union.

Rapture wells in the base of my spine, the serpent stirs and the *kundalini* surges through my body. The fire of an inner sun burns my skin and purifies my mind and I hold on to her, never wanting this to end. We're lost in a dream we've made real and our feet no longer walk on this plane.

Tangled in each other's arms, we cling on to each other for an eternity and I catch a glimpse of our shadows silhouetted against the wall. We appear as one like the comet frozen in space, like the holy svastika. Like a blessing, heralding the promise of good fortune.

The thirst of our five senses has been quenched and we recline on the pillows beneath the window. I gaze on Suvali with wonderment until the sun hovers on the horizon, sending spears of its life-giving energy into our room. We raise our trembling eyelids to the kiss of day, squinting in its warm, golden glow and something tells me there will be soon three hearts beating in our house.

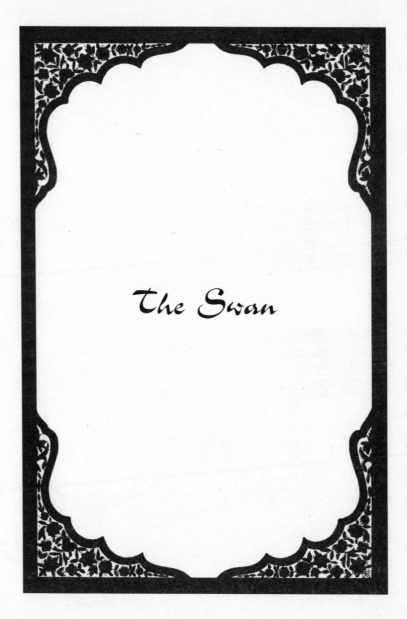

The Swan

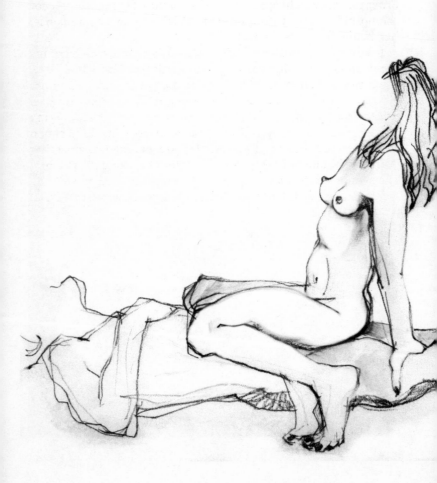

The Swan

Hansabandha
Srngararasaprabandhadipika

The swan glides over her lover's body, dominating him, her grace and beauty as she sits astride him creating irresistible images in his mind. Sometimes he simply feigns being tired in order that she might spring up on top of him. He realizes it's not the normal order of things but, for both of them he imagines, her being on top is a novelty.

Like a woman possessed, she suddenly needs him to wrap his hands in her long, luxuriant hair and pull her head back. He is often worried about hurting her but she goads him on and on. She sits on top of him with the straight-backed posture of a queen from another realm, and throws her head back, crying out in ecstasy as she pushes his *lingam* deeper inside her than he's ever felt before. His testicles are crushed against her painfully but he can't stop. Then, without breaking the rhythm, she swings her feet and legs so they are on one side of his body only, and his hard shaft is still inside her, pushing her to climax.

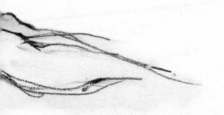

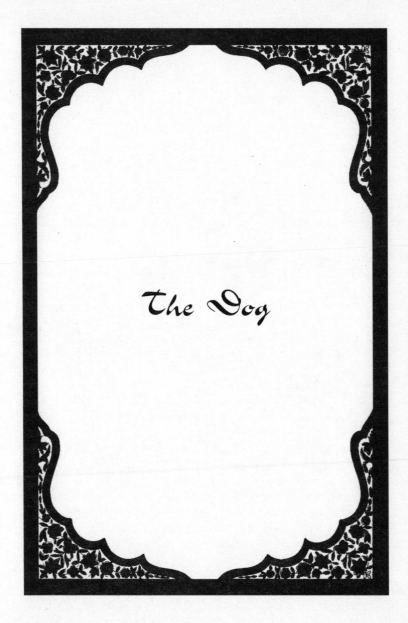

The Dog

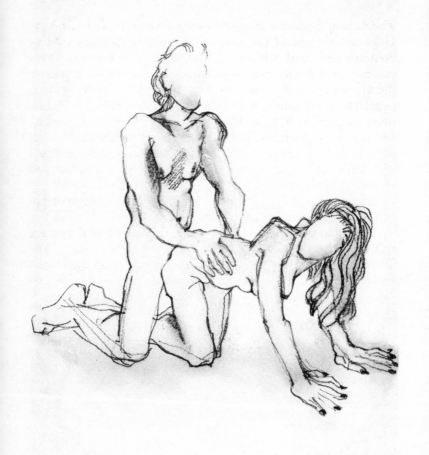

The Dog

Svanaka

Srngararasaprabandhadipika

The animal positions are games of pure theatre and mimicry. Dogs are not one of the more noble beasts; they are wild or domesticated, and without many redeeming features. This position allows the man to dominate and seem to subjugate the female. This is a rear-entry position that allows for deep penetration and quick, hard strokes by the man. She is on all-fours in front of him, and he grips her by the waist fiercely, causing her to turn and glare at him over her shoulder. Like dogs, both are to give in totally to their passions and claw, thrust and howl, and seem to be overcome. The woman should remember to keep her buttocks high as this allows easy access to the man. He should reach around and cup her breasts from behind to complete this posture.

Keep hold of the woman during this position as if you are unable to be physically parted. Hold on to her hair if she attempts to get away. Let her look back at you in anger and enflame your passions further. This is all part of the theatricality and the pleasure of the animal postures.

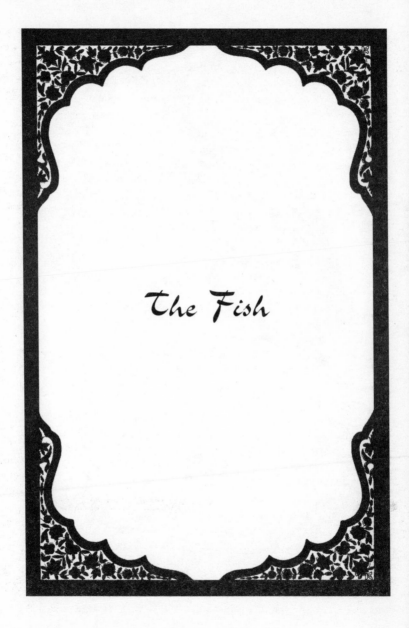

The Fish

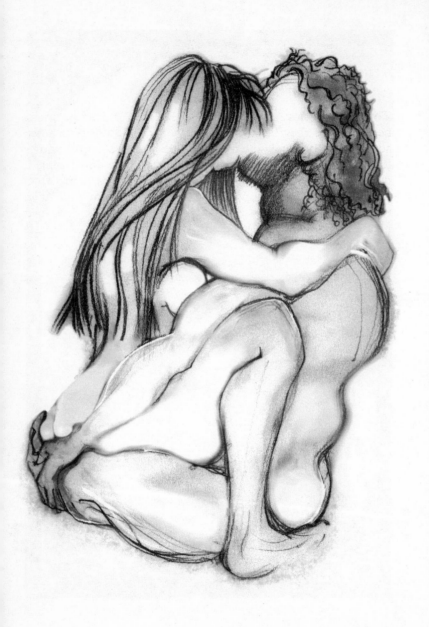

The Fish

Matsya
Srngararasaprabandhadipika

The medieval love texts created many other sexual positions besides those they found in *Kama Sutra*. The "fish" is a fun addition to the catalogue of gymnastic sexual postures with a foundation in yoga. This position is best done with a small, deer-like woman because the man is going to have to support all her weight. After getting into the lotus position, the man motions to the woman and signals his readiness. She then places her feet on his thighs and squats down so her breasts are crushed against his chest. She must be low enough to be able to be penetrated by the man's *lingam*. This may take some manoeuvring on her part. When penetration is achieved, the posture is achieved.

The Tale of the Drowning Man

as told by Maxim Jakubowski

Rajiv sat by the banks of the mighty river, dreaming, mourning.

The waters flowed with impeccable majesty, draining the streams from the faraway cloud-soaked high mountains on their long journey to the still distant sea. The sky was pure blue, the weather was mild but comforting, the harvests had been bountiful; so all was good in the mundane world. Though not at the core of Rajiv's heart. But was it really his heart that felt broken, or was his soul merely steeped in deep melancholy? He couldn't truly tell the difference. The pain was like a constant, nagging him every idle second that made up the night and day through which he now navigated like a dead man walking, like a lost and hollow soul.

Without her he was nothing.

That was all he knew.

First she had abandoned him. It was at the turn of the previous year. She had once said she loved him and the gods had smiled from high above in their accidental union, but eventually her wanderlust had somehow got the better of her. He had been her first man, but now she wanted to know more about the world out there, she craved further adventures, the reassurance that life could be more than just him. And he had been unable to change her impetuous mind, her youthful selfishness.

He had begged on his knees, shed tears, summoned all the poetry and tenderness his imagination could muster. But all to no avail.

He had visited temples and shrines and prayed to every god in the pantheon. If someone had suggested it might do the trick, he would have even promised his eternal soul to all the demons of the underworld if only to see her, hear her, feel her body again. But no one answered from that problematical other side. If it even existed. Or maybe his soul was worth nothing at all and was a poor bargain to the unholy powers that regulate the flow of hearts and minds.

He wrote her letters on the most delicate of papers, thin as silk and almost transparent sheets that shimmered as he consigned his pitiful words to them. He sent her the most beautiful flowers from fields and gardens, carried across towns and provinces by beggars he had instructed in the art of pity and modesty. But she just would not respond, as if the act of acknowledging his existence after her would betray her determination that they should become two forever. Not a word. Not a sight of her beauty. And he was bound by respect not to travel to her village and confront her with the sorrow of his despair, the deep wound of his longing. She had made him promise not to try to see her again, and he had ever so reluctantly agreed. And as he did so he also knew he would regret it forever. So all he now had were words.

She had once marvelled: "You talk like a poet . . ."

Or, the first time they united in holy congress of the bodies: "You're so well endowed . . ."

Or, on other numerous occasions: "You are my man . . ." or "My professor of love . . ."

But when he tried to remind her of those past feelings and intimate emotions, she now drew back and would not reply. Did she now think she had done wrong? Ah, the folly of youth can have such a cold, merciless heart.

And his talent for words was now totally useless in the face of her terrible indifference.

A year after their bittersweet parting of the ways, she appeared for the first time in his dreams. Normally, he was not a man who often dreamed of real people. His dreams were more incongruous sequences of phantasmagorical events and irrational fears which made no sense and felt more like a celestial puzzle of unlinked sequences he had not the power to understand.

In the dream, he was at a seasonal village feast and suddenly found himself in a room with a floor of sand, reclining on a soft bed with an unknown woman lying by his side, and he sensed that he was soon to bed this woman, even though he felt no attraction to her, slave that he was to the mating call of his penis.

He was about to raise a hand towards the sweetness of the mysterious woman's breasts when he suddenly saw the face of his lost love peering through the thin curtains that separated this bedroom from the outside. His heart jumped a beat or two. Then she was gone.

Still inside the dream, he jumped to his feet and ran after the love of his life, across fields, across plantations and then – in dreams there is no logic or sense of time – he caught up with her. They were in the room of a palace and she was standing by the balcony, smoking. Even though there was no sense of smell in this dream, he somehow knew that she was smoking the weed that makes you go mad. He rushed towards her, words as ever spilling from his mouth, frantic babble, imploring her to stop, to come back to him, to forgive him, to accept his undying love and forsake all the others who might have succeeded him in her bed, but she took fright and moved to avoid him and accidentally plunged to her death from the balcony onto the faraway ground below.

He woke up with a shock, in sweat, fevered.

And sobbed uncontrollably.

So now he had even killed her in his dreams.

Later that day, the news reached him from her village that she had drowned in the mighty river. No one knew how or why or had witnessed the event. Most likely it had been a tragic accident.

He couldn't even attend her death ceremony, harvest some of her ashes. No one had known of their love affair and her family and friends would have been too shocked to hear about it in such sad circumstances.

So, now, he sat by the river, with the ghost of his lost love floating in the spring air next to him, reminding him every single minute of the day like a knife in a wound of the sheer magic of her eyes, her body, her breasts, the flavour of her genitals where he had drunk like a madman of her essence, of the warmth of her insides when he had ploughed her hard with softness, of the sound of her voice as she had moaned like no other before in his arms.

He missed her.

So much.

He closed his eyes.

The pockmarked moon rose above the river, its rays high-lighting the ruins of a nearby, semi-abandoned temple, whose ravaged stones were gradually being swallowed whole by the creeping advances of the exuberant jungle.

He had once thought night and its curtain of darkness would help soothe the pain but it made no difference. In fact, there were times when he hovered between sleep and wakefulness and memories of their togetherness would stab his heart every single time his eyelids faltered and he sought forgetfulness in the embrace of the sandman. And the silence of the night was so heavy and full of desolation that he would feel like tearing out his eyes, his heart, his penis in a vain attempt to seek some form of merciful oblivion.

In the night, the sound of insects punctuated the silence. Did they never sleep? Strange, muted sounds, of animals, trees, clouds, phantoms, crept above the darkened land.

The water shone in the weak light of the faraway moon.

He forced himself to close his eyes as he sat there, wide awake and clothed in the bleak silence of yet another night without her; like every night in his life still to come, enough to make him wish for death, if that was the only escape. Grief has a subtle way of bearing down on the unwanted.

A shimmer of a sound reached his ears. Close, subtle. Like a wing grazing skin. With a sigh, he opened his eyes. It was still dark all around him. It took a few minutes for his vision to get accustomed to the penumbra. The waters of the great river glistened like melted ghee in the moonlight, a sliver of wind brushed against the trees in the distance, a minor key song of silences and secret whispers.

A concentric circle of thin wavelets broke against the shore where he was sitting morosely. His gaze stretched in the direction of its point of origin further towards the middle of the river. An anaemic bubble of air broke the surface tension. A frog? A fish? Rajiv rose and stepped closer to where the water merged into thin sand. Another series of delicate waves spread across the thinning shore. He squinted. Caught the hint of a movement out there on the waters.

The lunar pallor captured a shape, a ghost? White against white against the curtain of dark night. No, it couldn't be a fish. A larger animal of some sort? Water buffalos would never come out at night, would they? Rajiv scratched his scalp. But from his vantage point there was no way he could see more. Impulsively, he threw off his sandals and tiptoed into the water. It was warmer than he had expected. It had been a hot, sultry day and, anyway, the Himalayas where the river birthed were thousands of leagues away and the current had slowed on its long journey towards the sea.

A bird somewhere chirped sweetly.

Rajiv advanced a bit further towards the river's geographical centre, away from the comfortable safety of the land. The water was soon lapping around his knees. He focused his gaze on the point where the wavelets had earlier begun their circular journey. The water's surface was now quiet and undisturbed. He took a panoramic look at the river from his new vantage point. Stood still. And waited.

The solitary night bird sang again and took flight from a tree branch, breezing into his sight line, and alighted gently on the bed of the great river, so light as it descended that it made barely a ripple, unlike the creature Rajiv was now lackadaisically running down. The bird's sticklike feet dipped into the water and, for a brief atom of a second, Rajiv thought the poor bird would sink further and drown in the dark depths of the mighty river. But the bird deftly rose again and flew away, disappearing against the silhouette of a distant cloud. Rajiv followed its path with his eyes until a shuffling movement somewhere to his left caught his attention.

He turned.

What he saw took his breath away.

It was a bottom.

White in the moonlight. Glistening with the sheen of the river.

The most beautiful bottom he had ever encountered.

It could only belong to a woman.

Surely not a eunuch?

Yes, a woman.

No, a goddess.

The perfect bottom disappeared once again into the river. Leaving but the circular ghost of its shape behind, like a subtle dent in the chutney of the waters.

Rajiv finally allowed himself to breathe again. Or rather his lungs made him do so in protest.

He stood there, his body lifeless, in stasis, planted like an alien tree in a liquid environment. Colour returned to his cheeks. Another movement now caught his eyes, just a few hands away to his right, as the sublime creature surfaced again. This time it was not a backside, but a crown of dark hair that broke the water's surface, followed by her face, dark brown eyes piercing the night's darkness.

As rivulets poured bountifully down her forehead and cheeks, the young woman, now one-third or so submerged, noticed Rajiv's motionless presence.

He opened his mouth.

She smiled.

Revealing the whitest of teeth.

He tried to smile back, all too conscious of the fact that he knew that his own smiles somehow lacked sincerity.

A moment passed.

"Who are you?" he asked.

She kept on smiling but remained quite silent.

"Are you a goddess?"

She laughed, crystal sounds of mirth rising effortlessly from her throat.

He was struck with awe.

She rose further out of the water.

He drank in the spectacle of her body. Small breasts for which the word delicacy was invented, a gently curved stomach that begged for a head to lean against its soft skin, her delta of love was a small jungle of ebony curls, generous, impudently enticing and wanton as she stood there with her legs apart.

Rajiv was, again, devoid of words. Was this a curse upon him that the beauty of women should render words useless?

The beautiful young woman extended her arms towards him, as if indicating that Rajiv should take a hold of her hands. He obeyed. He was about to say something but the woman of the river pointed to her own lips in a gesture of silence. As their fingers made contact, Rajiv felt a surge of obscene desire course through his whole body and his *lingam* harden under the thin fabric of his tunic bottom.

She kept on smiling blissfully and it was better than words; it spoke of happiness, lust, desire, life itself.

She began to move back towards the nearby shore, and it was as if the light of the moon followed her like an aura. Hand in hand, Rajiv followed her, his gaze fixed on the exquisite curve of her naked rump, as pearls of the mighty river trickled down her inner valley to her thighs and legs. His *lingam* was now fully hard and poking like a snake through his meagre clothing.

They waded onto the shore and she turned to face him again. She noticed his unmissable and proud hardness, and for a moment Rajiv felt he should look away. But she displayed no disapproval and with wonderful immodesty let go of one of his hands and shamelessly took his fiery shaft between her supple fingers.

"Touch me," she ordered.

He hesitantly moved his free hand to her breasts, thinking aloud all along that the moment he dared to invade her privacy, all the gods from heaven would rush down to earth and strike him dead.

But what a wonderful way to die, he also thought.

As he caressed her tips, they hardened imperceptibly. Their other hands separated and his fingers ventured straight towards the apex of her *yoni*, parting her thick curls and gently invading her inner fire with the tip of one finger. While he did so, her own now free hand lovingly moved against his cheeks.

Their lips came together. He tasted her, tongues mingling, breaths combining. The night breeze that surrounded them quietened to a standstill, exiled away by the warmth that radiated from their bodies. The river streamed on by, oblivious to their embrace. When they came up for breath, she still held his *lingam* hard in her grip and he knew she could feel his heart beat frantically through the veiny currents of its stem. He realized they were magic creatures of the flesh and there could never be any shame between the two of them. Ever.

Later, she took him into her mouth and it was like dipping into a velvet volcano of pleasure, as she drained his juice for the first time, feeding herself on his unbound desire, lapping every single drop of his cream as if it were none other than the very food of life. She licked him clean from glans to balls, her tongue like the caress of heaven across every square of skin, even dipping towards his anal aperture across his perineum, every slip and slide like an arrow directed straight to the heart of his lust. He was hard again within minutes as the serpent of her tongue rimmed his sphincter and he almost begged her to grow herself an instant penis and impale him there and then – could witches or goddesses grow new limbs at will?

Still later, she crouched in front of him and spread herself open, revealing the blinding red of her innards to his lustful gaze and bid him lick her, tongue her, finger her until she squirmed with pleasure around his bunched and wet fist.

"Who are you?" he kept on asking between embraces and caresses.

But her only answer – indeed the only words she would ever speak in his presence, apart from delightful moans and deep contented sighs during their later congress – proved quite enigmatic: "I am only a fish from the mighty river, just here to keep men from drowning."

Finally, she indicated he should crouch on the ground on a bed of leaves. He sat in the lotus position, as erect as ever, and she lowered her body against his, facing him as she settled on his lap and his protruding *lingam*, her small but regal breasts brushing sensually against his own chest, and in one swift movement allowed him to enter her in a single upwards thrust, burying her cave on top of him to the hilt.

Rajiv cried out loud and the sound disturbed a flock of birds in the forest, who set off against the pale moon as daylight made a shy, early appearance.

On and on, drawing strength from each other, they plunged into the frenzy of the flesh, his shaft relentlessly exploring her inner depths and folds in search of untold ecstasy. They say the act of love is often a desperate quest for the essence of nothingness, that pure moment of nirvana when the whole surrounding world disappears and you are but a conduit for pure, unadulterated pleasure and for a brief instant manage to transcend your own body. If that is the case, the two ardent lovers of that river dawn flew away from the earth where they were making love several times, and possibly even ventured as far as the fading moon or the approaching sun.

They came in both silence and in loudness time and time again until finally there was nothing left to spend and their bodies, raw, scorched, torn but ebullient, could stand no more. The young woman from the river unsteadily rose from his shuddering *lingam*, and stood above him, his seed pouring quietly from her ravaged opening onto his chest where it mingled with his sweat.

Again, Rajiv was at a loss for words. But on this rare occasion, this was no cause for despair. Anything but. He tried to say something, a gesture of thanks or deep appreciation, but once again the beautiful young woman put her fingers to her lips and turned towards the river and, as the sun rose above the river and the forest beyond, she slowly made her way back to the shore where she entered the green water, her majestic buttocks swaying invitingly yet again, every curve in her body a symphony of allied perfection.

He watched in silence as she reached the middle part of the mighty river and slowly lowered herself and disappeared under its tremulous surface.

She never rose from the river again, although Rajiv sat there naked and exhausted, for a few hours more, his mind in turmoil.

Finally, his energy returned and he was able to rise and dress. As he slipped the tunic on, he could smell her all over him and his ragged clothing. He brushed his fingers against his still damp shaft and brought them to his nose, the fragrance of her inner core wafting gently towards his brain cells.

She smelled of the river.

"A fish," he said and smiled.

And, for now, the longing was gone, his lost love was in heaven and forgiven, and all was well with the world.

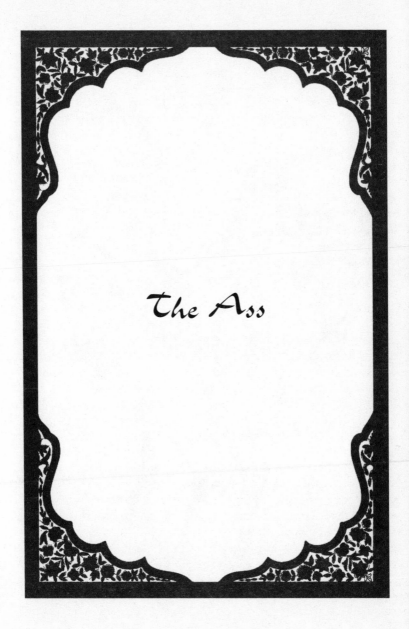

The Ass

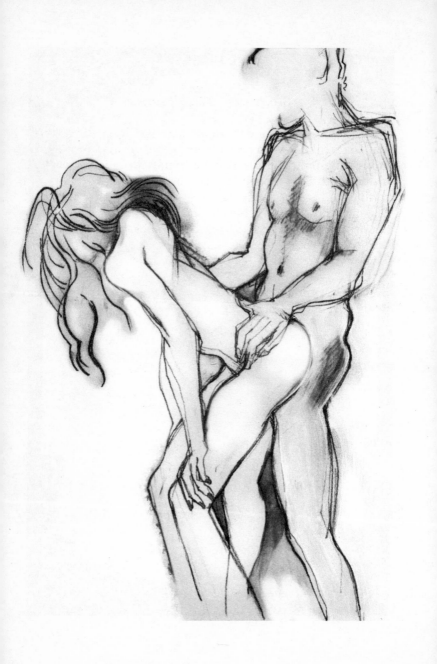

The Ass

Gardabha
Srngararasaprabandhadipika

The vision of the ass and its animalistic mating should inspire a man to take the woman he has chosen on their first meeting. He holds her from behind when she comes closer for a kiss, and instead turns her cruelly to face in the other direction and cuddles her, rubbing his hardness against her firm buttocks. She may try to protest, but the man is well aware how hollow her protest is. He takes her like an ass would take his mate, from behind. She spreads her feet apart and the man bends her with his hands, turning her pelvis until she is in a high squat. She places a hand on each thigh and he whisper words of love and passion into her ear to soften her, and then drives into her from behind with a thrust to make her cry out.

Ratirahasya

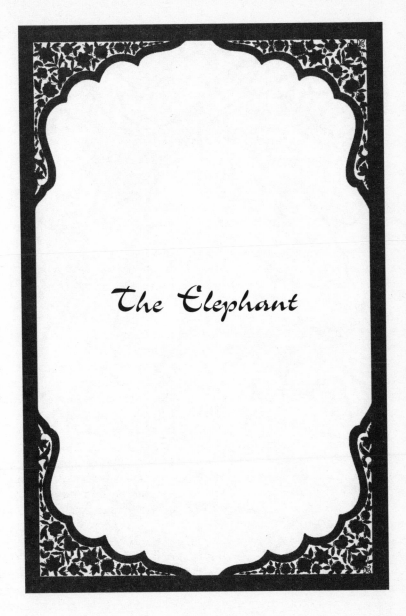

The Elephant

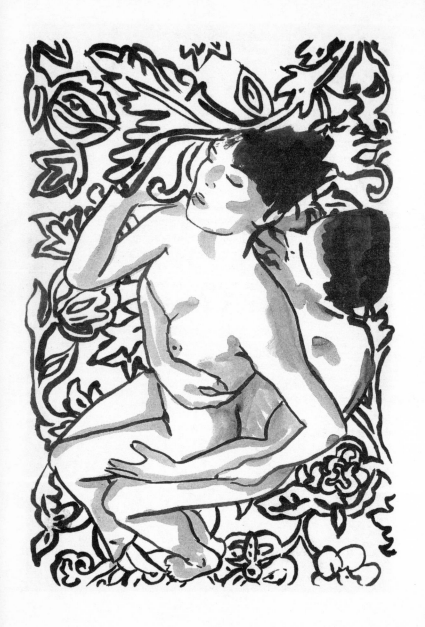

The Elephant

Aibha
Ratirahasya

This rear-entry position from a *Kama Sutra*-inspired love text involves the woman moving from her side to her stomach with her cheek pressed to the floor. The whole front half of her body is relaxing on the ground, however her hips and buttocks are raised slightly (this may also be a case of the man helping her to raise her buttocks by lifting them for her). From this position, the man has a lovely view of his lover's posterior and the closed bud of her *yoni*. When he penetrates her, he thrusts deep and pulls her hips up further. She should compensate by holding the front half of her body firmly on the floor. The man can employ the greatest variety of strokes in this position, all nine strokes if he is so inclined. The penetration can be very deep, and any discrepancies in size should be alleviated.

The Tale of the Elephant

as told by Lisa Elkind-Gardiner

Long ago in the ancient kingdom of Ayodhya, where the land was scented with honey and cardamom, lived a man who was always happy. This man was named Nidhish.

Nidhish was a successful merchant who sold costly oils and perfumes. Every day, when the early morning sun made the dewdrops shine like pearls on the lotus flower, Nidhish took his wares to market.

He would load his bullock carts with bottles of rose oil, ylang-ylang, sandalwood, jasmine and the precious patchouli oil that is known to increase sexual desire.

Happy Nidhish loved the marketplace with its myriad of colours, sounds and scents. He smiled at the men who sold fish, and at the children playing games. He smiled at the man who sold bronze and iron carvings and the men who sold lentils and rice. Most of all he enjoyed his friendly contact with the women who swayed past in their brightly coloured saris, their gold and silver jewellery glinting under the hot sun.

Before his marriage Nidhish had taken his pleasures where he found them. He knew many secrets about the women in the marketplace. He knew that the lovely Ramani had a birthmark in the shape of a heart on her thigh and that Tanvi had a waist so slender a man could span it with his hands.

All the women loved Nidhish, whose smile was like the sun breaking from behind the clouds. Some of the men liked him too, but others were jealous and became bitter.

"Why is he always so happy?" they would ask their wives. "Is it his wealth? Why does he sell so much perfumed oil? Perhaps he cheats his customers?"

But the wives would shake their heads and say, "He sells his wares because they are of good quality and because he is friendly. It is not his wealth that makes him so happy, rather it is love."

Nidhish was indeed in love. He loved his wife, the beautiful Salila, whose black hair shone like the sky spangled with stars and whose firm curvaceous body delighted him beyond measure.

She was not the only joy of his heart however for he also loved his mother deeply and always showed her the utmost love and respect.

One sad day Nidhish arrived at the market without a smile on his face. The other merchants, women and children whispered amongst themselves wondering what was wrong with him. They had never seen him look sad before.

"What has happened to your smile, Nidhish?" the men asked.

"Alas," cried Nidhish, "my mother Padma has fallen ill. The medicine men say she may die. I am miserable."

All that long day Nidhish did his usual job calling to all the people in the streets to come and smell his aromatic oils. The women's eyes lit up as they hoped to catch a glimpse of his gorgeous smile. But no smile came and they were confused and did not buy his wares. That night he went home with little to show for his day's work.

Nidhish lived in a fine bamboo and wood house with nine rooms and a balcony. He lived with his wife, his mother, his brother and his sister-in-law. His mother's room was the closest to the front door and when he came home from work in the evenings he would always go straight to her room and check on her.

This evening Padma lay on her bed, her complexion paler than he had ever known it, her dark eyes glassy. He knelt beside her and held her hand. Her skin was cold and clammy. He waited for her to open her eyes and say something, but in the end he just held her soft palm against his cheek and wished he could will away the haze of her pain.

It was still very hot weather, so he called his sister-in-law to fan his mother. Then he went to his own bedroom.

In his room Salila was fanning herself. She stood with her back pressed against the wall. Her eyes were made up with kohl and she wore his favourite thin red sari and his favourite silver anklet around her slender ankle.

In the dim light of dusk her fawn eyes looked almost too big for her face. He knew what she wanted, what she expected.

He knew she wanted him to come to her and pull her sari down at the front until he could see the soft curves of her breasts, to cup and fondle her soft peaches until her nipples hardened into little pebbles.

She expected him to push the thin silk of her garment up her smooth brown thighs until it bunched around her waist, his thumb exploring the fuzz of her pubic mound, his fingers slipping over her labia and the moist cleft between them, until she writhed and begged him to slide inside her tight *yoni*. They often made love in this way standing against their bedroom wall.

But for the first time in his life Nidhish could not bring himself to make love to a beautiful woman.

He walked right past her and lay down upon the bed. Salila opened her eyes wide in surprise. She moved away from the wall and climbed into bed beside him. Slowly she reached out with one hand and lightly touched his chest.

"I can't, Salila . . . because . . . Mama . . ."

She understood and pulled back. He closed his eyes and became the patient, soothed by the cool ministrations of her tiny, delicate hands.

"Salila," he said, "my back aches and I'm in pain."

"Husband," she answered, "I think you have fallen prey to self-pity and guilt over your mother's illness. Your first and second chakras are blocked. I can massage your back and then we can meditate together."

Salila went to heat the oils. When she came back she lifted the covers and began to make long deep strokes down his back. As she massaged she moved her body in a sensuous way designed to arouse.

But Nidhish pleaded tiredness and fell asleep and Salila lay awake worrying about him.

Meanwhile the Rāja of Ayodhya had heard tales of Nidhish, the happiest man alive. However he had not heard about Padma's sickness or Nidhish's recent sadness.

The Rāja's advisors had told him a false rumour. They told him Nidhish's happiness came from his magical perfumed oils. When the Rāja heard this rumour he ordered that Nidhish be summoned to the castle.

The next morning Nidhish went to the temple to honour Dhanvantari, the goddess of medicine and an avatar of Vishnu.

"Oh, Dhanvantari," he prayed, "your body is shining like the sun. You are present in the form of sparkles in the moon which is full of amrita, the elixir of immortality. Oh Hari, by the nectar of Vishnu's names Achyuta, Ananta and Govinda, please destroy my mother's illness completely!"

When he left the temple he met one of the Rāja's men. The messenger handed him a letter with the seal of the Rāja upon it. The letter told him he must bring his perfumed oils and visit Rāja Dhusyanta at once.

At this Nidhish smiled. He thought his summons to the Rāja might be the result of his prayers at the temple. Surely such a strange occurrence had been arranged by the gods. Somehow the Rāja would help him find a cure for his mother.

So the next day he and Salila loaded his bullock carts with the oils and, leaving his mother in the care of his older brother, they set off for the palace.

They rode the short distance to the capital city where the streets were paved with stone bleached white as bone in the sun.

Between the fine buildings in the city were channels formed of chiselled stone. Nidhish and Salila passed the great elephant house where the royal elephants were kept and became very excited knowing that they were nearing the palace.

They noticed the merchants here sold roses of all varieties and also pearls, rubies, emeralds and diamonds in the public bazaar. The couple were awed by such wealth.

At last they came to the palace. Nidhish's hands shook as he gave the letter with the Rāja's seal to the palace guards. The

guards looked the two of them over severely before nodding and
leading them in.

They were led through a grand entrance hall filled with ivory
carvings of lions, tigers and elephants to the Rāja's throne room.

The room had nine pavilions each magnificently ornamented.
The Rāja sat in the fifth pavilion. He wore a *dhoti* made of white
silk and a collar around his neck made of pearls and rubies. He
sat on an enormous throne of gold enriched with precious gems.

The Rāja beckoned Nidhish to his side and asked him about
his fine wares.

"Oh, Rāja I sell ylang-ylang. It has a heady exotic scent. It
calms the nerves. I have rose oil that acts as an aphrodisiac; it
relaxes and warms the senses. My precious sandalwood helps
increase sexual awareness and my patchouli oil betters sexual
desire."

Then he explained to the Rāja about his sick mother and how
the medicine man in his town had said there was no cure for her
and he asked the Rāja for his help.

The Rāja did not believe Nidhish had told him the truth
about the oils. He looked at Nidhish's smiling face and at his
lovely wife Salila and he believed the rumours his men had told
him. He thought the oils must be magical to make an ordinary
man so blessed.

The Rāja had many burdens in his life and did not much
enjoy ruling his kingdom. He longed to feel true happiness. So
he made an offer to Nidhish.

"My loyal subject, if you give me all your fine oils I will give
you a map to the Lake of Ambrosia. Anyone who drinks from
this lake will be cured of sickness and have eternal life. Your
mother will be cured. Sleep on my offer for an evening and
decide what you think. You must give me all your oils and tell
me the source from which you acquire them so I may continue
to have them all my life."

So Nidhish and Salila spent the night in a fine chamber in the
palace in an exquisitely soft bed. Salila, eager to make love,
reached for Nidhish. He grabbed her waist and pulled her
tightly to him. She moved her mouth across his shoulders,

kissing each spot of skin as though she had never touched him before. It had been weeks since they made love. But all day he had been feeling a pain in his lower back. He realized he still did not feel able to make love. The idea of taking his own pleasure when his mother was so ill made him feel guilty.

"I'm sorry, Salila, I can't, not until we have cured my mother." Salila rolled on her back and gave a deep sigh.

"Very well, Husband, you must meditate instead and begin work on cleansing your chakras. That should cure your backache."

But Nidhish did not meditate. He wanted to please his wife even if he could not take pleasure himself. He turned on his side and caressed her breast through her sari, playing with her nipples until she whimpered. He kissed her, inhaling the sweet scent that was distinctly Salila. Then he slid his hand beneath the silky fabric of her sari and up between her legs. He felt the slickness of her sex, and rubbed the hard little nubbin within until she rocked against his hand. Soon it glistened with her cream.

The scent of her arousal filled the air. Nidhish was almost ready to pounce on her. But the image of his sick mother came into his mind and he softened.

He continued to play with his wife's body until she shook and arched her neck. Her high-pitched cry finally made him hard. He watched pleasure ripple through her body and leaned over to give her a passionate kiss as she came. But he did not enter her *yoni*.

Salila woke her Nidhish early the next morning.

"We need to talk about the Rāja's offer, Husband. I want Mama Padma cured as much as you do but I'm worried about our livelihood. We will all go hungry without your oils. You must haggle with the Rāja."

Nidhish was unsure. He had not become a successful merchant without becoming good at haggling, but to haggle with a Rāja was a frightening prospect. Nevertheless he formed a plan.

Later that morning he stood alone before the Rāja's throne.

"Your Majesty, I have my answer. I appreciate your generous offer greatly and I long to cure my mother's illness. But a man needs his livelihood. I must be able to support my family."

The Rāja nodded solemnly. "What do you propose to do then?"

"I would like to ask that in exchange for the map to the lake I give you all my oils save one. The patchouli I must keep and continue to sell in order to feed my family."

The Rāja stroked the hair on his chin and thought. Finally he said, "You may keep the patchouli and good luck to you."

Nidhish bowed before him and kissed his hands.

The Rāja's servants helped Nidhish bring all the oils up to the throne room and set them beside the Rāja.

Then the Rāja presented Nidhish with the map and was rewarded with the younger man's stunning smile. The Rāja gave the couple three sealed copper pots to collect water in. He told them to leave their bullock cart with him and gave them a horse-drawn cab. Their new horse was Rama, a majestic creature the colour of a pitch-dark night.

After they left the Rāja began to feel guilty for he had not told Nidhish about the wicked demon who lived near the lake. This demon was the reason he himself had never been there, despite the fact that the lake was not far from the palace.

The next morning, Salila and Nidhish began their journey to find the Lake of Ambrosia. The map's directions led them along the banks of the River Ganges.

The air was invigorating, the river clear and green. Nidhish loved to watch each rush and surge of the river's current over the rocks. The spell that nature cast upon Nidhish that afternoon brought him peace and created within him a new rhythm, a new spirit. For the first time in weeks he felt able to meditate. He tuned in to the pounding sound of Rama's hooves and he focused on his breathing, imagining a white light streaming through his body cleansing him of negativity.

They rode for three miles south along the edge of the river until they came to a shrine dedicated to Shiva as marked on the map.

There was no temple here just a *lingam* made of white stone surrounded by bilva trees.

Nidhish pulled on the reigns of his horse and Rama tossed his head back breathing heavily. He led the horse down to the river feeling the creature's hot breath on his face.

Once his horse was watered he returned to the *lingam* and said a prayer.

"I bow before this *lingam*, which is the eternal Shiva, which is served by gods and other beings, which is the doorway for devotion and good thought, and which shines like billions of Suns. Oh three-eyed Lord Shiva thou art the saviour of all distressed. Oh Shiva, grant those I love freedom from dreary diseases and all the evils of mortal life."

Once he had finished his prayer, Nidhish noticed other worshippers had been by. There were boat-shaped baskets made from stitched leaves floating down the river. The baskets held rose petals, marigolds and white sweets. In the shallows, snow-white egrets were prodding for frogs.

Salila and Nidhish picked bilva leaves from the trees and wet them in the river. They placed these upon the phallic stone symbol of Shiva as an offering.

They climbed back in the cab and continued on.

The sun was now high and hot in the sky. In the distance they could see the silver Lake of Ambrosia where it met the river.

A mated pair of elephants were bathing in the sacred water. Nidhish had never seen elephants so relaxed. The male rubbed his back against a rock, having a good scratch, while the female lay on her side swishing her trunk back and forth with joy.

Nidhish alighted and tethered his horse to a tree. Then he fetched a copper pot and filled it with ambrosia for his mother Padma. He positioned the pot carefully in the cab and then grabbed one of his bottles of patchouli oil, thinking he might give Salila a massage in return for the one she had given him days before.

The elephants stepped out of the water and lay down side by side on the banks falling into a peaceful sleep. It was a sweet sight.

Salila and Nidhish smiled at each other. Careful not to disturb the elephants, they held hands and walked towards the silver water as excited as children.

But they had only taken a few steps when a terrifying demon magically appeared before them. He was as tall as an asoka tree and had eyes as big as saucers. He had the face and wings of a hawk with two tusks like an elephant and his hands and feet were blue.

He leapt up and down shouting, "That's it! You are walking in my land, near my lake. I allow no humans near the Lake of Ambrosia but you two will make a tasty meal for me."

Nidhish trembled and fell to his knees. "Demon, do not eat us," he cried.

But Salila said nothing and appeared calm.

The demon frowned at her. "Why is it that a young woman like you shows no fear in the face of a demon?"

Salila laughed. "You foolish demon, have you never heard of us? We are the thunderbolt people. We have thunderbolts in our bellies. If you eat us we will tear your innards to bits and all three of us will perish."

The demon looked frightened then he whimpered, "You tricked me. You are not a human, you are a goddess. Only a goddess could have a lightning bolt in her belly."

The demon flew off into the sky leaving a clear path to the lake.

Nidhish stared in awe at his clever wife and shook his head in astonishment. She merely smiled at him and ran towards the water.

In the full light of the sun, Salila's thin sari was almost transparent, showing all her lovely curves.

Thirsty from the long hot drive, she bent to drink from the silver water. Nidhish watched the gentle slope of her buttocks and for the first time in weeks he felt a real longing to hold her.

Salila stood tall and removed her sari. She stepped into the silver lake to bathe.

Nidhish set the bottle of patchouli on the banks. He tore at his *dhoti*, so eager was he to taste both the ambrosia and his wife.

She greeted him with open arms. Her fingers on his skin were as light as butterflies yet the impact of her touch was like a bolt of lightning streaking through his body. He wondered if it was the magic of ambrosia. He kissed her again and she laughed.

"Drink of the lake, my husband, there is no sweeter taste."

He kissed her throat, sipping from the inviting hollow there, then licked the droplets from her shoulders and breasts.

"Drink more, drink deeply," she cried, bending down to fill her own mouth with the liquid.

He took her in his arms and kissed her fiercely, inhaling the ambrosia she held in her cheeks.

He moved his hands down to clasp her sweet buttocks but she suddenly swayed and he had to grasp her hard to keep her from falling.

"I feel a strange drowsiness, Husband I think it is the magic of this lake. I need to go and lie down."

She went to lie on the bank curling on her side like the two sleeping elephants. Nidhish felt the power of immortality flowing through him. He went to join her, but as he did so he knocked over the bottle of patchouli oil, the oil that increases sexual desire and it spilled its contents over his wife's skin.

They both inhaled its musky scent.

Nidhish looked over at the elephants lying side by side. Then he looked at his wife curled up on her side facing away from him.

He slipped behind her until they fitted together like a pair of spoons lying in a drawer. The hot sun felt thick on his back like honey. He ran his hands over her glossy hair.

Salila moaned and pressed her buttocks against him. "Husband, I think we could make love in this position and I think it might unblock your chakra. It may even help the pains you have been having in your back."

Never had he thought to enter her *yoni* in this way before but it appealed to him. He felt a great tenderness for her as she lay in his arms, her soft buttocks pressed against him. He hoped the position made her feel cherished and protected. She was right. He had been feeling sorry for himself. He had thought he could not enjoy himself when his mother was so sick but he realized he had been foolish. He should never have neglected his wonderful wife.

He inhaled the familiar smell of her body and they both groaned as he slipped deeply into her *yoni*. Salila fitted him like no other woman ever had. Her *yoni* loved him tight and hard as he pulled out and thrust in again.

He found that in this new position he could easily caress her full breasts and stroke her clitoris with his hands. Each thrust made her mewl with pleasure. He continued to stroke her hard nubbin and her mewls became throaty cries. Her muscles clenched around his shaft. She began to caress her own breasts and play with her nipples and the beautiful sight made him groan louder. Her *yoni* was a silken sheath, gripping his body and filling him with so much pleasure it rode the edge of pain. As he thrust deep within her she bucked back against him, egging him on with whispered praise and encouragement. He closed his eyes as incredible pleasure engulfed him, then he pushed harder, thrusting all his length inside her one last time. A high scream of pleasure tore from her mouth. Together they reached a blissful climax. And thus the position *Aibha* (the Elephant) was born.

Nidhish gave the sacred drink to his mother Padma in a bronze cup. No sooner had she drunk it than a smile formed on her lips and she lay back and fell into a deep peaceful sleep. Nidhish saw lines disappearing from her skin almost immediately.

From that day on Salila and Nidhish often enjoyed the position of the Elephant. This position, coupled with regular meditation, helped cleanse Nidhish's chakra. His back pain was completely cured.

Nidhish learnt to make sealed copper pots for carrying sacred water from the Lake of Ambrosia and from the River Ganges. This gave his family a new source of income that replaced the oils he had given to the Rāja. He and Salila lived the immortal life of gods and he became known as Nidhish, the happiest man alive.

Panchasayaka

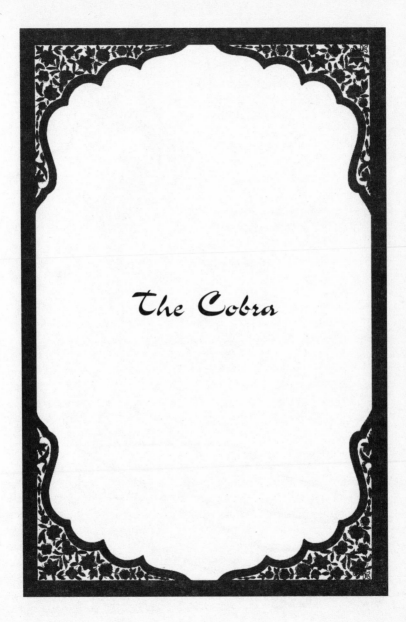

The Cobra

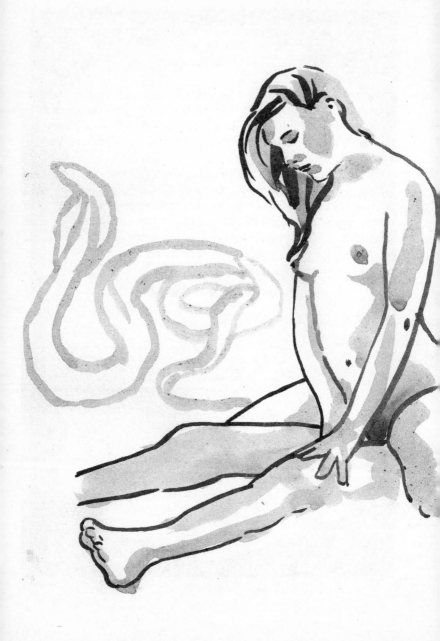

The Cobra

Nagabandha
Panchasayaka

Panchasayaka is a work from the fourteenth century whose translated title is *The Five Arrows*. It is a love text composed by Jyotirishvara Kavishekhara, which calls the *Kama Sutra* an ancestor, and is itself another addition to the tradition of Indian erotic science.

In this variation of the woman-on-top position from the *Kama Sutra*, the woman faces away from her lover so that he has a beautiful view of her buttocks as she moves up and down his shaft, as sinuously as a cobra. This is a sensual position of great visual delight for the man and he is able to touch her buttocks and her waist and see her hair cascading down her back, all at the same time.

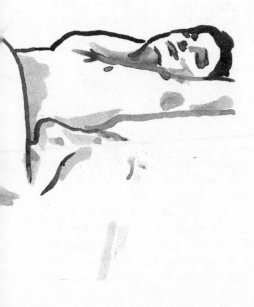

The Tale of the Legend of the Cobra

as told by Robyn Alezanders

The rivers had whispered they were about to overflow. To a casual observer, it merely seemed as if the waters were quite full, but to the seers, to the ones who knew how to read Prithvi's elemental children, the waters were raging. Eager to spill over the land, eager to spread.

And sure enough, just as they were about to wave through the ground, the wind blustered in and brought the Moon. She called upon the Sun and didn't wait long for a response to her coo. She grabbed her coveted, enveloped him in her luminescence, and brought sudden darkness to the work day. The waters halted their siege; they too were distracted by the celestial awe.

It had been a very dry hot day, typical of the season. The men had had to stop every few minutes to wipe their faces, take sips from their flasks. That's how talk had turned to the rivers' abundance; the workers were grateful that there looked to be an abundant amount to refill from. As the Moon continued her dalliance with the Sun, the men felt drops fall upon their sweaty shoulders. It had started to rain, and soon enough the pelting beads stimulated the rivers enough for them to finally let loose. Soon the villagers were wet from their heads to their feet, a storm whipping up amidst the blurred sky.

They stuck their tongues out to taste the rain and realized it wasn't water pouring down – it was milk. Out of curiosity they bent down and wet their hands with what was running over their toes, lapping up their ankles. Velvety, slightly sweet . . . milk. The condensation had churned into milk.

And up from the waves rose the *nāgas*.

Narmad often wrote about those magical eclipses in his poetry. The dances between Surya and His Lady were commonly recounted around the family tables. Moontide always seemed to bring the *nāgas* out from their alcoves, to slither out and join the festivities, weave through the mazes of feet. This also brought particular fascination to him.

His poetry came from the wondrous animals cohabiting the country. Every manner of each creature's being carried so much song; each carried their very own legend that was still evidenced by their present day character. Beauty and stealth could be found in all of them, whether they were predator or prey. He felt very blessed to have the intuition to understand their many languages, what made each of them so unique. As early as he could recall, somewhere around the toddler years, he could decipher the leopard's purrs, the elephant's grunts, the rabbit's mews. People from all parts of the continent knew his work well – his talent of comprehending the wildlife extended to the eloquent flow of language imparted throughout.

To the fervour of admirers he had, Narmad's writing must have reflected his own persona – wise and sensuous. To translate the ways of the animals so meaningfully must have meant that he was in tune with his animal self. But alas, when it came to hints of his manner, the poetry was a ruse. He had had no shortage of lovers; in fact he had been privy to the delights of numerous women. All types of shapes and skin tones – it wasn't unusual for a lady to spy him cosied up near a monolith of stones or under a tree, observing a particular creature for hours, taking meticulous notes that would later transform into another striking verse. The captivated lady would bring Narmad a pot of tea, a plate of sweets, sometimes a blanket or fan, depending on the weather. If conversation led to him accompanying her back to her home, or if the excitement could not wait and was consummated right there in the open desert land so be it.

He always brought pleasure to these consorts, and they always gratified him. To a point. Even though he enjoyed exploring their bodies, cupping breasts and rosy nipples, tickling that feathery spot where the navel led to their sacred flower, using fingers and tongue to partake of their wetness before entering them completely, there still remained the slightest sense of something missing. He mixed up positions, wrapped himself against the woman's body according to her shape, let her moans and quivers guide him along. Words floated through his mind, sensory stimulations that went towards spending great attention on his lover's desires. He treasured every experience, and took additional contentment knowing what joy countless women could relate him to. He just wished he could reach that one plane of bliss that persistently eluded him.

Indrakshi certainly embodied her name "beautiful eyes". Her eyes were a divine swirl of violet and chocolate, as if the gods had given her one shade, the goddesses another, and no one could break up such a lovely palette. Perhaps there was more than simply the aesthetics behind her sight, for she had an incredible sense of imagery that most likely was the foundation behind her talents as a painter. She would spend at least one full day a week grinding up the minerals and plants needed for the rich tones used on her canvases, and then the next four to five creating her wares. Once she had a fair amount of art completed, she would participate in the bazaar, often sitting near the snake charmers. Their music seemed a perfect accompaniment to her depictions of the deities, those which inhabited her dreams and compelled her to these visions.

She loved the dance between the Moon and the Sun, loved how the Moon had such a strong hold on the Sun, and how that magnetism affected the rest of the world. How the water especially echoed that tempo, how similar the water was to the sky, in shadowy motions and shimmery hues. Indrakshi was fascinated by the synergy that seemed to permeate between all living beings, and how the more she allowed the paintbrush to take on strokes of its own, the more she felt connected to those energies. There was something stirring within, something in her blood that was beginning to resonate with her portraits.

She had caught the fancy of many a man during her travels. As if her paintings weren't attention grabbing, as soon as she made eye contact and a gentleman saw that sparkle, sure enough there would be conversation, maybe a bit of wooing, whether it turned into a courtship of considerable length, or a brief affair, she was no stranger to earthly delights. No stranger, and not wanting to be.

Indrakshi was extremely comfortable with her body and what it could do. How the subtlest of movements, the tiniest bit of how she could roll her hips or arch her back, could keep a man's notice. She never avoided the rain, for it only tightened the sari's cling to her more, gave her more reason to run her tongue along her lips. She could easily bring about the pleasurable waves through her body herself, but it didn't compare to how a man could move inside her. How a man could use imagination and ingenuity to bring about the greatest of sensations. All of the great goddesses had that zeal, and Indrakshi felt a sadness for any woman who could not recognize that inherent strength.

Yet that strength came with one distinctive weakness. There wasn't one lover she regretted, nor one experience she rued. With every one of them she felt climax, just not as intensely as she expected. She had yet to enter that space that no doubt the goddesses employed at every whim – that of when a lover was synchronized in absolution. She felt the rivulets become pools, well up in her as a consort brought her to peaks, rode that release for as long as possible, but always at a distance. A measured distance. Not one man ever knew that she didn't reach as far and as deep as she should. They could release themselves when with and inside her, they could feel her quiver and sigh in pleasure. That a man could reach satisfaction and bring her along was enough.

She held all of the Mothers dear, but if pressed, was particular to Lakshmi. Often she imagined herself as a chosen maiden of the great deities, and how not to be fond of the gentle and endearing goddess revelling in the ocean of milk, swimming in that comfort.

Chaos was a slow visitor to the ways of Prithvi, the venerated Earth. Oh, Chaos had his moments to shine, when He managed to sneak up on the general layout of the kingdoms, but he just wasn't allowed as much freedom as in the primer times. The apparent battles between creatures, the divisions that called for allies and foes, were actually carefully plotted. It was the necessary order, that which need be in accordance for the general ebb and tide that defined the Heavens.

And so it was that the mongoose and cobra were clear representatives of those divisions. The sinuous ballet between beings either resulted in love or death – theirs was of the lethal step. To watch them engage in this dance was fascinating, each nimble toe of the mongoose responding to the cobra's lithe sway and warning hiss. The mighty *nāga* relished this combat, every instance becoming another opportunity to fine tune the senses, sharpen the reflexes, compose new variances of coiling around its intended.

Narmad couldn't believe that it had taken so long for him to witness such a spectacle. He had seen snakes before, had mentioned them in his verses, though not in this splendour. He had seen babies break through their eggs, the glint of that tiny fang. The envious comfort of them sunbathing on a niched rock. He had seen rainbows of colours slither under- foot, into the dusky waters, chasing frogs and fish. How mistaken he had been, categorizing the cobra as merely an- other type of snake – yes, Sheshnaga coiled at Vishnu's feet, the magnificent protector of the Holy One. The cobra was the amalgam of physical and mental licentiousness, its repertoire of movements calculated to incite and awaken. To emulate the cobra's majesty was to converse with the gods.

Indrakshi's dreams had been repetitive of late – Lakshmi tending to Vishnu and Sheshnaga, rubbing Her hands in soothing circles, while Kaali skipped along the clouds wrapped in a snake's layered hood. There was much revelry, the Mothers smiling and laughing as the Great Snake and His Father nibbled on their lavish attention. Kaali had replaced Her necklace of bones with one of lotus flowers, shifting from Her trembling guise to one of pure seductress. Indrakshi had awakened each time in a sweat, her fingers between her legs, heady thoughts wishing she could go where the goddesses did in these visions. As a result of these nightly hungers, her interest in the snake charmers' cobras had taken on a new attraction – even if she was in the middle of negotiating for her artwork, when she heard the flute notes, her attention wavered. Her peripheral vision noted the slim shadows rising and falling, drawn to the godly melodies. The cobras' flaired hoods brought to mind the way she wanted to be embraced, to be covered and consumed by an overwhelming passion.

She did the next best thing to walking in this mirage: she sketched and painted it. Those dreams were etched upon her soul, and they poured from her heart through her hands through the brushes. These new creations brought about a noticeable increase in admirers, professionally and personally. More women asked about buying pieces for their companions; more men either asked about series of the decor, or about obtaining private time with her. Indrakshi hoped that one of these new would-be suitors would finally be the key to her desires. The pleasure she did receive was obviously better than no pleasure at all, but now she saw Kaali when she closed her eyes during lovemaking, beckoning that more still waited for the right man to bestow.

Word spread about this latest set of renderings and Indrakshi was approached about contributing some of the canvases to the upcoming Serpent Festival. The *swamis* who came to talk to her did not hide their lascivious appreciation for her body, quickly deviating their grins from her eyes to her breasts. They believed that a woman who could draw like that had to elicit such inspiration from her own dalliances, and found themselves quite feverish speaking to her. Their robes barely hid the effect she had on them, and they could not wait to see even more of her during the ceremonies. If thoughts such as the ones in her portraits resulted from everyday life, what would the revelry bring?

True to form, the summer heat was broken by the monsoons. The winds roared through the villages, speaking in the same tongues as the snakes. Hissing chatter passed beneath window sills; through trees, people heard it hovering at their ears and most took a break from work to prepare for the festivities, for the more put into it, the grander the outcome. The *nāgas* were of such a special order that their gifted presence proved more fortuitous every year. Anything could and did happen during the celebration.

Narmad felt especially delighted to attend this year – a few of his poems were going to be recited by musicians. A couple of his last companions had gone on to form relationships with priests who oversaw the rites, and suggested he become an actual part of the holy day. Destinies were up to sly trickeries already – turning him on to the mighty cobra in time for him to add another animal to his compositions, and mould words to pay homage to them during such a tribute. After observing the cobra's grace and magnitude, he decided to take respite from the ladies. He had become so enthralled by the creature that he felt he needed time to reflect upon himself and perhaps choose his next consort the same way the cobra chose where he lay – methodically, intuitively, symmetrically.

The first month that passed without release was tough – the flirtations he encountered were plenty, and brought him to erection quickly. He learned to deflect by telling himself that such an immediate convenience would only make his drive worse because he knew now that there would be a substantial aura to the one who held the key to his awakening. These little caresses and grins and giggles that came his way were welcoming and assuring, just not indicative of the one. The more prominent displays – the bunching up of dress to thigh, the blatant solicitations – were a bit more difficult to resist, but he learned to turn off by considering that such overtness was not a truer revelation of connection. The second month spent quelling gratification was slightly better, because he had a wealth of poetry now boiling within him, and he had developed more of a routine to rid the erotic thoughts. His responses gradually lessened so that by the time Nagapanchami, the Serpent Festival, loomed, he knew that the goddess incarnate would be the only one to make his thoughts stray from his art.

Indrakshi chose a wine-coloured sari interwoven with silver and gold threads, and silver undergarments for the ceremonies. Her toenails were a fresh shade of toffee. A streamlined dab of kohl at each eye played up their vibrant hues, and a metallic serpentine clip pulled her hair back enough to further show off that dazzle. She wanted to savour everything about her first time at the ceremonies, and knew that her paintings at the shrines could be even more fantastic once people associated her appearance with her name. She also knew that despite Nagapanchami's propensity for unleashing the wild, she would be focusing more on the professional aspect of her art. She still appreciated the ogles in that she took pride in her carriage as a woman, but lately her lust for the common invitation had been diminishing. The winds were bringing change.

It was the night of the Cobra king; the Moon put Surya to sleep early, the sky in turn pierced by torchlight. All across the country, the drums reverberated, the cadence summoning the guests of honour. The mystics swarmed upon the temple grounds with large baskets of their adored, taking extreme care as to not misstep and upset their precious charges. The air draped heavy with the musky incense, the splendour of the evening penetrating everyone's psyche – how intoxicating the women were in their finest array of silks and satins, their hair whipping through the bustle as the dancing became more frenzied. The men in their cool cotton *dhotis*, their hips gyrating in tune with the ladies, mimicking the majestic cobras.

Descending from the temple's pillars were the *Nāga* effigies in resplendent scales, balanced so that the devotees could lay their lips upon the heads, pay greetings face to face if too shy to do so with the flesh and blood ones. It was due course that the netherworld dissolved its portals so that after so much time of imbibing the wine, the smoke, the fragrances, there was little notice of who were the Nagini and who were mortal women. At what moment did Nakamal rise from Her shrine beneath the nim trees to flicker between the shadows and enthral the local mortal men with Her exotic amusements and the hopeful maidens for introduction to more womanly delights?

Indrakshi didn't realize how much she would be aroused by the hedonism. She had attended many festivals before, and considered herself to be well in tune with her country's openly expressive manners. This though, this was what Mother Kaali had extended Her palms to, this is what gave such providence to the squalls that blistered the land, and fostered the *nāgas'* magic. She watched how the candles drew out her paintings, how the flames moved to the pungis' whistles, and as the cobras awoke from their baskets, their eyes turned towards her – their eyes acknowledged her paintings as the greatest of offerings, that born of her soul.

She heard something new amidst the chanting, words that seemed to speak for her canvases. It was as if someone had been able to transcribe what went through her mind as she chose images as her primary language. There seemed to be a subtlety missing in the performer's recitation, as if the eloquence was a little unfamiliar. Then she noticed the young man who stood near her paintings, mouthing the words – he must be the original artist. The way his lips glistened over each passage, he was speaking for the *nāgas* as they so deserved.

Narmad revelled in his fortune, that he was standing before canvases that elaborated on Sheshnaga's charms in a way he could not express solely through words. He heard mention of the artist, Indrakshi, and knew that she carried the true spirit within her. She had to be the one to bring him into that higher plane.

The Cobra King whispered, the same way the rivers had whispered so long ago. The sibilant mantras drew Narmad and Indrakshi to the sacramental hall where the cobras slithered free, where the pots of creamy *dugdha* and saccharine *madhu* spilled onto the floors, where the cellophane petals of the *utpala* released aromatic wafts as the cobras crushed them in their paths to enshrine the columns.

As only an attentive courtesan can incite, her body bent beneath his hands, and each was shocked into the greatest tactile sensations. He lavishly devoted himself to every part of her, his fingers leading his mouth to envelop inches below and above her waist, keeping her dripping. He chose a long voluminous sapphire feather from the treasure trove that was bestowed upon the snakes, and told her to show him how to move. Kneeling nude save for her jewellery, she imagined the plume as his tongue, as the snake's, trailing from her ears to deep into the delicious swirl between her breasts, and then across her buttocks, back and forth, back and forth . . . She pictured herself atop a magical carpet nestling down in a royal bedroom, the spice-scented candles reminders of the silken skies travelled for sensual discoveries.

The feather descended upon her backside, rising and falling upon the skin, making her thighs convulse in pleasure. She stood to meet his embrace and they moved along the floor in their own private court. The cobras sensed their movements, and flared their hoods, stimulated by the lusts. Backing Indrakshi into a corner, Narmad dripped milk along her golden skin. She wrapped against him, wanting, thirsting. His hands dug into her upper thighs, massaging them, her escalating moans urging further exploration. He took one of the feather's quills and applied a milk and honey blend to her belly, for his to slide upon. She was under his hands, drawn into a frenzy, aching, the sheer thoughts of what one could do to induce that delicious prickly blush across the skin.

He became the Cobra King, rose above her, writhed within her. His thrusts kept note with those of the mighty cobras that curled behind them, engaged in their own mating circles. Looking down upon her rapturous face, his release was slow, drawn out in such a forceful elicitation.

Her eyes flickered briefly, to see his muscles pulsate as he wriggled his hips and thighs to mesh with her demands. He was elongated, regal. He was the cobra in human form. He was what the gods and goddesses promised could come forth from the *paataala*, when the rains unlatched the other plane's doorway. She felt herself floating far beyond the temple's construction, into that ocean where Lakshmi frolicked.

They rolled over, shooing off the snakes that had come so very close to observe this spark. He took her again, this time from behind, his upper thighs pressing against her buttocks, as they rubbed in winding motions. She met his thrusts by drawing back up on her knees, giving herself over to the call of the Nagini to let the human and serpent spirits meld . . .

Thus the way of the cobra, that of the majestic *nāga*, was born.

It was the way she moved her hips. Undulating from the nest of plush cushions, responding to the serpent master's call, she entered into spontaneous trances at musical whims. Slow seductive murmurs, enticing growls, she slid back and forth, never losing a step in whatever hypnotic world occupied her mind.

Easy to be spellbound, watching her. The long wavy mocha hair streaked with black, the illuminating eyes framed by arched brows in a heart-shaped face. A ravishing figure perfectly accentuated by full breasts and ample hips. One could know she smelled like the night, by breathing in her bewitchment from afar. She was the elusive goddess who artists throughout time dedicated themselves to catching, to hold long enough to inhale her beauty, for all the world to appreciate.

How inspired they must have been.

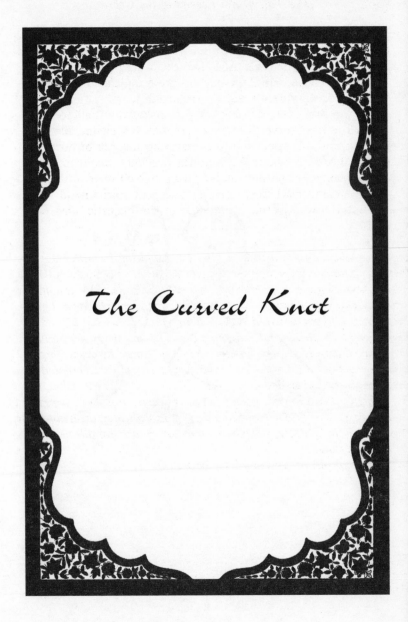

The Curved Knot

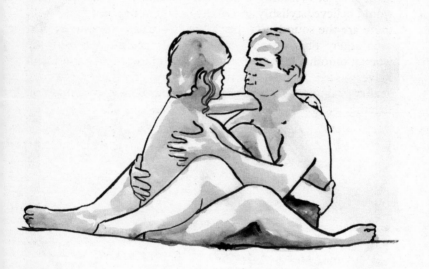

The Curved Knot

Kirtibandha
Panchasayaka

Deriving pleasure from sounds is a big part of the sensual aspect of the *Kama Sutra*. Everywhere there are sounds of moaning, slapping, yelping, cooing. The participants are encouraged at every step of the text to be vocal and reciprocate every sound the lover makes, including mimicking the noises of animals (one would believe, stylishly and to the best of your ability). As well, there are the sounds that positions create as bodies hit against each other. This sitting position, which has the man pull the woman onto his lap for penetration, alludes to these sounds in its very *sutra*. It mentions that the sound of your sex slapping against your lover's will sound like the continuous flapping together of the ears of a herd of elephants.

The Tale of the Curved Knot

as told by Monica O'Rourke

Ashok took them because it was his will. They obeyed because he was the master, but also because he was beautiful: dark hair draped his shoulders, and his eyes were so cocoa brown they were almost black. In his strong arms he held his lovers tightly, whispering in their ears even when he could have remained silent. He took them against their will but soon it became their will to have him. Ashok was a generous lover, but he had no desire to love. Once they succumbed, they no longer were of interest.

Rishabh was Ashok's manservant who served him well in matters of the heart and mind. "You anger Kali," he warned. "Your servants beseech her."

"My servants?" Ashok asked. He smiled and shook his head. "My servants are faithful. None would betray me."

"You take them against their will."

"It is *my* will! Mine is the will that matters. They have no say in how I run my household."

Rishabh bowed his head and knelt before his master. "I have angered you. I beg forgiveness."

Ashok *had* been angered. Had he not given his servants everything they desired? Had he not fed and housed them, sired them when they were fertile? Yet Rishabh spoke of betrayal, and Ashok knew there could be no forgiveness. He would discover the blasphemer and she would be punished. But he would not change how he ran his household. He would do as he wished, take who and what he wished.

He took Nalini by the black of sky, on a night when no stars shone and the moon offered no warmth. She begged for his mercy, and this angered him more. He had shown her tenderness before and she had loved him for it. Now she screamed as he forced himself inside her, taking her from behind like the dog she was. Ashok bit her shoulder, raking his teeth along the flesh, leaving his mark on her.

"Please, Master!" she cried. "Don't hurt me."

He pushed her face into the ground beside the riverbank and lifted her legs higher, thrusting harder, driving her deeper into the rocks and mud. When he finished he left her sobbing in the dirt.

Ashok's reputation as a kind and gentle master changed quickly. The girls hated and feared him and often tried to hide when he came. But the one who ended up caught paid the price for the others as he took out his anger on the treacherous girls.

Chandrika was sold to Ashok's household and brought with her two daughters. Indumukhi was the elder, and she was plain of face and plainer of mind. Sadly, she looked like her mother, Chandrika. Tall and bony, features sharp and hard, like a man. Ashok's only desire for Indumukhi was for her to feed the animals and wash his clothes. No desire of the flesh existed where Indumukhi was concerned. Ashok was angered that Rishabh had brought these women to his dwelling and considered replacing his manservant. This was not the first time Rishabh had upset him. Ashok's tolerance grew smaller by the day.

Chandrika managed to hide her younger daughter from Ashok by sending her on errands when she knew the master was searching for a girl. Rishabh also knew of the other daughter's existence and knew his master would be pleased if he brought the girl to him.

But Chandrika knew what Rishabh was planning, had seen the look in the man's eyes when he noticed Chandrika's youngest girl.

"I beg you," Chandrika told him one night. "Master can have any girl he chooses. Please do not betray my daughter."

"There is nothing special about your daughter," Rishabh said. "Our master can have her if he wishes."

"Mohini is special. She is untouched, and she is only a child."

"Mohini?" The name startled Rishabh. He shuddered, but quickly shook his head. "Bring her tonight. Our master will decide for himself."

Chandrika chewed her lip. "I cannot allow that."

Rishabh turned quickly and faced the woman. He slapped her mouth and she fell to the ground. "Allow?" He grabbed her hair and pulled her to her feet.

Chandrika cried out, begging for mercy.

Rishabh slapped her again and again until her lips bled, until she crumpled to the ground at his feet.

"Bring her tonight!" he bellowed. "Or you will both die."

Rishabh found Ashok and told him what had happened. "The girl is beautiful," Rishabh said. "Not like her mother or sister. Her face is soft, her hair dark and lovely, like spun silk."

"You have done well," Ashok said. "I do wish to have her."

"As you desire." Rishabh turned to leave, but hesitated. "There is one thing . . ." He swallowed, regretting his words. His master would have eventually learned the truth. He wondered if he would have been wiser to remain silent.

Ashok cleared his throat, a sign Rishabh recognized as impatience. "Her name is Mohini," Rishabh said in a hoarse whisper.

"So?"

"Sire, it's her *name*."

"Names mean nothing to me. You speak nonsense, Rishabh."

"But the meaning of her name is *bewitching*. It could be a sign."

"A sign of nothing! Your superstitious beliefs are not mine. Do you believe I have achieved my status by believing in nonsense?" Ashok considered himself a benevolent master but also a shrewd one. If he listened to the nonsense his servants spoke, he would be afraid to leave his bed.

"If she is such a beauty, then of course I want her. I demand you bring her to me." Ashok left then, not wanting to discuss this any further. He wandered down to the river and sat beneath the shade of a tree. The branches hung low, dropping an occasional leaf, and he sat mesmerized, entranced by the leaves, thinking about his servant girls. He would bring Mohini here, to this wonderful place in the shade, and he would be tender with her. Maybe.

When night came, Rishabh found Chandrika and demanded she produce her daughter, Mohini.

"I do not know where she is."

Rishabh raised his hand to slap Chandrika and she cowered. "I speak the truth! When I told Mohini what she must do, she ran away. She is afraid."

"You will find her, and you will bring her," Rishabh said, "or you will both die."

Chandrika stepped back, away from Rishabh's hands. "I beg you. You must not allow this to happen. The gods will be angered if anything happens to her. Mohini is a special girl."

"Special? She is a servant girl! She may be special to you because she is your child, but she is not special. Another word and I will cut out your tongue!"

Chandrika bowed her head. "I will find her."

Chandrika ran into the woods to the place she had hidden Mohini. The girl was sitting quietly beneath a tree, playing with a clump of moss. She was startled by the appearance of someone in the darkness, until she recognized her mother's voice.

"Mohini? Where are you?"

"Here. I'm here." The girl smiled, fearing nothing now. Her mother would take care of her, as she always had. Her mother would protect her from harm.

Chandrika knelt beside the girl and stroked her hair. "I'm sorry," she whispered. "There is nothing else I can do. They will kill us both if I do not bring you to Ashok."

Mohini shook her head, and tears dripped from her eyes. "But why? Why do I have to go to him?"

"It is his will."

"It is not my will!"

Chandrika grabbed Mohini's shoulders and shook her. "Don't ever speak those words aloud! They will kill you if you say such things."

"It isn't fair."

"Fair or not, it is what it is. His will is the only one that matters. I have tried to protect you, Daughter. It is not worth our lives to remain stubborn. Do you understand?"

Mohini nodded and bit back her tears. She was afraid, but she was angry, and she needed to know why there was such injustice. Ashok should not have the right to take her if she did not want to be with him. Such was the way where she and her family came from. It was this strange, unforgiving land she had grown to hate. A strange land with strange men and strange customs. Mohini couldn't understand why she had been brought here, against her will, to do the bidding of a man she despised.

"I'll go with you because you wish it," Mohini said. "But it is *not* my will. And he will be sorry."

"Mohini, listen to me –"

"I will have all that is his," she said. "He will be sorry."

Chandrika had promised Rishabh she would return with the girl. She had not promised the girl would be co-operative.

They returned home a short while later, and Rishabh ordered Mohini wash herself and dress in clean clothing. She stank like the woods, he told her, like dirt and bugs, and she was not suitable to be presented to their master.

"This is how I am," she said defiantly, but Chandrika dragged the girl away to wash her.

"Are you trying to get us both killed?" she asked her daughter at the edge of the river. They sat together in the grass and Chandrika wiped the dirt from her daughter's hands and face.

"Pray with me," Mohini said. "Pray to Kali."

"Do not invoke the name of Kali!"

"Kali will protect me. Kali will not allow this to happen."

"Kali will punish you if you invoke her name."

"No," Mohini said. "She will punish him. For taking what does not belong to him. For making servants of women who want to be free."

"Our freedom is not for Kali to decide. We will find our own freedom."

"How?" Mohini cried. "With our deaths?"

"I beg you," Chandrika said. "Do not do this. Just be with him one time. Then he will leave you be. This is his way."

Mohini's dark eyes narrowed, but she nodded. Chandrika gently tucked the girl's hair behind her ears. "You are beautiful, Daughter. Now go to him. Do what you must."

They walked back and were greeted by Rishabh's whip. He struck Chandrika in her legs until she fell to the ground and begged for mercy. Mohini tried to help her mother but was yanked back by Rishabh.

He grabbed Mohini's arm and dragged her away, until she could no longer hear her mother's painful wailing. "She will live," he said, "unless you disobey. Do you understand?"

"Yes. I understand."

Rishabh shoved her inside the room where Ashok was waiting. Ashok smiled and held out his hand. "She is beautiful."

"You are pleased." Rishabh smiled.

"That remains to be seen. She is pleasing to the eye, but that does not mean I am satisfied."

Ashok took Mohini's hand. "I wish to have you."

"I have heard."

"This does not please you?"

"I have been told it does not matter what pleases me. Only what pleases you."

Ashok grinned. "You have been taught well. Do you know what pleases me?"

The girl remained silent for a moment. "I think I will learn what pleases you."

Ashok studied her before speaking again. "Do you not wish to be with me?"

Rishabh cleared his throat. "Sire, what does it matter what this peasant thinks? She is here, and she will do whatever you wish."

Ashok glanced up, having forgotten Rishabh was in the room. "Leave us."

"But —"

"I do not wish to repeat my words, Rishabh."

When they were alone, Ashok cradled Mohini's face in his palms. "Answer my question."

"Your manservant was right. It does not matter what I wish. If I did not come to you, my mother and I would be killed."

Ashok shrugged. "Such is the way, little Mohini. But you may find being with me most pleasurable."

"Perhaps if we had met properly. You are most handsome. But I do not wish to be with you, so I know I will find no pleasure."

"We shall see."

He brought her to the riverbank and spread her beneath the tree, her garments a blanket in the grass and dirt. His caresses were gentle, his mouth eagerly suckling her breasts. His fingers explored her wetness, and despite her reluctance she found herself wanting him, eagerly anticipating his touch.

"Lift your legs," he said, shifting her weight, bringing her ankles to rest on his shoulders. He bent into her and licked her, tasted her. She writhed beneath him, and despite her wishes found herself wanting him more with each passing second. He lowered her legs.

She cried out in pain, at first, feeling him inside her for the first time. He slid in gently, slowly, until he was thrusting, soft at first and then faster, harder, until Mohini's pain was unbearable, until she thought he would tear her apart.

But then she came, and the pain became pleasure. She wrapped her arms around his neck and clawed at his skin.

When he pulled out she turned away, breathing hard, hating herself for feeling the way she did, hating that she had betrayed herself.

"I told you there would be pleasure," Ashok said.

Mohini refused to look at him. There had been pleasure, but she still hated him. Hated what he had done to her. There would be no forgiveness. She would have revenge.

She stood up.

"Where are you going?"

She pointed towards the house.

Ashok shook his head. "We aren't finished."

Mohini was inexperienced and could not imagine what else was left to do. "Sir?"

"You had your pleasure. Now I have mine."

It was as if a demon had possessed him. The gentle lover disappeared. Ashok grabbed her and pulled her back down to the ground, pinned her against the soil.

He bit her breasts until she screamed, and stroked himself until he was hard again.

"Please!" she cried. "It hurts!"

He thrust himself inside her, pounding hard, until her head banged into the tree behind her. She sobbed, reaching between her legs, trying to push him away. He pulled out and dragged her closer, roughly turning her onto her stomach.

"Hold still," he panted, pulling her towards him, lifting her buttocks and shoving himself inside her again, pounding roughly at her flesh.

"You are mine," he grunted. "You would be wise to never forget. I take what I want!"

"Please," she sobbed. "Please stop." Her cheek dragged against the dirt. Fingernails scratched at the ground, and she waited for what seemed forever for him to finally finish with her.

"Kali, hear my prayer!"

Ashok finished, and pulled quickly away. He grabbed Mohini by the throat and yanked her to her feet. She clawed at hands, at the grip choking her breath away.

"How dare you pray to Kali?" he yelled. "I should kill you now!"

She dropped to her knees, gasping for breath. "Please," she begged. "I did not mean –"

He slapped her across the face and she fell back, smashing her head against the tree trunk. He dropped to his knees and grabbed her ankles. "Do you think Kali would help such a pitiful wretch? Do you think you can cause me pain?"

"No!"

"I will show you pain!"

But Kali had heard Mohini's prayer. She appeared before them, eyes wild, tongue darting in and out of her mouth like a serpent tasting the air. Tied to her waist was a belt of severed heads.

Ashok scrambled away but Kali grabbed his hair and yanked him back.

"Please," Mohini cried. "I meant no harm! Please spare my life." She fell back and hugged the tree trunk and sobbed into her arms.

Kali lifted her sword above her head. "There will be blood."

"I beg you," Mohini said. "Spare us."

Kali lowered her sword and stood silently before them. "I will spare you."

Mohini gasped, "Oh, most merciful—"

"But there will be blood," Kali said, pointing towards the house. From the distance Mohini could hear a sudden, piercing wail in the darkness. She recognized the terrified voice of her mother, Chandrika.

"No!" Mohini sobbed, burying her face in her hands, knowing she had killed her mother. "Forgiveness! She has harmed no one, Kali."

"You dare speak my name?"

Mohini shook her head, realizing her indiscretion too late. "I only wanted justice," she whispered.

"Justice for who? For you? Who are you to deserve justice?"

"Against the man who wronged me! He took me against my will."

"You did not seem to mind earlier, little girl. When you received your pleasure."

"It was still against my will!"

Kali looked down at Ashok. "And you. What do you have to say?"

"I did not invoke you. I would never have disturbed you."

"But you *have* disturbed me."

"I only took what was mine. I paid for her. I paid for all of my servants. I own them and do what I please with them."

Kali smiled, an evil sneer twisting her lips. "Then you shall have what you wish." She turned to Mohini. "And you. I do not wish to give you freedom, because you are most undeserving."

"But why?" Mohini pleaded. "Why am I undeserving? What have I done wrong?"

"You were asked to do this one thing, and then it would have been over. A selfless sacrifice would have saved your family. But you offered nothing, and you planned his death. You would have taken everything that belonged to him."

"No," Mohini said. "I never—"

"Do not lie to me!" Kali yelled. "I know what is in your heart, girl."

"You of all beings must understand revenge! I only wished to harm him the way he has harmed me."

"Then you shall."

Kali brought Mohini and Ashok together beneath the tree, forcing them to face one another. They shifted, unable to control themselves, unable to resist limbs moving to Kali's will. With bent knees they slid closer together, until he was inside her again, their arms resting against their sides, holding each other's hands. Ankles rested against each other's ribs. Ashok pulled Mohini closer, hot breath gasping in her ear.

"You will remain together for eternity," Kali said.

And in this position they became a tree, branches growing inward to forever clasp one another, rocking gently with the wind, a curved knot of bark and branches and leaves. It has been said that if the trunk of the tree is pierced, it leaks not sap but the blood of Ashok and Mohini, forever doomed to share this existence.

Ananga Ranga

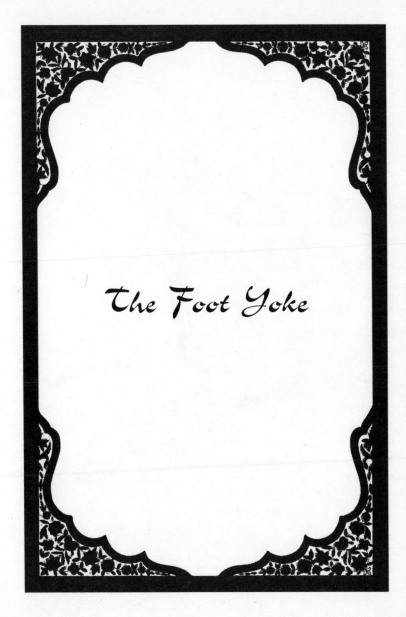

The Foot Yoke

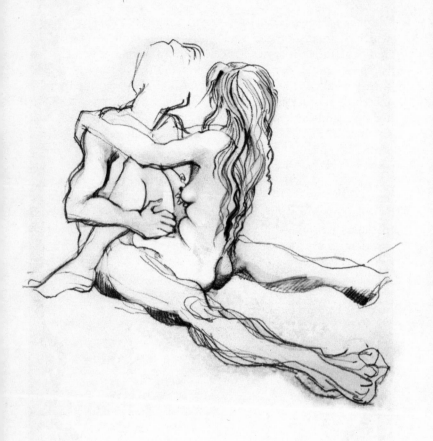

The Foot Yoke

Yugmapad-asana
Ananga Ranga

Yugmapad-asana is a name given by the poets to that position in which the man sits with his legs wide apart and, after insertion and penetration, presses the thighs of his woman together. This is a pleasurable, rhythmic position from the *Ananga Ranga* for loving couples. The man and the woman mirror each other and match each other stroke for stroke, pulling with their arms in a forward-and-backward see-saw motion, ensuring enough steady friction for both the man and the woman to reach orgasm. Both can have their knees drawn up against their bodies, providing the other with a view of the genitals, aroused and ready for love. The couple in this position should be of an equal passion so that the rocking motion is well balanced and neither is doing more work than the other. It is also important that the passions are somewhat equal so that the intense male (or female, for that matter) doesn't injure the other partner by loveplay that is overly boisterous and rough. An unequal balance also means that the female, if somewhat hard to satisfy, might be unable to reach a climax or take any satisfaction from the union whatsoever.

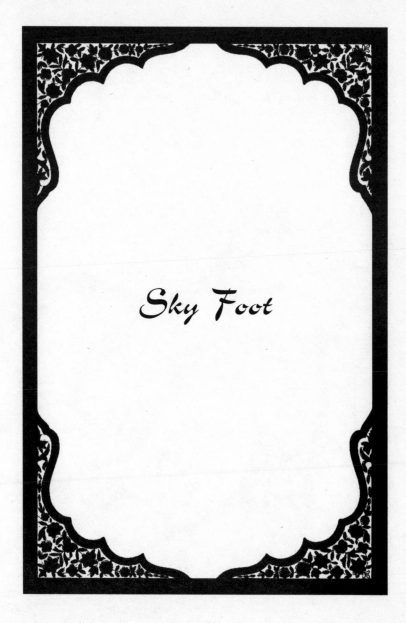

Sky Foot

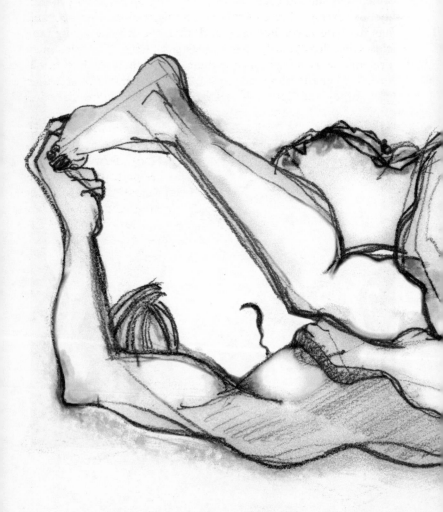

Sky Foot

Vyomapada
Ananga Ranga

Sometimes congress between a husband and wife can be filled with loveplay and eroticism. It is not all duty, you know. He watches as she lies back, waiting, opening up her thighs to him for his caresses. Pretend this is a transgression. The husband lets his wife know her role, and after she stops giggling, she closes her legs tightly and evades his kisses. The man may pretend he is an admirer and he has crept into her bridal bedchamber the night before she is to be married to someone else. Enjoy the delicious transgression, as Krishna cavorted with his married milkmaids.

Vyomapada-uttana-bandha is when the woman, lying upon her back, raises her legs with her hands, drawing them as far back as her hair; the man, then sitting close to her, places both hands upon her breasts and enjoys her.

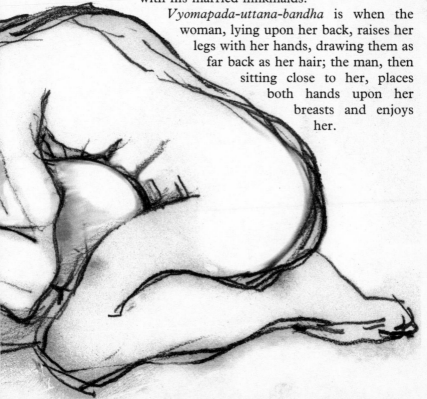

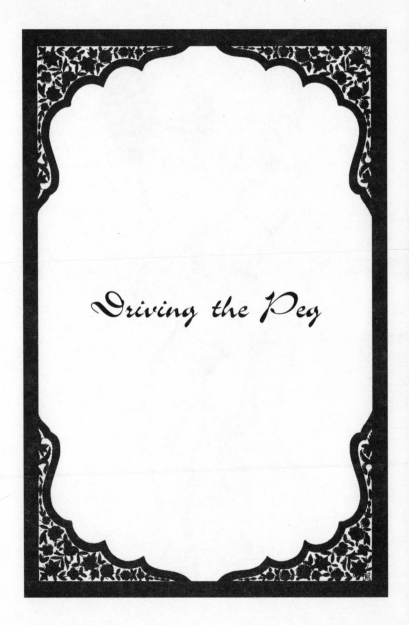

Driving the Peg

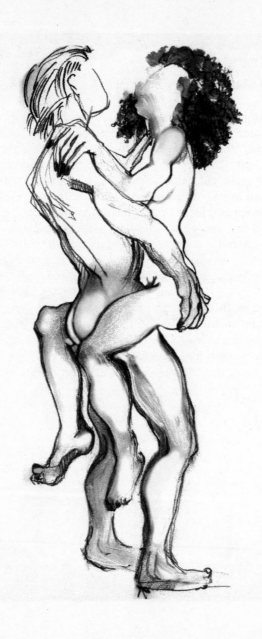

Driving the Peg

Kirti
Ananga Ranga

When a woman grasps her lover around his neck with her hands and straddles his waist with her supple legs, locking them around him, it is the position mentioned by Kalyana Malla in his sixteenth-century love text, *Ananga Ranga*, called *Kirti*.

If the time is right, and the man's desire is strong, he lifts his lover up and quickly impales her on his shaft, so that he can see her eyes widen and feel her *yoni* contract with delight. The man looks down into her eyes as he enters her with his rod, so that she seems literally to be hanging from his shaft with no other visible means of support than her desperate, clinging arms around his neck. Her *yoni* contracts around him while she hangs and bounces against her lover. Kisses and bites are appropriate at this time. She should try to raise herself to his neck in order to leave a line of points or other love mark. Her struggle may be in vain, however, as she's overcome with the pleasurable sensations cascading over her body as the man drives her towards orgasm. She will then desire him even more.

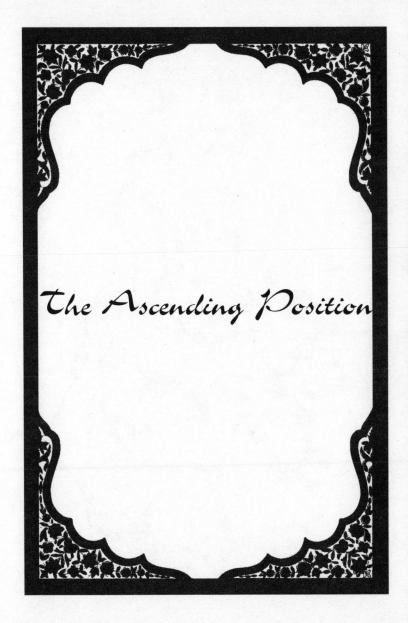

The Ascending Position

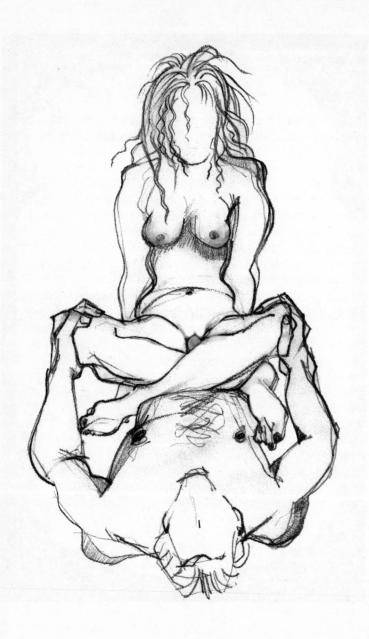

The Ascending Position

Utthita-uttana-bandha
Ananga Ranga

If the woman's passion has not been satisfied by her session with her lover, she should take control and make him lie on his back, as she has been made to many times before. If she then perches on top of him and crosses her legs, she can take his erect *lingam* and insert it in order to finish pleasuring herself. This will be a novel position for her lover because she is effectively taking control, and using him to satisfy herself selfishly. He enjoys gazing on her as she perspires between her breasts and works herself back and forth on his rod, touching all the best places in her *yoni*, the secret places she touches herself when she needs pleasure but is alone.

When she gets a little quicker in her movement and begins lifting herself faster and faster on her man's *lingam*, he will know that her orgasm is near but should refrain from touching her or helping her along. Instead, he should just enjoy her desperation as she pumps back and forth on him, trying her best to reach her climax. If she catches him smiling at her as she does this, she might scowl at him with good humour. Or she might go so far as to put her hand over his eyes so he can't look at her any more. If he lifts her off him, interrupting this posture and not letting her finish, she would then show him all her displeasure, until he lay down again and allowed her to resume her slow, cross-legged sliding along his *lingam*. She's so close, she tells him, so close. Just lie there and be still like a good boy. And that makes him smile again, but he lies back and does what he's told.

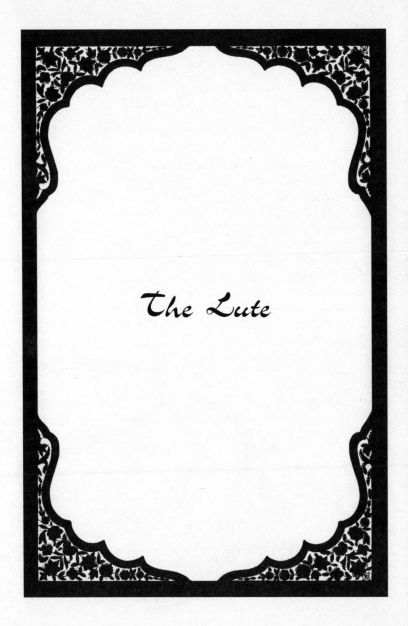

The Lute

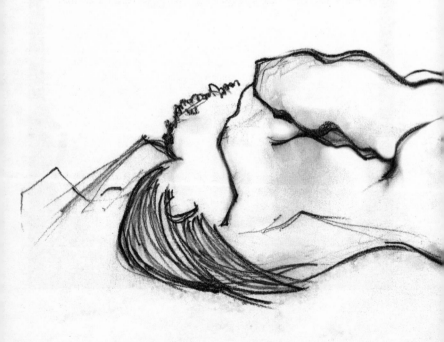

The Lute

Vinasana
Ananga Ranga

A woman has been known to leave a good man because of the sexual pleasure provided by a low man skilled in this position. This position is also called the "transverse lute". The woman, while on her side facing her partner, should lift her leg slightly to let her partner gain access to penetrate her. At this time, he can position his leg on her thigh so he is better able to make thrusting motions while inside her. Because the *yoni* is almost pressed closed, and the *lingam* has to open it up to push inside, this position is great to minimize any size discrepancies between the man and the woman.

There is another variation of this position where the man raises one of the woman's feet to his heart, while leaving her other leg stretched out straight, tracing the length of his.

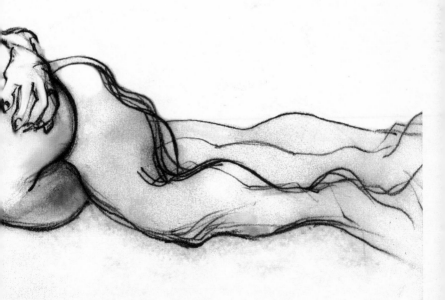

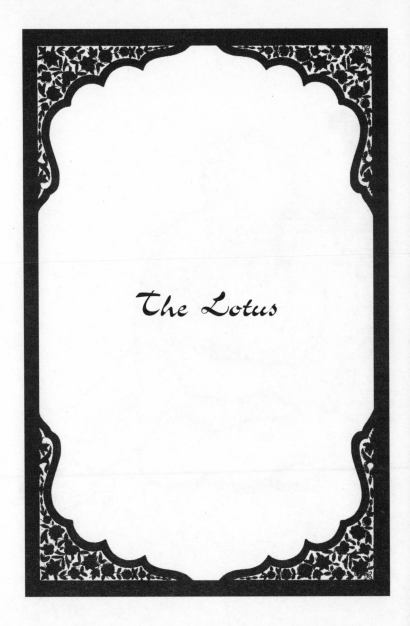

The Lotus

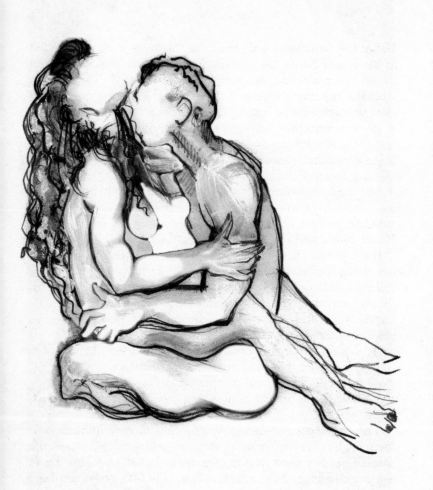

The Lotus

Padma
Ananga Ranga

Using the same yoga foundation as the lotus position detailed in the *Kama Sutra*, the *Ananga Ranga*'s lotus position instead calls for the woman and man to both be seated. The woman straddles the man's hips and seats herself in his lap, snuggling close enough against him to feel her breasts against his chest. A chest connection between the lovers means they can feel each other breathing, and monitor the quickness of the breath that signals that orgasm is close. They then have the option of slowing down if one partner is speeding ahead of the other. It is this kind of conscious technique, this ability to control the pace and drive of the sexual act, that lifts it from the instinctual animal level to the civilized congress found in the *Kama Sutra* and other love texts.

If the woman is very young, or if it is your first time coming together, consider this position as almost a tender, loving embrace. This position is very relaxing and easy, and allows the woman a bit of freedom to move her pelvis along the man's *lingam*, while he embraces her round the back. He is also able to help with her movements, and can pull her further onto his shaft to gain deeper penetration. The couple has the ability to lean back while supporting each other round the back and waist, close their eyes and give in completely to the sensations. Or they can admire each other's bodies and leave kisses in the appropriate places.

The seated face-to-face positions can be very intimate and loving. They are perfect for the longer-lasting couple, where the woman needs a good deal of time spent in foreplay in order to achieve climax, and the man is able to hold off orgasm until she is ready.

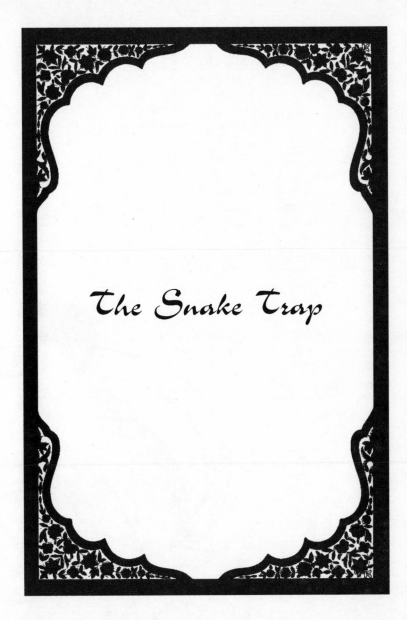

The Snake Trap

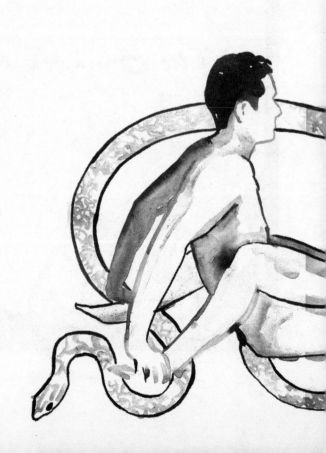

The Snake Trap

Panipash-asana
Ananga Ranga

An *asana* means a "sitting posture" in Sanskrit. The "Snake Trap" is an *Ananga Ranga* posture in a traditional yogic form. In a sitting posture, both husband and wife (her legs outside his, almost as if straddling him) grab and hold each other's feet and begin congress. It is a posture that allows only little, subtle movement, but the intensity is made up for by the constant contact with the lover's gaze and the full view of the each other's bodies. Penetration is not as deep as in other postures but the position itself is relaxing and pleasurable. The translated title of "snake trap" might mean the trap that your feet are in, wrapped in the hands of your lover. It is a perfect position for whispering to your lover and feeling the intimacy that only comes from this kind of face-to-face position.

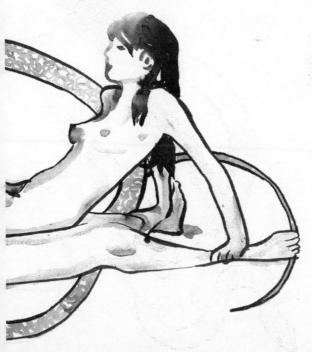